Parish Nursing

Development, Education,
and Administration

Parish Nursing

Development, Education, and Administration

EDITED BY

Phyllis Ann Solari-Twadell, PhD, RN, MPA, FAAN
Assistant Professor
Marcella Niehoff School of Nursing
Loyola University Chicago
Chicago, Illinois
Formerly Director, International Parish Nurse Resource Center

Mary Ann McDermott, EdD, RN, FAAN
Professor Emeritus
Marcella Niehoff School of Nursing
Loyola University Chicago
Chicago, Illinois

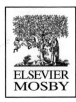

ELSEVIER
MOSBY

ELSEVIER
MOSBY

11830 Westline Industrial Drive
St. Louis, MO 63146

PARISH NURSING: DEVELOPMENT, EDUCATION, AND ADMINISTRATION   ISBN: 0-323-03400-4
First Edition

Notice

Knowledge and best practice in this field are constantly changing. As new research and experience
broaden our knowledge, changes in practice, treatment and drug therapy may become necessary or
appropriate. Readers are advised to check the most current information provided (i) on procedures
featured or (ii) by the manufacturer of each product to be administered, to verify the recommended
dose or formula, the method and duration of administration, and contraindications. It is the
responsibility of the practitioner, relying on their own experience and knowledge of the patient, to
make diagnoses, to determine dosages and the best treatment for each individual patient, and to take
all appropriate safety precautions. To the fullest extent of the law, neither the Publisher nor the Editors
assume any liability for any injury and/or damage to persons or property arising out or related to any
use of the material contained in this book.

International Standard Book Number 0-323-03400-4

Executive Editor: *Darlene Como*
Managing Editor: *Linda Thomas*
Publications Services Manager: *John Rogers*
Senior Project Manager: *Cheryl A. Abbott*
Senior Designer: *Bill Drone*

**Working together to grow
libraries in developing countries**

www.elsevier.com | www.bookaid.org | www.sabre.org

ELSEVIER   BOOK AID International   Sabre Foundation

Printed in the United States of America

Last digit is the print number: 9 8 7 6 5 4 3 2 1

About the Authors

Phyllis Ann Solari-Twadell

Phyllis Ann Solari-Twadell, RN, PhD, MPA, FAAN, received her bachelor of science and her master's degree in nursing and her doctorate from Loyola University Chicago. She received a master in public administration from Roosevelt University, Chicago. She was employed for 25 years at Advocate Health Care in Park Ridge, Illinois. For 10 of those years she worked in addiction treatment. For the last 6 of those 10 years she held the position of director of nursing services at Parkside Lutheran Hospital, a specialty hospital for addicted patients. From 1984 to 1988 she was president of the National Nurses Society on Addictions. For the last 15 of the 25 years Dr. Solari-Twadell held the title Director of the International Parish Nurse Resource Center, Advocate Health Care, Park Ridge, Illinois. In that capacity she was the editor of *Perspectives on Parish Nursing Practice*, a regular publication of the International Parish Nurse Resource Center. Dr. Solari-Twadell coordinated the annual Westberg Symposium on Parish Nursing for 15 years. She coordinated the development of a standardized core curriculum for parish nurses in collaboration with Loyola University Chicago Marcella Niehoff School of Nursing and Marquette University School of Nursing, Milwaukee. This included the preparation of faculty to offer the standardized core curriculum in over 70 sites in the United States and Canada. Dr. Solari-Twadell co-edited the texts *Parish Nursing: The Developing Practice* and *Parish Nursing: Promoting Whole Person Health within Faith Communities*. She is a fellow in the American Academy of Nursing. Currently, she is assistant professor at the Loyola University Chicago Marcella Niehoff School of Nursing and has responsibility for the development of the Center for Spirituality Leadership in Health Care.

Mary Ann McDermott

Mary Ann McDermott, RN, EdD, FAAN, is Professor Emeritus, Marcella Niehoff School of Nursing, Loyola University Chicago. She has served in a variety of roles at Loyola since 1969: department chair, maternal child-health nursing; assistant dean and director of the undergraduate program; acting dean in the school of nursing; director of the University Center for Faith and Mission; and most recently as the faculty coordinator for University Ministry's Lilly grant: Project EVOKE on Vocation/Call. Dr. McDermott is a fellow of the American Academy of Nursing and was named Loyola University Chicago Faculty Member of the Year in 1994 and in 2002, Illinois Nurse Leader of the Year. From 1981 to 1987 she served as the director of a university sponsored – nurse managed center in a Roman Catholic congregation, a program she co-founded with two other faculty members. She has participated in many community activities and served as chairperson of the boards of Lutheran General Hospital (1994-1995) and Advocate HealthCare (1998-2000). For much of the last 2 decades, her research, grant involvement, curriculum development, speaking, consultation, and publications have been in the areas of parish nursing, health ministry, and nursing and the arts. A graduate of both the baccalaureate and master's programs at Loyola, she has a doctorate in education from Northern Illinois University in curriculum and supervision.

About the Contributors

Kathleen Cleary Blanchfield, RN, PhD

Chapter 6, Parish Nursing: A Collaborative Ministry

Dr. Blanchfield is currently with the suburban Chicago Parish Nurse Ministry at St. Michael's Parish, which is affiliated with Advocate Health Care. She has a BSN from Loyola University Chicago, an MS from St. Xavier University, and a PhD from the University of Illinois. She is on faculty at Lewis University and serves as a basic parish nurse preparation educator. She has a master in pastoral studies from Loyola's Institute of Pastoral Studies, with an emphasis on spiritual care for the elderly and a certificate in spiritual direction from the Claret Center. Dr. Blanchfield is a member of the Chicago Archdiocese's Advisory Committee on Priests' Health. She is a nationwide presenter on congregational health ministry, and the author of articles of parish nurse ministry.

Jayne Britt, RN, BS, CIC

Chapter 13, Competencies in Parish Nursing Practice

Ms. Britt currently manages the Parish Nurse Program at Holland Hospital in Holland, Michigan. This position includes management of parish nurses in 10 faith communities in partnership with the hospital, as well as affiliations with Western Theological Seminary and Hope College Nursing Department. It also includes the promotion of community health ministry as part of Holland Hospital's Department of Community Outreach, and coordination of the Holland-area Parish Nursing Network. Ms. Britt's nursing experience includes medical-surgical nursing; nursing management; quality management; and infection control in acute, long-term, and home healthcare settings. She completed the Basic Preparation for Parish Nurses and the Basic Preparation for Parish Nurse Coordinators courses in 2001.

Joan M. Burke, RN, MSN

Chapter 21, Parish Nurse Coordinator: Working with Congregations and Clergy in Fostering the Ministry of Parish Nursing Practice

Ms. Burke earned her bachelor of science and her master's degrees in nursing from Loyola University Chicago Marcella Niehoff School of Nursing. She began her nursing career in general medical/surgical nursing and obstetrics. She also has worked as an occupational health nurse for a large corporation and in long-term care, acute care, telemetry, and in critical coronary care. She also held a head nurse position on a 40-bed medical unit. After receiving her MSN degree in home health administration, Ms. Burke first began her work in home health as a staff nurse and later as a director. She has experience in home health and has taught Medicare regulations to new staff. Most recently she has held the position of coordinator of a parish nurse ministry for a large Roman Catholic healthcare organization in the Chicagoland area.

Lisa Burkhart, RN, MPH, PhD

Chapter 8, The Growing Accountability in the Ministry of Parish Nursing Practice

Dr. Burkhart, a PhD graduate of Loyola University Chicago, is currently an assistant professor in the Marcella Niehoff School of Nursing, Loyola University Chicago. She is co-developer of the Center for Spiritual Leadership in Health Care,

Marcella Niehoff School of Nursing, Loyola University Chicago. She is the author of Integration, a documentation system for parish nurses developed through the International Parish Nurse Resource Center, Advocate Health Care. She is also the author of the documentation portion of the standardized Basic Preparation in Parish Nursing course, distributed through the International Parish Nurse Resource Center, Deaconess Foundation. Dr. Burkhart's areas of research include development of spiritual nursing diagnoses, interventions, and outcomes for standardized taxonomies (NANDA, NIC, and NOC) used in computerized documentation systems and in measuring patient outcomes in parish nursing practice. Additional areas of research include studying spiritual care in nursing practice and health systems.

Sheryl S. Cross, RN, MSN, MDiv

Chapter 12, Developing Dual Competencies: A Personal Perspective

Rev. Cross became an ordained minister in the United Church of Christ (UCC) in 2003 and is now serving as the pastor of a rural Illinois congregation near St. Louis. She has more than 14 years of experience in health ministry as a parish nurse, parish nursing associate director, educator, consultant, author, and pastor. She was previously with Deaconess Parish Nurse Ministries and the International Parish Nurse Resource Center in St. Louis. Rev. Cross is a contributing author to *Assuring Congregational Health and Wholeness for the 21st Century*, the standardized core curriculum developed through the International Parish Nurse Resource Center, and editor of the 2002 reprint. She was a contributing author to *Women at the Well*. She is the author of "Developing Worship Services" and "Increasing My Comfort with Leading Prayer and Worship" in *Conversations in Parish Nursing* by J. Halsey. She is a frequent retreat leader and speaker for health ministry groups including the Westberg Parish Nurse Symposium, the Health Ministries Association Annual Conference, and other ecumenical and denominational gatherings. As chair of the UCC Parish Nurse Network since 1995, Rev. Cross has served as a consultant for the development of health ministry resources and activities as an adjunct to national UCC staff.

She is active in the Health Ministries Association as a board member and chair of the Clergy Network.

Karen Egenes, RN, EdD

Chapter 2, A Historical Perspective of Parish Nursing: Rules for the Sisters of the Parishes

Dr. Egenes is an associate professor in community and mental health nursing at Loyola University Chicago, Marcella Niehoff School of Nursing. She received a baccalaureate degree in nursing from Marquette University and a master's degree in psychiatric nursing from Rush University. She received a doctorate in curriculum and supervision from Northern Illinois University. She also holds a master's degree in United States history from Loyola University Chicago. Dr. Egenes is a research fellow at the University of Pennsylvania, Bates Center for the Study of the History of Nursing. Dr. Egenes has conducted research both in Great Britain and the United States about topics related to the history of nursing. She is presently first vice president of the American Association for the History of Nursing.

Janet Wall DiLeo, RNC, BS, MPH

Chapter 24, Working with Underserved Congregations: A Case Study

Ms. DiLeo was director of the Congregational Wellness Division of the McFarland Institute in New Orleans, Louisiana, from January 2001 to April 2004. In that position she was responsible for the development of the Church Nurse Program, which primarily addresses the needs of underserved church populations in the metropolitan area. She is a registered nurse, with a master's degree in public health from Tulane School of Public Health and Tropical Medicine. Janet is currently serving as a community health consultant to local non-profit organizations in New Orleans.

Cassandra Scott Graham, RN, BSN, MAOM

Chapter 24, Working with Underserved Congregations: A Case Study

Ms. Graham is director of the of the Congregational Wellness Division of the McFarland Institute in New Orleans, Louisiana, where she is responsible for the design, establishment, and support of programs promoting wellness and health in local congregations. She has 16 years experience in various aspects of nursing: case management, acute care, and community nursing. She is an experienced advocate of healthcare for underserved populations, through her long-term relationships with faith-based communities. Since 1995 she has partnered with neighborhood churches, community policy units, the judicial system, schools, and community-based organizations. She has presented sessions on inner-city African-American churches and parish nursing at various conferences. Among Ms. Graham's honors are her award as one of the Great 100 Nurses from the New Orleans District Nurses Association and the Mayoral Certificate of Merit in 2000 for community service. She received her diploma of nursing from Charity School of Nursing in Louisiana, her bachelor of science in nursing from the University of South Alabama, and a master's in organizational management from the University of Phoenix.

Cynthia Z. Gustafson, RN, PhD

Chapter 17, Distance Delivery of Parish Nurse Education

Dr. Gustafson is chair of the nursing department at Carroll College in Helena, Montana, and is also the founder and director of the college's Parish Nurse Center. In Montana in 1998 she established one of the first distance education programs for parish nurse preparation. She has been active in parish nursing since 1990, establishing the Parish Nurse Center at Concordia College in Moorhead, Minnesota, and working on the national level to assist with the development of the core curriculum for basic parish nurse preparation. Cynthia also assisted with the establishment of parish nursing in Swaziland, Africa, in 2000. She serves as a parish nurse for her home congregation.

Annette Langdon, RN, BS, MA

Chapter 14, Learning to Pray

Ms. Langdon is parish nurse and director of health and caring ministries at Calvary Lutheran Church of Golden Valley in Minneapolis, Minnesota. She has her master of arts in pastoral theology and ministry from Luther Northwestern Theological Seminary in St. Paul, Minnesota. Ms. Langdon has worked as a parish nurse since 1978, the last 17 years of which were at Calvary. She is also adjunct faculty for the Parish Nurse Center of Concordia College, Moorhead, Minnesota, where she has taught the basic parish nurse preparation course since 1992. She developed the curriculum on prayer and worship leadership for the parish nurse preparation course through the International Parish Nurse Resource Center.

Rosemarie Matheus, RN, MSN

Chapter 15, Mentoring the Parish Nurse

Ms. Matheus was a professor in the Marquette University College of Nursing, in Milwaukee, Wisconsin for 25 years, until her retirement in 2002. She created the Parish Nurse Institute Preparation Program at Marquette University in 1991 and prepared over 1600 parish nurses in 40 states from across the United States through that program. She has presented on parish nursing at numerous nursing conferences, religious conventions, and health institutions, including an international nursing conference in Amman, Jordan, and several annual Westberg symposiums. Ms. Matheus has co-authored articles in *Public Health Nursing* and the *Journal of Geriatrics* and has authored a chapter on parish nursing education in the International Parish Nurse Resource Center's text on parish nursing. She was a participant and contributor in the creation of the standardized curriculum created by the International Parish Nurse Resource Center. Ms. Matheus developed the parish nursing services program at Aurora Health Care Systems in southeastern Wisconsin and has served as its paid consultant for the last 3 years. Care Systems in southeastern Wisconsin and has served as its paid consultant for the last 3 years.

Edward McLaughlin

Chapter 6, Parish Nursing: A Collaborative Ministry

Reverend Edward McLaughlin is pastor emeritus of St. Michael's Parish in Orland Park, Illinois. He was ordained a Catholic priest for the Archdiocese of Chicago in 1959 and served several congregations in associate pastor and pastor roles, as well as teaching on the seminary faculty at Quigley South and St. Mary of the Lake. He served most recently for 18 years as the pastor of St. Michael's Parish and has been a champion for parish nursing.

Faith Bresnan Roberts, RN, BSN, CRRN

Chapter 25, Grant Writing for Parish Nurses and Parish Nurse Coordinators

Ms. Roberts is currently coordinator of the Community Parish Nurse Program at Carle Foundation Hospital in Urbana, Illinois. She is co-author of the AACN *Core Curriculum of Sub-Acute Care* and has also published articles on the socialization of nurses into the profession, burns and sexuality, spirituality, parish nursing, prayer, and presence. Ms. Roberts speaks across the United States and Canada on topics close to every nurse's heart, having given over 1000 presentations on state, national, and international levels. She has been named a Visiting Scholar by Texas Medical Center. She has been a nurse for 29 years and holds her certification in rehabilitation nursing.

Annette D. Stixrud, RN, MS

Chapter 23, Building a Parish Nurse Network: A Case Study

Ms. Stixrud has been executive director of Northwest Parish Nurse Ministries in Portland, Oregon, since 1991. Her current outreach project is working with Maternal Life International to help develop and expand parish nursing in Swaziland, Africa. She served 18 years as nurse/teacher in three developing countries (Tanzania, India, and Egypt). During this time she gained experience working with Christian, Muslim, and Hindu communities.

Elizabeth Johnston Taylor, RN, PhD

Chapter 4, Spiritual Formation for the Ministry of Parish Nursing Practice

Dr. Taylor is associate professor at Loma Linda University School of Nursing in Loma Linda, California. She earned her doctorate in nursing from the University of Pennsylvania, where she studied the psychosocial and spiritual aspects of living with illness. Her expertise in researching spirituality and health-related quality of life was further developed during a 2-year postdoctoral fellowship at the UCLA School of Nursing. In addition to academic studies, she has obtained two units of Clinical Pastoral Education and training in spiritual direction. She has received funding for her research and training from the National Cancer Institute, the Agency for Health Care Policy and Research, the John Templeton Foundation, the Oncology Nursing Society, the ONS Foundation, and the Hospice Nurses Association. Dr. Taylor has numerous publications, including articles and book chapters, on topics such as quality of life, ethical decision making, pain management, and spiritual responses to illness. Her book *Spiritual Care: Nursing Theory, Research, and Practice* is published by Prentice Hall. She serves as a member of the *Oncology Nursing Forum* editorial board, as a collateral reviewer for Sigma Theta Tau and Oncology Nursing Foundation research grants, as president of the Iota Lambda chapter of Sigma Theta Tau International, and as coordinator for the ONS Spiritual Care Special Interest Group.

Carol S. Tippe, RN, BSN, MPH

Chapter 16, Encouraging the Heart of Parish Nurse Ministry: The Sabbatical Renewal Leave

Ms. Tippe has been the minister of health/parish nurse at St. Mark's United Methodist Church in Iowa City, Iowa, for 15 years. The poetry in her chapter for this book was written during her 4-month congregationally-funded sabbatical in 2000. Ms. Tippe received her BSN from the University of Iowa in 1979 and her master in public health nursing from the University of North Carolina-Chapel Hill in 1983. She celebrated 25 years of professional nursing practice in 2004, having taught nursing, worked in community health, nursing homes, student health services, hospice care, and most recently parish nursing.

JoVeta Wescott, RN, MSHA

Chapter 25, Grant Writing for Parish Nurses and Parish Nurse Coordinators

Ms. Wescott works as a consultant and grant writer. She is the project director for a grant on clergy nutrition and sabbath education. She was previously a parish nurse consultant for a large health system. In this position she served parish nurses, health ministers, and clergy throughout Kansas. She served on the advisory committee for the 2004 Parish Nurse Curriculum. She is a faculty member for the Basic Preparation for Parish Nurses course. Ms. Wescott has published on the topics of spirituality, advance directives, and parish nursing. She is a member of many local and state coalitions.

Lisa M. Zerull, RN, MS

Chapter 19, Administration of Parish Nursing: Describing the Roles

Ms. Zerull is currently the program director for Community Case Management, Outreach, and Wound Ostomy and Continence Nursing Services for Valley Health System in Winchester, Virginia. In addition, she is the parish nurse coordinator for the Northwestern Virginia Parish Nurse Coalition. Ms. Zerull has been the parish nurse for Grace Evangelical Lutheran Church since 1996. She received her bachelor's degree in nursing from Ohio State University and her master's in nursing from George Mason University. She has received the Excellence in Nursing Practice Award from Sigma Theta Tau, Rho Pi chapter, and was designated Outstanding Nurse in Virginia by the Virginia Nurses Association in 1999.

Deborah Ziebarth, RN, BSN

Chapter 22, Policies and Procedures for the Ministry of Parish Nursing Practice

Ms. Ziebarth is currently the manager of Community Benefit Outreach Nursing at Waukesha Memorial Hospital in Waukesha, Wisconsin. For the last 10 years Ms. Ziebarth has also served as a parish nurse and a parish nurse coordinator, managing 21 parish nurses in 36 community sites. Previously she served as a missionary nurse in a large village in Somalia, East Africa, for 3 years. Before these experiences she worked for 13 years as an intensive care nurse. Ms. Ziebarth is currently enrolled in the MSN program at Cardinal Stritch University in Milwaukee, Wisconsin.

Wendy Zimmerman, RN, BSN

Chapter 7, The Public-Private Partnership: Expansion of the Ministry

Ms. Zimmerman has been involved in parish nursing since 1987, when she served as the parish nurse for Carter-Westminster Presbyterian Church in Skokie, Illinois. She currently serves as the parish nurse coordinator for Washington County Health System in Hagerstown, Maryland, a program that partners with 43 faith communities and over 100 unpaid parish nurses. Ms. Zimmerman has been a speaker at the Health Ministry Association and the Westberg Symposium national conferences and presents regionally at parish nurse retreats and educational gatherings. She received her bachelor's degree in nursing from North Park University and Theological Seminary in Chicago and has done graduate work at DePaul University, also in Chicago.

My life with Granger was not going to be ordinary. That was clear from the beginning of our relationship. Long before he was ordained, I knew that his ministry would be different, although neither of us could foresee the direction it would eventually take.

Still, when we moved to Bloomington, Illinois, our first (and only) church, I had dreams of raising our family in this lovely community. Surely, this church offered plenty of challenges to keep Granger busy for years.

We moved to Bloomington in 1939. The results of the Depression still abounded. The First English Lutheran Church had a large debt, so big that the mortgage company put the building up for auction. Buying back the church was Granger's first challenge.

His ministry was not limited to raising money to pay off the debt and recruiting new members for the church, though. Far from it. Granger's tendencies to reform – to try to improve how things were done in many areas – blossomed. He developed relationships with the other clergy in town, even those whose theology forbade them to walk into a Lutheran church. He had a church member, who was a physiology professor, teach sex education to the confirmands. He challenged the custom of ministers marrying couples "on the spot" and proposed that all clergy do premarital counseling. In Granger's mind there was always a better way to make God's presence known.

When we had been in Bloomington for just a little over a year, Granger and I went to the old Majestic Theater in town. Granger spotted the pipe organ that had not been played for 10 years. Granger and I missed the music of a good pipe organ. English Lutheran had a little reed pump organ that was powered with a vacuum cleaner motor.

Never one to pass up an opportunity, Granger decided that the pipe organ was perfect for English Lutheran. By Thanksgiving he had convinced the brother of a friend, who was an organ builder, to investigate whether the theatre organ could be rebuilt in our church. Sure enough, after Fred did a little research, he declared that the organ could be restored. The church purchased the organ for $600. It took 18 months to rebuild the organ. In the meantime, the pipes were stored in the parish hall basement and every other available corner of English Lutheran.

Getting the organ assembled was a lot of work for everyone. On the day after the dedication, the president of the board, Fred Anderson, who was a dedicated person, drove into our driveway. I said to him, "Well, Fred, you can all relax now." He shook his head and looked at me so pitifully. "No," he responded, "Granger will think of something else." How true that's been all through the years.

In 1941 Granger had the opportunity to fill in for a week as the chaplain at Augustana Hospital in Chicago. He had been instructed to visit every patient, every day, in that 300-bed hospital. Typical of Granger, he turned a deaf ear and came up with his own plan. He looked for the friendliest nurse he could find and told her that he was pinch-hitting for the chaplain. He asked her to find the people who really needed what he had to give. After clarifying what it was he "had to give," the nurse directed him to a man who had two teenagers who were driving him nuts. After a short time the man said something like, "You know, chaplain, I've done more serious thinking in the last few days in the hospital than I have done for many months, even years." That was a theme that Granger heard all week long.

Granger was excited by the endless possibilities he saw for the church and for himself in healthcare.

Talking with patients about profound life issues was just the beginning. I knew after that week at Augustana that we would not live in Bloomington much longer.

Throughout Granger's years in healthcare, in both the hospital and clinical setting, he came to respect the innate ability that nurses had to care for the whole person: the body, mind, and spirit. He realized nurses were pivotal in the care of each patient. From 1944 on, after he accepted the job of full-time chaplain at Augustana Hospital, he became more convinced than ever that nurses were key to the quality of care patients received. He wanted them to play a more prominent role. As usual, he was not content with the way things were.

When he moved on to the University of Chicago in the 1950's, he involved nurses in religion-medicine case conferences. In the 1970's at the Wholistic Health Centers, nurses were equal members of the team. Forty-two years after his initial contact with hospital chaplaincy and nursing, he fine-tuned his vision for nurses and came up with the idea of the parish nurse.

So on target was the concept of parish nursing and so right was the timing that within a few years there were more than a thousand parish nurses across this country and others. Fortunately for parish nursing, many capable people became involved on all levels. Because of this, parish nursing became a credible profession rather than just an interesting idea. The people who were involved in the early days were the ones who saw to it that parish nursing was taken seriously in the academic community, as well as in the medical community and the church community. Although there was always room for experimenting, they made sure that nurses held to the basic model.

The editors of this book were pioneers in the development, implementation, and education for parish nursing. Many of the contributors were also with parish nursing from its early years. The book draws on the expertise of people in nursing and related fields.

Over the years parish nursing has evolved, and so this updated book is needed. This book reflects current practices and research in parish nursing. It is aimed at healthcare professionals, clergy, educators, students, and everyone else who might need an in-depth perspective on parish nursing. It covers many aspects including spiritual development, interventions, collaborative care, accountability, competencies, and continuing education.

I am very impressed with the strides made in the specialty of parish nursing. Parish nursing made sense to me from the very beginning, and I am so glad that it thrives. Granger would be proud that parish nurses continually test out new possibilities and that they build on his dream.

Helen Johnson Westberg

Introduction

Unfortunately, most readers of this book will be nurses and pastors.

Now that I have your attention, given that crabby opening line, let me say what I mean by that opening word "unfortunately." Certainly it does not imply lack of respect for members of the nursing and clergy professions. They are *key* to the development of the parish nurse concept and to realizing it. And – now let me use the second person pronoun – *you* nurses and nursing educators, *you* ministers and priests who have this book before your eyes, may not represent a congregation of the "converted." *That* means that the authors of this book do not assume they are only "preaching to the converted."

You may not be only half-converted. That is, if you are a nurse, you are almost certain to be tantalized by the vision of parish nursing offered here, but you may immediately lose heart when you picture how hard it is to realize the role. Again, you may be only converted – converted as a pastor because, although you will see at once where this concept fits into the theology and mission of a congregation, you may have a hard time summoning energies to add "one more thing" to the complex institution to which you minister in the name of Jesus Christ. Your table and agenda are full.

Yet, I am convinced in both cases that you will be convinced by the arguments, inspired by the vision, and informed by the practical details of this book. The worry is that neither you nurses nor your pastor, without whose support the parish nurse project will get nowhere, will be lonely, apparently self-interested promoters. "Unfortunately," you cannot carry it by yourself. Now let me drop the second-person language and start talking also to other readers who, one hopes, might be looking over your shoulder or might respect your recommendation.

Fortunately, for example, this *is* a book for finance committees and stewardship committees of congregations. The late Pastor Granger Westberg, in his lucid and memorable account of how the parish nurse program was invented, tells how he worked his way around congregations, making the case. All went well until he reached the finance committee. There the trouble started. How can an item costing $10,000 or more be fit into a congregational budget? In his story, they are not villains but realists. Some of his best friends, and mine and yours, are no doubt on finance and stewardship committees, or should be. They simply know how hard it is to get busy congregations and their members to give priority to something new.

One could say that the parish nurse program is a great money-saver, but that does not work well, because most members will never know it. A young politician doing some apprentice or intern work for a U.S. senator once told me of his work on a piece of legislation. As I recall it, the law would simply seek to enforce the demand that freight trains come equipped with a certain kind of flashing strobe light that would serve as a warning to cars approaching crossings. From studies made in the states that enforced and did not enforce such laws, it was estimated that about 20 lives would be saved every year. "Unfortunately, those 20 people will not ever know that this law, and the action by this senator, saved their lives, but, still, their lives will be saved."

There is no doubt, no doubt at all, that a parish nurse will similarly save people money. They help teach "preventive medicine," which is the least expensive form of care there is. Through their counseling, their referrals, their "brokering" and "fixing," there is no doubt that they will help individuals, insuring agencies, and governments save money in a time of a healthcare financing crisis.

One could verge on the point of overselling by reminding us that healthy congregants are more free to give more woman-hours and man-hours through their congregations to the service of others, and that the parish nurse program will help keep more of them healthy. But I use the fiscal theme here at the beginning only to symbolize the fact that there are large potential audiences for this book and to express the hope that it reaches them.

Why make such a fuss about the locale for the recently developed form of service? Why focus on the congregation, when, historically, people have connected through the nursing profession with hospitals, "visiting," or home care – but not with places that have steeples and domes, altars and high steps, which made things hard for people in wheelchairs? Why?

Some years ago while writing about health and medicine in our part of the Christian tradition, I interviewed the presiding bishop of a denomination in that tradition. What advice could he give to someone who has just been given medical bad news? His answer: "My advice is that that person should have been an active member of a vital congregation for quite a few years." Meaning? Meaning that when misfortune comes, it is important to be part of a community of care. A congregation enfolds one in intercessory prayer – loving one's neighbor on one's knees. A good congregation provides care and casseroles, rides to clinics, and cards for the bedside table. It represents a gathering of people who have heard and keep on hearing the word of the Healer, who are busy interpreting the message of wholeness in a world of brokenness. By their own stumbling words, halting actions, and only sometimes distracted thoughts, they help the person who is ill come to terms with some of their problems, to cope, and, in a way, to transcend them on the pilgrimage to triumph.

So – the congregation is important. It will become more so as people realize its vital role in a time when healthcare in traditional institutions is simply beyond the range of more and more people, in a time when expenses grow. Not too long ago, a veteran physician who cares for aged people told me that he visited his 90-year old father daily in a Jewish senior citizens' home. This physician can afford the best of care, and provides it, for a man whose dignity is threatened along with his memory, which fails him thanks to a disease. "I have to say," said this Jewish physician, "that for all the professionals in his range, the person who treats my father as a dignified and worthy human being and who seems to get some response, is a young black aide who probably will tell you she does that for him because she loves Jesus." The doctor went on to use that as an illustration of a resource in the believing community. "You folks spend too much time working on the religious angle in hair-raising, urgent, sudden healthcare crises-like 'shall we pull the plug?' Religion has most to offer in terms of long-term care, of sustained relations, where year in and year out people have to be motivated to take care." Congregations exist for that, and the parish nurse program helps them realize such care intelligently.

In a way, the invention of the parish nurse concept is part of several revolutions going on before our eyes but hard to define and grasp.

First, it is part of a revolution in understandings of health and medicine. For 2 centuries we had been moving, usually unwittingly but sometimes wittingly, into accepting the model – the jargon has it "paradigm" – which saw that only conventional science could cure. Invest enough in research, make enough discoveries, develop enough professionals, build enough institutions, spend enough money, show enough awe, and such science would take care of our problems.

Today that model or paradigm is very much in question, not least of all among many scientists, researchers, discoverers, professionals, institution builders, and appropriators. They are coming to recognize that humans have or are "healing systems" that come into positive effect only when they are seen in the context of the larger systems around them. Westberg reminds us that the parish nurse program was nurtured by a hospital that believes in human ecology. Believing thus, it promotes the idea that we humans have to be seen in the delicate web and fibers of our contexts, which include God, nature, others and the self.

Of course, the search for a new paradigm can lead to many devices or prescriptions which can delude and misuse people. Some uses of the term "wholistic," for instance, are connected to ideas that connect the individual to the universe, its forces and energies, in such a way that the individual is "part of God" or "becomes God" or is offered complete transcendence of suffering and care. Often this goes by the code word "New Age" holistic care. Without needing to contend that nothing good comes from disciplines connected with such an approach, we can observe its limits. People do keep suffering, falling ill, and dying in spite of their beliefs of that sort – of, for that matter, their belief in the God beyond the gods who is the Creator, the Healer, the One who cares and weeps with us on the path to fulfillment.

The parish nurse concept is born in an entirely different context of "wholistic" care. It knows that in congregations people hear messages and try to realize them – messages directed to a world in which hate and misery, limits and pain, and doubt and despair threaten almost as much as love and joy, boundary-breaking and pleasure, and faith and hope are promised and realized.

Not many seasons ago, I presented an essay by a Christian neurosurgeon to a secular group of physicians, humanists, and social scientists. He told what the service of "Christ crucified" meant to him when he interpreted his vocation, his life in respect to patients. Of course, the author reminded readers, he stayed within the bounds of his profession and kept the physician's covenant that one keeps in a pluralist society. That is, although he may use "invasive" techniques in brain surgery, he is not "invasive" in respect to patients' belief systems, not disruptive of their patterns, and not ready to be distracted from what they have sought by coming to him. It was a nice, important distinction, without which he could not function and help in healing.

One of the participants in the group spoke up in response. I suppose a stereotyper would call him a latter-day Marxist social scientist. That is, he uses Marxist techniques of social analysis to call into question the professions and structures of our society. (He does have a good mind and does not offer Marxian therapy, simply "socialized" care, at this late date.) But he spoke up for others in the group when he said he hoped that the surgeon was not engaging in a new version of the body-mind distinction. That is, when this Christian deals with the body, he is nothing but a scientist and when he deals with the mind, his mind, he is a believer. Without spelling out *how*, this professor said he hoped that the physician

was more "wholistic." He should use his faith to engage in critical analysis of how his profession works and through what institutions he works and toward what end they are all directed.

This is not the place to follow up on what all that means and can mean. It is the place to remind ourselves that, in even the most apparently remote corners of "scientific" and "academic" life, thoughtful people are giving second thoughts to the place of faith in the provision of healthcare. It may take a few minutes to work such people around to understanding the vital role of congregations in the ecology of the lives of half of Americans. It may take a few hours to help them come to see the promise of the parish nurse program in respect to that role. This book will certainly help in such tasks.

Most readers, however, are not going to be Marxist sociologists, scientific skeptics, or secularists whose spiritual imaginations have atrophied if they were even given a spiritual vision at all. Most readers will be nurses and pastors, church committees, and, one hopes, theologians – people whose own imaginations may have been atrophied or whose visions have not yet been caught. They are people for whom constraints of time and money will be in the front of the mind, but in whose hearts the Holy Spirit, who "calls, gathers, and enlightens" the congregation is also active.

One of the great advantages of parish nurse work, in contrast to that of the neurosurgeon in a high-tech hospital or the employee in a tax-supported institution, is that nurses work in a context where certain meanings are allowed to be developed explicitly. Theologian James Fowler has written on the two languages of pluralist society. On one level, out of respect for each other, in a spirit of tolerance and deference, and to keep civil peace, we do not always "unload" the whole focused theme of our beliefs. Often we may feel that those beliefs could be of direct aid to someone else. Still, the rules of the game call for some holding back. For example, one doesn't enter into an interfaith dialogue and then suddenly change the rules of the game midway and try to pounce on partners with pitches for conversion.

At the same time, says Fowler (I am rephrasing a bit), sometimes this situation makes us feel as if we are biting our tongues, choking to hold back what we might utter, holding our breaths, or stepping cautiously because we know there is a particular story, a special language of faith, and a distinctive grasp of God's grace, which would be of greater aid than the language we would elsewhere use.

The parish nurse program works chiefly in congregations or communities where a certain language of faith is ready at hand. This does not mean that the nurse becomes preacher, has to be an explicit teacher, or a theological expert. It means that she or he knows that the Christian story is privileged and can not only be brought up but is also expected to have its place. It means that the nurse works in an ecology of meanings and care that promotes drawing on that message of grace and the practices and habits the message encourages.

One of the rules of etiquette for writers of forewords to books is that they should not give the plot away. There were many times as I read this manuscript when I wanted to steal more than the single Westberg story of his encounters with finance committees, in order to lure readers on.

But these authors can and do speak for themselves. One of my marginal notes on the manuscript of a practical essay in this book – and there are several – is "these authors think of everything." This is "how to" literature of a high order. Maybe what makes it all hold together is that it is also "why to" literature. We have needed that and will need it if we accept the "risk" about which Westberg speaks and dreams. We might risk helping discover and invent something new in human care at a time of great need, when hearts grow faint but the message of God in Christ does not.

Rev. Martin E. Marty, PhD

Martin E. Marty is the Fairfax M. Cone Distinguished Service Professor Emeritus at the University of Chicago and a columnist for The Christian Century. *He is editor of the semimonthly* Context, *a newsletter on religion and health, and a weekly contributor to* Sightings, *a biweekly electronic editorial published by the Marty Center University of Chicago Divinity School.*

Preface

The creation of this book is the result of the work of many. The contributors, who have a rich experience in the ministry of parish nursing practice, have generously taken the time to work with the editors making this book a reality. The title of the book is simple and straightforward. The intention of the writing is to focus in three primary arenas: continued development of the ministry, education, and administration as it relates to the ministry of parish nursing practice. For some, the use of *the ministry of parish nursing practice* to describe parish nursing will be new. The intent in using this terminology is to stress that parish nursing is both ministry and practice. It is not solely one or the other, but both. Therein lies the challenge: to demonstrate and offer a ministry that intends to minister to the soul with the integrity and accountability of the professional practice of nursing.

There have been a number of books published about parish nursing since our previous book, *Parish Nursing: Promoting Whole Person Health Within Faith Communities*, was published in 1999. Consequently, we did not want to provide still another book on setting up a parish nurse program or to simply update our previous work. This book has several intended audiences: those interested or involved in the ministry of parish nursing practice; directors and/or coordinators of parish nursing for a cluster of hospitals, a healthcare system, or a regional network of parish nurses; and hospital administrators/managers, trustees, or physicians. The expanding parish nurse educator community is another audience. This includes deans and trustees or members of advisory boards of universities and/schools of nursing. Seminary faculty and clergy represent still another potential readership along with other lay ministers or members of health cabinets.

This book represents the work of so many, not just that of the chapter authors. Behind every chapter author stands the work of many others who have pioneered the development of the ministry of parish nursing practice in their congregations, schools of nursing, healthcare institutions, or community agencies. Several of the authors will be familiar to the parish nurse community; others will be brand new.

Organization of the Book

The book is divided into three sections. **Unit I, Development of the Ministry of Parish Nursing Practice**, addresses some of the unique aspects of the ministry ingrained in this practice. The reader will be acquainted with a historical perspective on parish nursing, as well as two very important issues that remain current in this ministry of parish nursing practice: research and accountability. Rationales for spiritual formation and for nurturing the self are explored, as well as helpful strategies for consideration. Detailed descriptions of successful collaboration and partnering will surely be useful to the reader. **Unit II, Educational Preparation for the Ministry of Parish Nursing Practice**, examines parish nursing education. Curricula issues are discussed: evaluating for competency, preparing for dual competencies, the distance learning format, and the role of mentoring. Three related chapters are included that examine the identity of the parish nurse educator: *Chapter 10, You Teach Who You Are: A Lesson Plan for the Parish Nurse Educator; Chapter 14, Learning to Pray;* and *Chapter 16, Encouraging the Heart of Parish Nurse Ministry: The Sabbatical Renewal Leave.* **Unit III, Administration of the Ministry of Parish Nursing Practice,** provides the reader with several very practical chapters on the role of the administrator, how to work with a congregation, setting up policy and procedures, building a network, the challenges of working with underserved congregations, and how-to tips of grant funding. The current issue of ensuring quality outcomes for parish nursing is meant to be provocative. The final chapter in this section describes and then challenges the reader to envision a model of spiritual leadership and consider embracing the identified capacities in leading others. Surely the proposed framework will elicit a great deal of discussion.

We have used the term *parish nursing* to refer to this ministry, although we are aware of the coming acceptance of the terms *congregational nursing* and *faith community nursing* as more inclusive. We have also used "he" and "she" interchangeably when referring to the parish nurse, because although parish nursing is a predominantly female ministry, we value and support the contribution of our male parish nurses.

At the conclusion of each of the three sections of this book, we have provided our prospective on the challenges that face the ministry of parish nursing in practice, education, and administration. Challenges can be seen as insurmountable problems or, from a more adventuresome perspective, opportunities for creative solutions. For some, the challenges will present endless frustration rather than opportunities for taking a risk, making a mistake, and hopefully learning a valuable lesson. Dealing with the challenges presented by the ministry of parish nursing practice will not be for the faint of heart. It is doubtful that there will be any single solution. That is not the nature of the ministry of parish nursing practice. It never has been! If the solutions become too simple, this should be a clue to all of us that we are probably compromising the nature of parish nursing and acquiescing to the culture of the medical model or the current healthcare system. Parish nursing has always been a catalyst for change. Challenges are inherent in the ministry of parish nursing practice.

Acknowledgments

There are a number of acknowledgments to be made. The editors first and foremost want to thank Rev. Granger Westberg for his inspiration, vision, tenacity, and charisma. His widow, Helen, and his children, John, Jane, Joan, and Jill, have not only continued to inspire both of us in our work on this book but have also contributed their writing skills to the project. We are deeply indebted to the many contributors who responded to our invitation to share their experience and wisdom. Our gratitude also goes to those individuals who served as external reviewers for this manuscript. We wish to acknowledge all those at Elsevier who supported this project. We want to especially thank our editor at Elsevier, Linda Thomas, who showed not only interest but also enthusiasm for the project from the start and guided the process through the maze of corporate publisher approvals. We appreciate the untiring work of Cheryl Abbott, senior project manager. Together we thank the dean of the Marcella Niehoff School of Nursing, Sheila Haas, RN, PhD, FAAN, for believing in the value of the ministry of parish nursing practice, along with the continuous support of our colleagues at Loyola University Chicago, especially those in the school of nursing. We are particularly grateful for the opportunity to develop the interdisciplinary Center for Spiritual Leadership in Health Care through the School of Nursing at Loyola University Chicago. This effort will allow us to continue to expand offerings for those in the ministry of parish nursing practice and other healthcare professions to enhance their own spirituality and care of others. Together we express our deep appreciation for the years we were privileged to be associated with Lutheran General Hospital, Advocate Health Care. The people we were blessed to know have enriched our lives personally and professionally and have brought us into contact with people who have left their footprints on our hearts.

There are also some individual acknowledgments to be made.

Phyllis Ann Solari-Twadell expresses her appreciation to the original staff of the International Parish Nurse Resource Center: Annette Mariani, Rusty McDermott, Denise Dowling, Eileen Klemundt, Olga Wegehaupt, Audrey Munger, and Karen Cornforth, who not only gave her the experience of spiritual leadership but who also provided dedication, creativity, and nurturing to the development of the ministry of parish nursing practice. Ann continues to be grateful for the presence of her family: her daughter and son-in-law, Kim and David Kuhlman; her stepson and his wife, Eric and Anne Twadell; her nephew and his wife, Joseph and Suze Solari; her grandchildren: Nathan, Clara, and Stephen Kuhlman and Kaitlyn and Lauren Twadell; and her grandnephews to whom she is Nona, Rowan and Vincent Solari who remain God's greatest blessings, lifting Ann up to be a "grandmother rich in the spirit." Ann also recognizes the richness of her life that was formed in relationship with her deceased mother and father, Phyllis and Archie Solari; her husband, Stephen Lacombe Twadell; and her brother and sister-in-law, Joseph and Jean Solari. She remains thankful for the life of her brother and sister-in-law, Robert and Patricia Solari.

Mary Ann McDermott thanks her husband, Dennis, for his love and his continuing encouragement for just about anything she does! For their support, she thanks her children Dennis and his wife, Tina; Michael; Sarah and her partner, Kerry Wong; and William and his wife, Wendy. To Ryan and Carly, she also says thanks for just being her grandchildren. Mary Ann

expresses deep appreciation to her spiritual director and friend of 25 years, Father Harold Bonin.

We would like to remember our deceased colleague, Anne Marie Djupe, RNC, MA, who was a pioneer in the administration of the ministry of parish nursing practice and co-editor of the first parish nurse text in 1990, *Parish Nursing: The Developing Practice*. We would also like to remember the contribution of Judith Ryan, RN, PhD FAAN, to the development of the ministry of parish nursing practice through her assistance with parish nurse educational colloquies and the development of the collective mission and vision for the ministry of parish nursing practice.

Finally, we are grateful to God for all the inspired direction and grace bestowed on the ministry of parish nursing practice.

To all the parish nurses, parish nurse coordinators, and parish nurse educators, past and present, who have given of themselves so generously to shape and develop the ministry of parish nursing practice.

Phyllis Ann Solari-Twadell
Mary Ann McDermott

Contents

UNIT II

Educational Preparation for the Ministry of Parish Nursing Practice, 109

Appendixes

UNIT I

Development of
the Ministry of
Parish Nursing
Practice

A Personal Historical Perspective of Whole Person Health and the Congregation

Reverend Granger Westberg

INTRODUCTION—BY JANE WESTBERG

This chapter, "A Personal Historical Perspective of Whole Person Health and the Congregation," was originally written by my father Granger Westberg in 1990 and rewritten by him in 1999 before his death in February of that year. In this chapter he begins his historical review in the late 1960s. Actually, he had begun grappling with the notion of whole person health in the 1940s, long before it was a generally recognized—let alone widely accepted—concept.

In 1944, convinced that the body could not be treated separately from the mind and spirit, Westberg, then a 31-year-old parish pastor, made an unusual career move. Against the advice of his colleagues who thought he was throwing away a promising career, he became one of the first full-time hospital chaplains. In those days the vast majority of chaplains at Protestant hospitals were elderly and worked part-time in relative isolation from physicians. Chaplains were expected to visit as many patients as possible, so their contacts with patients were often limited to passing out pamphlets and offering prayers. Westberg felt that clergy could offer much more and that they could work effectively with physicians and nurses in providing whole person care, particularly if they had the opportunity to acquire some new understandings and skills being taught outside of seminaries in relatively new, hands-on "clinical training" programs. To prepare himself for his work at Augustana Hospital, Westberg attended several such courses in which he studied with Russell Dicks, Anton Boisen, and other pioneers in clinical pastoral education.

Only a few physicians at Augustana grasped Westberg's vision of clergy, nurses, and physicians working together in caring for the whole person. However, nurses usually understood and were excited about this concept. One barrier to whole person care was the fact that many physicians treated nurses as second-class citizens rather than full partners on a health team. Westberg, however, recognized that nurses were potentially one of the most valuable members of the health team because they were in a unique position to help patients with physical and psychological problems as well as problems of the human spirit (Westberg, 1955a; Westberg, 1955b).

In his first month at Augustana, Westberg created and taught a for-credit course in religion and health for student nurses. The course included the "art of conversation," which he taught in part by asking students to write up their encounters with patients using the verbatim case-based write-up method that he learned from Russell Dicks. In the course, he also addressed the needs of the whole person, the use of prayer and sacraments in the sick room, the parish pastor in the hospital, and the chaplain-nurse team. Westberg's first book, *Nurse, Pastor, and Patient* (1955), grew out of this course, which was one of the first of its kind in the country.

3

In a 1945 letter to his colleague O.V. Anderson, Westberg said he wanted to teach a course on religion and health to medical students and interns. He knew that such courses were absent from the medical curricula. This dream, however, had to wait.

Aware that most seminaries, including his own, did not offer courses that prepared clergy for their work as counselors and members of the health team, Westberg and Dicks jointly created clinical pastoral education courses at their respective hospitals for parish pastors and theological students. Westberg urged seminaries to offer clinical education. Westberg also worked with Dicks and others in establishing the Association of Protestant Hospital Chaplains (APHC), which developed standards and guidelines for chaplains. (APHC is now the interfaith organization known as Association of Professional Chaplains.)

In 1952 Westberg accepted an opportunity to move toward more whole person healthcare by bridging the worlds of medicine and religion. As chaplain of the University of Chicago Clinics and associate professor of pastoral care in the federated theological faculty, he set up courses in which theological students and pastors had clinical experiences that included being part of health teams, along with physicians, residents, and medical students. In time he realized his goal of teaching courses in religion and health to medical students. He also held religion and medicine case conferences that included physicians, clergy, and some nurses. Reflecting later on these conferences, Westberg described the nurses as intermediaries between clergy and physicians:

> In those case conferences, we pastors and physicians attempted to learn how to talk with each other. We soon learned that we lived in two different worlds and spoke two quite different languages. It was the nurses who helped in the translation. As we gradually got over the language barrier, with the help of nurse interpreters, our discussions became more valuable (Westberg, 1979).

Westberg's inroads in medicine became evident in 1956 when he was given the first joint appointment in any major university at the University of Chicago's School of Medicine and Divinity School. That year in a keynote address at the annual meeting of the Association of American Medical Colleges, Westberg asserted, "There has been growing interest in the patient as a person, a whole person, with physical, mental and spiritual needs" (March, 1957). "Seminary professors," he said, "were beginning to invite physicians to participate in the instruction of theological students because they recognized that clergy could never minister to a soul apart from a body and had blind spots in regard to the physical and psychological needs of people." Westberg suggested that physicians, in turn, "have blind spots in terms of the philosophical or theological dimensions of the lives of their patients," so he recommended involving clergy in the education of medical students (Westberg, 1957).

Westberg felt that some progress was being made in providing more whole person hospital-based care. However, he was becoming increasingly convinced that to make a real difference in the health of the nation, more attention needed to be given at the community level to preventing illness and to identifying it in its earliest, most easily treatable stages (Westberg, 1956). He argued that clergy, who have a key to every home in their parish, were in an excellent position to identify and help people who were "a little bit sick" (Westberg, 1958; Westberg, 1979).

Westberg also envisioned congregations having a key role in prevention and whole person healthcare. In a sermon at Rockefeller Chapel, he declared, "There is a magnificent rebellion against a religion that only preaches and fails to heal" (Westberg, 1960). Preaching and teaching is not the minister's task alone; nor is healing restricted only to physicians. It is "entirely probable," said Westberg, that properly educated Christian lay people "can provide a quality and range of healing services beyond anything ever imagined." They can provide "pastoral healing of troubled individuals as well as the healing of troubled homes" (Westberg, 1960). Westberg continued:

> The Church has not assumed its share of responsibility for the health of the community. It has defined health in too narrow a fashion.... It has taken two world wars, a depression, the influence of Sigmund Freud, the development of social work, the establishment of a new denomination (Christian Science), to shake us who belong to the Church out of our

complacency and to make us rethink the command to heal, which our Lord gave to us 1900 years ago.

In other talks Westberg said, "Church buildings, especially parish houses stand vacant a large part of the week" (Westberg, 1956-62). Instead, during the week, some of the space could be used for a clinic, for counseling services, or for "day hospitals" where people in distress could come for pastoral care and other services. Therapy groups of various sorts could be conducted. The various services could be related to an individual church or a council of churches.

While he was at the University of Chicago and later, from 1964 to 1967 as Dean of the Institute of Religion in Houston, Westberg set up congregation and community-based clinical education programs for interfaith groups of clergy. In the late 1960s, Westberg, then Professor of Practical Theology at Hamma School of Theology at Wittenberg University, created the first prototypical wholistic health center. He begins the following chapter by saying that the Wholistic Health Centers began spontaneously, but clearly he had done a lot of groundwork that clarified his vision, focused his thinking, and prepared the way first for Wholistic Health Centers and then for parish nursing. The remainder of this chapter is the original as submitted by my dad.

IN THE WORDS OF GRANGER WESTBERG

It all happened quite spontaneously. A group of us had been experimenting since the late 1960s with "Wholistic" Health Centers that were family doctors' offices in churches. Our aim was to see if we could bring about whole person healthcare in a church setting by having spiritually oriented family doctors, nurses, and clergy working together as a team.

It was a project enthusiastically sponsored by the W.K. Kellogg Foundation and the Department of Preventive Medicine and Community Health of the University of Illinois College of Medicine. More than a dozen of these Wholistic Health Centers were begun in neighborhood churches in upper-, middle-, and lower-income areas in cities around the country (Holistic Health Centers, 1976; Holistic Health Centers, 1977; Tubesing, 1976).

The evaluations of these doctors' offices in churches over a period of 10 years indicated that the quality of care offered when these three professions worked together under the same roof was measurably more whole person oriented than the average doctor's office. Further, it was clear that the nurses in each of these centers were the glue that bound these three professions together in a common appreciation of the healing talents of each.

Critics of the project doubted that scientific medicine and religion could collaborate in the care of patients. Over the years, however, they saw that it was working very well. As they tried to ascertain why it worked, they gradually came to the conclusion that most of the nurses employed in these clinics could speak two languages: the language of science and the language of religion. The nurses were acting as translators. They helped the doctor and the minister communicate in ways that were helpful to a whole person approach to healthcare.

Parish Nurses: A New Idea

As inflation swept America and it became more and more expensive to start new Wholistic Health Centers in churches, someone said, "If the nurses in these clinics have proved so valuable, why not try placing a nurse on the staff of a congregation and see what happens?" When we asked individual nurses about this idea, the response was immediately favorable. We decided to give it a try.

I went to Lutheran General Hospital (LGH) in 1984 because I had a long-standing relationship with several of the founding leaders of the hospital. LGH, located in Park Ridge, Illinois (a northwest suburb of Chicago), was founded in 1959. The hospital had long been a leader in pastoral care for its patients, and it showed immediate interest in participating in a pilot project. LGH describes its philosophy of "human ecology" as "the understanding and care of human beings as whole persons in light of their relationship to God, themselves, their families, and the society in which they live" (Norstad, 1994, p. 3).

Trying to Bring the Dream to Life

An administrative team from LGH was organized to plan and implement the first institution-based program. I was asked to go out and meet with pastors and congregational members. We were seeking six churches as our initial participants. We also decided to go to large churches of various denominations that might be able to afford hiring a nurse. Initially we were asking the church to pay the full half-time salary of about $10,000.

As I met with the pastors and described the concepts, about 75% showed great interest and 25% some interest. They readily recognized that the nurse would be a person to assist them in their ministry to people who were hurting and many whom they felt they couldn't adequately serve by themselves.

I then asked each pastor if there was a group of people to whom I could describe the concept on some evening. In many cases, this group consisted of nurses and other health professionals from the congregation. The response was immediately positive. Next I was invited to a decision-making board, such as the church council. I described the overall picture of health and the role of a nurse in the church. Again, the response was very positive.

All responses were positive until I met with the finance committee. They immediately expressed concerns about their budgets and finding the resources to support additional positions. Many felt that they couldn't fit the position into their current budget. Each of the churches I talked to had good reason for its financial concerns. Many were involved in building or renovation projects. It was then that I realized something very important. None of these large churches had a line in their budget with funds appropriate for risk taking. Consequently I had to go elsewhere to find funds. I went back to the hospital and explained that none of the churches, regardless of size, were willing to risk a salary of $10,000. This was 1984.

With the help of LGH administrators, who were eager to respond to the churches' willingness to participate in such a program, a plan was developed: LGH agreed to pay 75% of the salary the first year while the church paid 25%. It was decided that in the second year, the church would increase its contribution to 50%, the third year 75%. In the fourth year the church would be making the full payment. The hospital would continue to pay for the nurse's benefits and liability insurance.

The Pilot Project Is Underway

With the new proposal that they would contribute 25% of the salary the first year, six churches were willing to participate and agree to a 3-year trial period. Four of these churches were Protestant, and two were Roman Catholic. They were located as close as six blocks away from the hospital and as far as 30 miles away.

In early 1985, the hiring process began. An advertisement in a local paper brought some 30 applications for these half-time parish nurse positions. Interviewers from both the hospital and the churches discovered hidden talents in these nurses, and the quality of the candidates was deemed to be amazingly high. By and large, they were women (no male nurses applied) who were in their 30s and 40s and whose children were in school. They all showed genuine interest in a type of nursing that would allow the kind of creativity they had always desired.

All of the candidates were stimulated by the potential of a whole person approach to their work with people. The fact that they would be working within the context of a congregation and actually serving on the pastoral staff of the church was of great interest to them. Most of the candidates indicated that their original motivation for going into nursing was influenced strongly by a desire to incorporate the spiritual dimension into their work.

Jointly Learning from Experience

After choosing six nurses to participate in the program, we decided not to superimpose upon them a course of instruction because we were not at all sure what direction such a course should take. Instead, we invited them to spend a half-day each week at the hospital in an informal discussion group where, in the presence of a teaching chaplain, a nurse educator, and a family practice physician, they could describe what they felt they needed in an ongoing educational process. The salary of the staff supporting these sessions was part of the contribution from the hospital.

Once a week, the nurses came to LGH for 3 hours. This time was part of their salaried workweek. We began each day by going around the circle comprised of these six nurses and asking them to tell of their experiences in the parish during the preceding week. In the early weeks it took anywhere from 1 hour to 90 minutes for these women to tell the stories of their ministry. The telling of these stories brought about all sorts of questions, spontaneous role-playing of situations, even tears and laughter. Everyone took part. At the end of every session, we were all exhausted but also exhilarated to think that these unusual happenings were taking place simply because a nurse had been added to the staff of a church.

The parish nurses told us of their many opportunities to talk with people informally between services, at coffee hours, at meetings of church organizations, at potluck suppers, and in home visits with the sick or shut-in people. We saw that in these informal sessions nurses had an unusual opportunity to talk with people in the early stages of illness. Before people ever thought of seeing a doctor about their very minor problems, the nurse, with her unique sensitivity to early cries for help, was already responding to them.

Identifying Five Roles of the Parish Nurse

During the first year or two of the parish nurse project, it became clear that parish nurses played the following five roles:
1. The parish nurse is a health educator.
2. The parish nurse is a personal health counselor.
3. The parish nurse is a referral agent.
4. The parish nurse is a coordinator of volunteers.
5. The parish nurse is a developer of support groups.

Church Leaders as Natural Leaders in Preventive Medicine

It gradually dawned on us that churches are actually the one organization in our society most suited to leading in the field of preventive medicine. Scientific medicine has not been known for its contributions to preventive medicine. Jeff Goldsmith, a national healthcare advisor, says that the nation's healthcare system still acts as if most diseases strike "like a fire in your home" rather than "like a fire in a pile of leaves." As a result, he says, healthcare is preoccupied with climbing ladders and chopping holes in roofs instead of keeping a bucket of water and a rake nearby.

The history of the parish nurse movement is closely tied up with an understanding that churches, when they are functioning at their best, are dedicated to keeping people well. This means tending the little fires in piles of leaves. But most people do not see churches and synagogues as an integral part of our present health system (Westberg, 1988). If a pollster asks the question "What are the health agencies in your community?," the usual reply mentions local hospitals and perhaps a well-known clinic.

Churches as Part of the Healthcare System

When we speak of healthcare, we usually mean "sickness care." That's where hospitals and doctors' clinics do such a good job. So we still have to raise the question "What are the institutions of our culture that keep us well?" At least five institutions can do this if they are functioning well: home, school, church, the workplace, and the public health department. We are well aware of the sickness that can follow if any one of these five is not contributing to a quality of life that builds up immunity to disease.

The churches and synagogues of America are becoming conscious of their role in keeping people healthy. They have never really seen themselves as part of the nation's health system because healthcare was believed to deal with a complex thing called "medical technology" that was becoming more technical every day. Almost with the same suddenness, society is now realizing that many illnesses are preventable.

Most illnesses come on slowly. It is as if our bodies are trying to tell us that something about how we look at life, or handle life's many problems, is making us sick. If we are not sick, we are at least more vulnerable to the germs attacking us. If a great deal of illness is related to our way of looking at life—our outlook on life, our philosophy of life—then, of course, religious institutions must be integrated into the healthcare system.

Nurses as Organizers

Parish nurses can play a key role in integrating religious institutions into the healthcare system. They are well suited to creating community-based health centers in churches. Almost two-thirds of the people in the United States have some tangible relationship to congregations. Churches of all sizes and shapes are to be found in all corners of the United States, and in almost every church there is a registered nurse. Most large churches have 25 or more nurses in their membership. Most of these churches, however, have never even thought to use these nurses in any creative manner, until recently.

The Christian Way as a Foundation for Healthful Living

Sixty years ago, a best-selling book by the famous missionary to India, E. Stanley Jones, titled *The Way*, contained the following quotations that help us understand that the Christian way provides an excellent foundation for healthful living (Jones, 1930):

> When we live the Christian way, we are living the way we were made to live...made in the inner structure of our being.

- Evil is a turning of the natural into the unnatural; it is a living against life.
- Self-love, the natural, can become selfishness, the unnatural.
- Self-respect, the natural, may be lured into pride, the unnatural.
- Love, the natural, can be beguiled into lust, the unnatural.
- Sexual desire, the natural, can be lured away from its God-intended creative function and become an end in itself.
- These simple, natural functions, dedicated to God and controlled by God, bring life to the whole person. But if they *become* god, become ends in themselves, there is one result: death – death to development, to happiness, to the whole person.

E. Stanley Jones and many other Christian divines through the centuries were remarkably aware of the wholeness concept that many of us are coming to see as a sensible approach to health. It gives validity to the entrance of churches into the health field.

Making Christian Faith More Relevant to Our Age

Many active, dedicated church members of all branches of Christendom are searching for ways to make the message of Christian faith more relevant to our age. They are fascinated by the way Jesus in his healing ministry always dealt with people as whole persons. They are disturbed that our present highly technical healthcare system tends to neglect the spiritual dimensions of illness. Just as the ecological movement has captured the imagination of youth throughout the world, whole person emphasis in healthcare also could be among the captivating concerns of a generation.

Many churches want to make a more meaningful contribution to society. They feel that they are stagnating because they spend so much of their time just talking. They want to become involved in action that leads to a healthier society. It is time to bring religiously oriented people into the discussion of what is meant by high-level wellness.

Facilitating Agreement on the Meaning of Health

If we can agree on a number of major religious concepts—stated clearly and succinctly—concerning health, our chances of getting church people and healthcare people to collaborate will increase greatly. I have suggested nine statements that could possibly be accepted by a wide variety of religious people (Westberg, 1982). They are the following:

1. Health is intimately related to how a person "thinketh in one's heart."
2. Physical health is not to be "our chief end in this life"—only a possible by-product of loving God and one's neighbor as oneself.
3. Health is closely tied up with goals, meaning, and purposeful living; it is a religious quest, whereas illness may be related to a life that is empty, bored, or without purpose or aim.
4. Our present disease-oriented medical care system must be revised to include a strong accent on modeling and teaching prevention and wellness.
5. Our present separation of body and spirit must go, and an integrated whole person approach must be put in its place.

6. Merely existing is different than living under God and responding to the prompting of God's spirit.
7. The body functions at its best when a person, who is the body, exhibits attitudes of hope, faith, love, and gratitude.
8. True health is closely associated with creativity by which we as people of God participate with God in the ongoing process of creation.
9. The self-preservation instincts of the human can be happily blended with the innate longing to love and to help others.

Health and Salvation

We who have been engaged in the parish nurse movement have found much meaning and challenge in the widespread determination to understand the meaning of the word *health* as much broader and deeper than ever before. It is a natural part of the vocabulary of the Bible and of Christian theology. "And the health shall spring forth" is a famous quotation from Isaiah. *Health* and *salvation* are words used interchangeably throughout the scriptures. Parish nurses are engaged in doing the Lord's work when they assist in encouraging people to move toward the whole person goals of the highest scriptural injunctions.

Parish nurses are now serving in hundreds of churches throughout the country, united in their desire to bring salvation to people, understanding that the basic meaning of the word *salvation* is *being made whole*. The Great Physician knows that not everyone wants to be made whole. Churches are in the motivation business. They understand how important it is to motivate people to want to live healthier lives. Christ himself asked that question of the man at the pool of Bethesda: "Do you want to be made whole?"

Taking Belief Systems Seriously

The whole person movement takes a person's belief system seriously. If one's belief system is faulty, it affects the way the body functions. If whole person concepts can be integrated with one's religious beliefs, each will motivate the other.

Today the Church is sorely needed to help motivate people to put body, mind, and spirit together and to convince them that the integration of these three can lead to truth, health, and wholeness.

Why Churches Are Natural Settings for Parish Nurses

The following are reasons for believing that churches provide a natural setting where parish nurses can do their most effective work as health educators, health counselors, coordinators of volunteers, agents of referral into our complex medical system, and integrators of faith and health:

1. Churches are to be found everywhere, out in the neighborhoods where people live—urban, suburban, rural communities—and their buildings are largely unused during the weekdays.
2. Churches have a long history of serving their communities through social activities and continuing education programs.
3. Churches symbolize our need to take seriously the problems of the human spirit that are so often related to the causes of illness.
4. Churches provide a remarkable reservoir of dedicated people who are willing to volunteer their services to assist in humanitarian endeavors.
5. Church members have a growing appreciation for the opportunity to model, in their own church buildings, the need for cooperation between scientific medicine and religious faith.

Basically the parish nurses' role is to reach out for more whole person ways of ministering to people who are hurting. Many healthcare professionals slowly have grown in their desire to integrate human caring with the achievements of high-tech medical care. Most of these professionals are under such restraints of time and bottom-line concerns that they cannot practice what they know would be better healthcare.

Parish nurses have the unique opportunity to demonstrate effective ways of combining the strengths of such collaboration between the humanities and the sciences.

REFERENCES

Jones, E.S. (1930). *The way.* New York: Association Press.

Norsted, F.M. (1994). *Presentations: Governance and philosophy.* Park Ridge, IL: Lutheran General Health System.

The Wholistic Health Centers: A new direction in health care (Experience Report). (1977). Battle Creek, MI: W. K. Kellogg Foundation.

Tubesing, D. (1976). *An idea in evolution: History of the Wholistic Health Centers project 1970-1976.* Hinsdale, IL: Wholistic Health Centers, Inc.

Westberg, G. (1955a). *Nurse, Pastor, Patient.* Rock Island: Augustana Book Concern.

Westberg, G. (1955b). "The nurse is the chaplain's ally." *The Modern Hospital,* 84(4).

Westberg, G. (1956). "A clergyman comments on the physician's role in the community. *Medical Bulletin.* Summer: 5-8.

Westberg, G. (1957). Religious aspects of medical teaching. *Journal of Medical Education* [Now *Academic Medicine*] 32(3): 204-209.

Westberg, G. (1958). The "new" field of religion and medicine. *Postgraduate Medicine* 23(6): 688.

Westberg, G. (1956-1962). Unpublished manuscripts. Avenues to health through religion.

Westberg, G. (1960). Unpublished, untitled manuscript (sermon) given at Rockefeller Chapel, University of Chicago.

Westberg, G. (1979). From hospital chaplaincy to wholistic health center. *The Journal of Pastoral Care* 33(2):

Westberg, G. (1982). The church as a health place. *Dialog,* 27(3): 189-191.

Westberg, G. (1988). Parishes, nurses, and health care. *Lutheran Partners,* Nov/Dec, 26-29.

Wholistic Health Centers. (1976). *Survey research report.* Hinsdale, IL: Society for Wholistic Medicine.

A Historical Perspective of Parish Nursing: Rules for the Sisters of the Parishes

Phyllis Ann Solari-Twadell
Karen Egenes

The historical perspectives for parish nursing have been well documented in the nursing literature (Bay, 1997; Clark & Olson, 2000; O'Brien, 2003; Patterson, 2003; Penner, 1997; Shelly & Miller, 1999; Striepe, 1993; Zerson, 1994; Zetterlend, 1997). Most of these works focus on the origins of parish nursing in the Christian tradition and emphasize its roots in the Protestant sects, specifically the work of Protestant deacons and deaconesses. The Kaiserwerth Deaconess program founded in Germany in the mid-nineteenth century by Theodore Fliedner, a Lutheran minister, repeatedly is presented as the prototype for modern parish nurses (Clark & Olson, 2000; O'Brien, 2003; Patterson, 2003; Shelly & Miller, 1999; Zerson, 1994; Zetterlend, 1997). Zerson notes that "Christian whole person needs were addressed in a variety of parish settings over the centuries. Notable among them were early Christian deaconesses; *Gemeindeschwestern* in nineteenth-century Germany; and Episcopal, Methodist and Lutheran sisters of the same period in the U.S." (1994, p. 20).

Although most histories of the parish nurse movement thus far have focused predominantly on protestant religious communities, the roots of parish nursing can also be found in a particular community of Roman Catholic sisters. In fact, the founders of this Catholic religious community composed rules for the sisters who worked in parishes that can continue to serve as guidelines for present day parish nurses.

The Daughters of Charity of Vincent de Paul: Roots of Parish Nursing from the Roman Catholic Tradition

Louise de Marillac lived in France in the 1600s. After the death of her husband in 1624, she sought out Vincent de Paul to serve as her spiritual director. Madame de Marillac had experienced a revelation from God earlier in her life that "she would serve God through assisting her neighbors," and she sought to develop a means to do so (McNamara, 1996, p. 482). In 1617 Vincent de Paul developed the first of his "*charites*" in his rural parish at Chatillon-en-Bresse. These Confreries de la Charite (usually called simply "*charites*") were societies of wealthy women called the "Ladies of Charity," who visited sick persons in their homes and provided both nursing care and spiritual comfort. *Charites* soon spread through rural France. In 1629 the first *charite* was established in Paris, with Louise de Marillac as its leader. However, the *charites* of Paris differed from those in rural areas. In the *charites* of rural France, the Ladies of Charity were accustomed to hard work and thus provided direct services to the infirmed, whereas in the French capital, the Ladies of Charity often delegated the care of the sick to their servants.

To aid the Paris association of Ladies in their work, Vincent recruited "good country girls," whom he called the med *Filles de la Charite* (Daughters of Charity). He also sent Louise de

Marillac on a tour of the provincial charites to oversee the services provided and to improve the standards of care. As a result of this tour, Louise de Marillac recommended that the Daughters be provided with a basic education in home-based care (Seymer, 1933, pp. 56-59). Thus on November 29, 1633, Vincent de Paul established a school of nursing at 43 Rue du Cardinal, Lemoine, Paris, which was one of the first formal schools of nursing in Western Europe. The direction of the school was entrusted to Louise de Marillac, who oversaw the formal classes that prepared the daughters to care for the sick either in hospitals or in their homes (Lefebre, 1933). The Ladies of Charity of Paris, in turn, supported the students and oriented them to life in the city.

The nursing school increasingly focused on preparing students for work among the urban poor. First de Marillac needed to teach her students to read and write so they would be able to document and report the care they provided. She also taught the students to administer simple remedies and to perform basic nursing skills of the time, such as proper use of a lancet to bleed a patient. Many of the students' lessons were related to the care of the poor in their homes. de Marillac instructed the students in basic principles of teaching and learning so they could provide their clients with basic instruction in household tasks such as mending, cooking, and cleaning. They also instructed clients in management of a household budget and in childcare. The students encouraged the poor to care for their neighbors, as well, and supported the clients in these endeavors (Calvet, 1959; Bertrande, 1956).

With time, de Marillac and Vincent de Paul worked together to develop the Daughters of Charity into a community of religious women who would create a "life of religion in the world" (McNamara, 1996, p. 482). This religious community differed markedly from other Catholic communities of the time because it was not monastic. As a Daughter of Charity, a woman religious usually lived with one or two daughters in a village community, "having no monastery but the houses of the sick and the place where their superior lived, having no cell but a rented room, no chapel but the parish church, no cloister but streets of the city, and no enclosure but obedience" (McNamara, 1996, p. 483). The daughters

were instructed to "go to the sick…having the fear of God for a grille and holy modesty for a veil." (McNamara, 1996, p. 483.)

In 1642 the first four Daughters of Charity took vows to devote themselves to a life of service to the sick poor. However, in keeping with their nonmonastic tradition, the daughters took vows for only one year at a time and made a yearly renewal of these vows. This tradition continues to the present day (Seymer, 1933).

Rules for the Sisters in Parishes

At first the Daughters of Charity had no formal rules but followed a few directives authored by de Marillac. The spiritual formation of the Daughters was entrusted to Vincent de Paul, who instructed them at weekly lecture conferences. de Marillac transcribed the talks, 160 of which survive today (Seymer, 1933). Each of these instructional sessions clarified the significance of serving the "souls as well as the bodies of the poor" (McNamara, 1996, p. 483). One conference held on August 24, 1659, was titled *On the Perfection Required for Sisters in Parishes*. Articles one and two of the conference addressed the "Rule of Parish Sisters" (Leonard, 1979, p. 1210). Although they originated over 300 years ago, the content of these rules relates to the current ministry of parish nursing practice. Each rule noted here is extrapolated from the guidelines developed by Vincent de Paul for the Daughters of Charity working in local parishes in the seventeenth century. Also included is an application of the rule to present-day parish nurses.

Rule One

"They shall call to mind that as their employments oblige them to be for the most part outside the house and in the midst of the world and frequently all alone, they should therefore be more perfect than those who work in hospitals" (Leonard, 1979, p. 1210).

Vincent de Paul called on the sisters of the parish to be virtuous. He was well aware that these sisters spent most of their days without the physical support of their colleagues or fellow religious women. Without their own development as virtuous people, the sisters could not best tend bodies and souls of those they served. The sisters of the parishes were expected to exceed members of monastic religious communities in their demonstration of the four virtues: "humility, obedience, detachment from creatures, and holy modesty" (Leonard, 1979, p. 1216). The sisters who worked in the hospitals and lived "in community" had the physical, emotional, and spiritual support of their fellow religious women. The sisters of the parishes worked alone and lacked this supportive presence. Therefore their self-development was imperative.

These words of caution could be similarly directed to the parish nurses of today who strive to care for the whole person. Parish nurses of today must continually strive to be virtuous and above reproach. This implies that parish nurses work on their own development—emotionally, physically, and most important, spiritually. This rule calls on parish nurses to create time for their spiritual development and prayer life, as well as their physical wellbeing. Self-care is not optional.

Rule Two

"Also be on guard against frequenting the society of men, taking pleasure in conversing with them, especially ecclesiastics—shun that and still more, their society, because, on the pretext of piety, you seek after self satisfaction and, as a rule, begin with good inclinations. Affection gradually begins through things that are spiritual. Then one begins to show it and say: 'Sir, in the Name of God, I beg you think of me; help me to become perfect; tell me what I should do and don't spare me.' That is very good, indeed. The confessor will say: 'I shall do so; I shall take care to let you see my affection.' And here too, the poor confessor is not thinking of anything wrong. Sisters, this little self-gratification by words, which has begun on the spiritual side, afterwards, becomes sensual, and, then he is the only confessor in the world that can please her …. As soon as you feel an attachment for a confessor, leave him; he will destroy you" (Leonard, 1979, p. 1211).

This admonition is especially pertinent to female parish nurses who must work closely with male clergy or to male parish nurses who must work closely with female clergy. The relationship of a parish nurse to the pastor or the relationship

of the parish nurse to a spiritual director is a very intimate, privileged relationship—one that must be guarded from any impropriety. In today's society the parish nurse cannot hold inappropriate feelings of affection for clerical colleagues that exceed the boundaries of a professional relationship. Such feelings compromise the parish nurse's ability to remain objective, adversely affect the nurse's ability to serve the congregation in the manner as intended, and ultimately destroy the sacredness of both the cleric's and the nurse's ministries. Often one can be blinded by affection for another. Many times concerned onlookers can recognize the affection two people have for each other even before those involved recognize it themselves. Attachments interfere with the ability to empty oneself, be present to another, and to serve in ministry with God and His will as the primary attachment. Vincent de Paul cautioned the daughters, "It is not the confessor who is the cause of your advancement: it is God" (Leonard, 1979, p. 1212).

Rule Three

"Think of the end to which God has called you. To serve the sick not only corporately, by giving food and medicine, but spiritually so that those that die will leave the world better prepared. Assist those you serve to die well and those who recover to lead better lives" (Leonard, 1979, p. 1221).

Parish nurses serve the whole person with particular attention to the client's spiritual needs (Solari-Twadell, 1999). Therefore parish nurses are directed to "be" with another to tend to the person's spiritual life for the purpose of helping the person to live a fuller life. The directive of Vincent de Paul is especially pertinent to the parish nurse's role in end-of-life care. The parish nurse often coordinates meals or caretakers for a person in the final stages of life, yet it is also imperative that the parish nurse helps the dying person to be well and at peace with this transition.

Rule Four

"Spiritual assistance should include consoling and encouraging instruction regarding things necessary for salvation such as acts of faith, hope and charity toward God and neighbor, teaching them to resign to the will of God. Be brief and do not fatigue them" (Leonard, 1979, p. 1222).

Vincent de Paul urged the sisters to be open, honest, and direct in their communications and to avoid belaboring issues. No matter what the point of time in history, persons who are ill and suffering should not need to be further burdened by a parish nurse or any other well-intentioned but boorish minister, tirelessly preaching on topics that the minister believes are important. In most situations, the nurse needs to listen and to be present and prayerful. The time with a client should be that of the posture of steward. The parish nurse is, above all, a steward of the gift of the sacred intimacy that is shared with another. It is important for the parish nurse to be present, to listen, and to respond thoughtfully using few words.

Rule Five

"Sisters in the parish must regulate their time according to the needs of the people to be served. Sisters shall not sit with the sick. Others in the family or friends should be asked to do so. Rely on others so that you shall not be delayed in assisting others" (Leonard, 1979, p. 1224).

Time management was important in the days of Vincent de Paul as it is in the present. Therefore recruiting a legion of volunteers in the parish to provide respite care, make meals, arrange transportation, and most importantly, relieve the parish nurse of these requests is crucial. One of the primary mantras of the parish nurse must be the "multiplication of the ministers," or creating opportunities for others in the congregation to serve. By providing willing volunteers with opportunities to serve others, the parish nurse can be available to others who require the unique skills that only the parish nurse can provide. In addition, this provides a time for members of the congregation to enrich their spiritual lives by being in service to others in need.

Rule Six

"General confession of one's whole life is important to one's own spiritual and religious growth" (Leonard, 1979, p. 1225).

As noted earlier, it is highly recommended that the parish nurse have a spiritual director or confessor. This will be discussed more fully in Chapter 4. The development of self-awareness is a persistent goal. The parish nurse must continually strive to be aware of personal attitudes and issues to avoid inappropriately transferring these sentiments to clients. Equally important is attention to religious practices or rituals that enhance the parish nurse's own spiritual and religious life. Discipline in attending to these matters will prepare the parish nurse to serve others better from a spiritual or religious posture.

Rule Seven

"The message of health and wholeness needs to be extended to those near the sick such as children" (Leonard, 1979, p. 1225).

The illness of a family member is particularly stressful for children, who may have difficulty comprehending all that is occurring. It is very important to remember the children.

Furthermore, children are our future. If, at an early age, they are given the insight to understand health from a whole person perspective, they can embark on a lifetime of health promotion activities that are based on body, mind and soul. Early belief in a good and gracious God can relieve anxiety, hopelessness and fear. The experience of participation in religious rituals can feed the soul and minister to the mind and body. What a gift for the young ones to be able to call on at any time on their lives. Although the parish nurse might be called upon to serve an adult family member, it is important also to seek out the children and offer them a prayer of comfort as well.

Rule Eight

"Remedies for the sick is the role of the physician" (Leonard, 1979, p. 1226).

Even in the 1600s a scope of practice was recommended for the Daughters of Charity in the parish. Parish nurses must maintain active nursing licensure in the state(s) in which they practice. In addition, parish nurses should be aware of the *Scope and Standards of Parish Nursing Practice* (ANA, 1998). This document clarifies the limits and boundaries of the ministry of parish nursing practice; it describes what parish nurses should be fulfilling in their service to others in their congregations. Maintenance of an appropriate scope of practice not only brings integrity to the practice of parish nursing but also allows parish nurses to focus on the essence of this role, leaving other physical care matters to the appropriate provider(s).

Rule Nine

"Be aware of resentment or irritation that may surface when those being cared for do not follow the recommended remedies" (Leonard, 1979, p. 1226).

Wouldn't it be ideal if everyone that was ill or recovering had the capacity to do all that was instructed in order for them to get well? Yet that is not always the case. When an individual is not actualizing behavior consistent with achievement of patterns of wellness, the parish nurse's work is to explore the deviation in the client's behavior. Hidden resentment, anger, hopelessness, or fear could be rendering the person powerless in following through on recommended regimen for treatment. The client's lack of follow-through is not something that the parish nurse can afford to take personally. If a feeling of resentment makes itself known, it is important for the parish nurse to recognize it and detach from it while serving the client. However, it is equally important to further explore the situation with a spiritual director or parish nurse colleague to understand one's own posture and inclinations in the given situation. A parish nurse must come to an understanding of one's own self to be emotionally, spiritually, and physically prepared to be able to serve another.

Rule Ten

"Sisters in the parish shall receive no presents for the care that they render. Instead they should be indebted to those they serve. Nor shall the sisters use for themselves anything that is appropriated for those they serve. In serving others only have God in view" (Leonard, 1979, p. 1227).

The parish nurse is not a fee-for-service provider. The services rendered by the parish nurse are offered on behalf of the congregation that has either hired or chosen this nurse to serve the congregation in the capacity of parish nurse. Today, if an individual or family wanted to show their appreciation for the ministry of parish nursing practice, the nurse might recommend that a donation be made to the congregation and dedicated to the parish nurse ministry of the congregation. Monetary gifts to the ministry of parish nursing practice can add up. Perhaps enough money could be accumulated over the period of a year to send the parish nurse to a parish nurse educational program or other classes that would enhance the parish nurse in serving the members of the congregation. The act of referring the grateful client or family to make a monetary contribution to the ministry of parish nursing practice will enhance their understanding that the parish nurse ministry is a service that comes forth from the congregation and is not just the efforts of a single individual.

Conclusion

History can offer many suggestions to enrich practices of the present time. However, if no attention is paid to lessons from the past, then we are locked into either repeating the mistakes of the past or relying only on our limited experiences. Each faith tradition historically has served the ill in some capacity. Many continue to do so today. However, many faith traditions are not assisting their members to enhance their well-being from a "whole person" perspective in a context of community. The ministry of parish nursing practice offers this opportunity.

The ministry of parish nursing practice has deep roots in the Roman Catholic tradition through services provided in the past by religious communities of women. The Daughters of Charity is one vibrant example. The community of the Daughters of Charity was founded at a time when France was besieged by epidemics, wars, and political unrest. Into this arena came a new breed of religious woman: one who functioned in a community, rather than in a cloister; one who visited the sick in their homes, rather than in hospitals; one who promoted care of the whole person by providing both nursing care and spiritual consolation.

The directives given to the Daughters of Charity who embarked on work in parishes seem to have served them well. The Daughters were able to enter the lives of the members of a congregation, provide a unique form of whole person care, and remain focused on their mission while simultaneously avoiding any hint of indiscretion. They can serve as helpful guidelines to those engaged in the parish nurse ministry at the present time.

REFERENCES

American Nurses Association (1998). *Scope and standards of parish nursing practice*. (9806st). Washington, D.C.: Author.

Bay, M.J. (1997). Healing partners: The oncology nurse and the parish nurse. *Seminars in Oncology Nursing* 13(4), 275-277.

Bertrande, Sister (1956). *A woman named Louise*. Normandy, MO: Marillac College Press.

Calvet, J. (1959). *Louise de Marillac: A portrait*. New York: P.J. Kennedy & Sons.

Clark, M.B. & Olson, J.K. (2000). Nursing within a faith community: Promoting health in times of transition. Thousand Oaks, CA: Sage.

Lefebre, J. (1933). French schools of nursing. *Trained nurse and hospital review.* 10(LXLI): 305.

Leonard, J. (1979). The conferences of St. Vincent De Paul to the Daughters of Charity. (Translated from the French). London, England: Collins Liturgical Publications.

McNamara, J.K. (1996). *Sisters in arms: Catholic nuns through two millennia*. Cambridge, MA: Harvard University Press.

O'Brien, M.E. (2003). *Parish nursing: Healthcare ministry within the church*. Boston: Jones and Bartlett Publishers.

Patterson, D. (2003). *The essential parish nurse: ABC's for congregational health ministry*. Cleveland: The Pilgrim Press.

Penner, S. & Galloway-Lee, B. (1997). Parish nursing: Opportunities in community health. *Home Care Provider* 2(5), 244-249.

Seymer, L.R. (1933). *A general history of nursing*. New York: MacMillan Company.

Shelly, J.A. & Miller, A.B. (1999). *Called to care: A Christian theology of nursing*. Downers Grove, IL: InterVarsity Press.

Solari-Twadell, P.A. (1999). The emerging practice of parish nursing. In P.A. Solari-Twadell & M.A. McDermott. *Parish nursing: Promoting whole person health within faith communities*. Thousand Oaks, CA: Sage.

Striepe, J. (1993). Reclaiming the churches healing role. *The Journal of Christian Nursing*. Winter: 4-6.

Zerson, D. (1994). Parish nursing: 20th century fad? *The Journal of Christian Nursing*. Spring 11(2): 19-20.

Zetterlund, J. (1997). Putting the care back into health care. *The Journal of Christian Nursing*. 14(2), 10-11.

Uncovering the Intricacies of the Ministry of Parish Nursing Practice through Research

Phyllis Ann Solari-Twadell

Westberg (Journal of Christian Nursing, 1989, p. 26) considered his work in parish nursing as the "culmination of my work in relating theology and healthcare." Westberg (1986) tracked the development of this ministry and reported that people in the congregation were responding to the parish nurse in four areas: health education, personal health counselor, teacher of volunteers, and organizer of support groups (p. 195). In another article (1988) Westberg reported five major areas of activities that were associated with the parish nurse role. Added to the first three functions identified in the 1989 article were the parish nurse as a liaison with community health professionals and the parish nurse as clarifier of the close relationship between faith and health (pp. 28-29). Interestingly, he had dropped the work with support groups. At the time this information was being gathered from parish nurses working in the original parish nurse project at Lutheran General Hospital in Park Ridge. In addition, Reverend Westberg spoke with other parish nurses across the country regarding their experiences in developing this role and serving others in the capacity of the parish nurse in their congregation. Holstrom (1999), who was one of the first parish nurses in the Lutheran General parish nurse project, identified seven functions of the parish nurse role: health educator, personal health counselor, referral agent and liaison with congregational and community resources, developer of support groups, trainer of volunteers, integrator of faith and health, and health advocate (pp. 67-74). Almost all articles on parish nursing include some report of these functions as central to the parish nurse role.

As the ministry of parish nursing practice has grown in the United States from the Midwest to include all states (Solari-Twadell, 2002), as well as Canada, Australia, Singapore, England, Africa, and other countries, understanding the intricacies of the parish nurse role has become more difficult. In addition, very little research on the parish nurse functions has been undertaken, perhaps because the parish nurse functions, as described, are not discreet. In other words, the content of the parish nurse functions overlap. For example, the function of integrator of faith and health can easily be actualized in personal health counseling and health education because it is so central to the parish nurse role. Health education can be part of personal health counseling and vice versa. What sufficed early on in describing the ministry of parish nursing practice does not help us learn today what parish nurses are actually doing. The lack of discreetness of the parish nurse functions prohibits understanding the parish nurse role. Comprehending the distinctiveness of the role of the parish nurse is important to the maturation of the ministry of parish nursing practice. Lack of role clarity can compromise its integrity. Furthermore, being able to document the complexity of the role is a problem. The inability to succinctly describe what the parish nurse does results in a lack of recognition for the service provided and the work done. Without a clear comprehension of the parish nurse role one cannot develop educational programs that sufficiently prepare the nurse for the parish nurse role. Furthermore, the parish nurse coordinator does not have sufficient information to assist the parish nurse in competency development, nor can clear boundaries for the ministry of parish nursing practice be established.

Use of the Nursing Intervention Classification System as a Means of Identifying the Work of Parish Nurses

The Nursing Intervention Classification System

The *Nursing Intervention Classification* (NIC) was first published in 1992, with later publications of the text in 1996, 2000, and 2004. NIC is a comprehensive standardized language that describes treatments that nurses perform (McCloskey & Bulechek, 2000). NIC was developed through seven years of funding from the National Institutes of Health, National Institute of Nursing. The development of NIC has occurred in four phases. They are the following:

- Phase I—Construction of the Classification (1987-1992)
- Phase II—Construction of the Taxonomy (1990-1995)
- Phase III—Clinical Testing and Refinement (1993-1997)
- Phase IV—Use and Maintenance (1996-ongoing)

This standardized vocabulary is recognized by the American Nurses Association, included in the National Library of Medicine's Metathesaurus for a Unified Medical Language, included in the Standard Nomenclature for Medicine (SNOMED), and incorporated into the indexes of the Cumulative Index of Nursing (CINAHL) and Silver Platter. It is also part of the Joint Commission on Accreditation for Health Care Organizations' (JCAHO) chapter on management of information as one classification that can be used to meet the standard on unified data (Iowa Intervention Project, 1996).

At the time this research was completed, the Nursing Intervention Classification System was comprised of 486 intervention labels grouped according to the NIC structure, including seven domains and 30 classes (McCloskey & Bulechek, 2000). The seven domains are Physiologic Basic,

Physiologic Complex, Behavioral, Safety, Family, Health System, and Community. An intervention is defined as "any treatment based upon clinical judgment and knowledge, that a nurse performs to enhance patient/client outcomes" (McCloskey & Bulechek, 2000, p. xix). Each intervention listed in NIC has a label, name, definition, a set of activities, and background readings. For example, the intervention label Spiritual Support is in the Behavioral Domain, and the Coping Assistance Class. NIC is "used for clinical documenting, communication of care across settings, integration of data across systems and settings, effectiveness research, productivity measurement, competency evaluation, reimbursement, and curricular design" (McCloskey & Bulechek, 2000, p. 3). A few interventions are found in more than one class. However, each intervention has a unique number (code) (McCloskey & Bulechek, 2000). The strengths of NIC are the following (McCloskey & Bulechek, 2000, p. xiii):

> Comprehensive
> Research-based
> Developed inductively based on existing practice
> Reflective of current clinical practice and research
> Easy to use due to the organizing structure
> Clearly and meaningfully written
> Based on an established process and structure
>   for refinement
> Field tested
> Accessible through numerous publications
> Linked to North American Nursing Association
>   (NANDA) nursing diagnosis, Omaha System
>   problems, and Nursing Outcome Classification
>   (NOC) outcomes
> Nationally recognized
> Developed at the same site as outcomes
>   classification
> Translated into several languages

NIC provides a means for clarifying what parish nurses do. It not only identifies the discreet interventions of the parish nurse but also clarifies activities associated with each intervention. In the following research on parish nursing, parish nurse activities were operationalized as output represented by the nursing interventions defined by the NIC system.

Other specialty nursing groups have used NIC to identify the work of nurses. The ambulatory nursing staff at a particular site was asked to identify the frequency of use of each intervention in NIC. The top 30 interventions used by the ambulatory nurses in that site were identified using the NIC system (Androwich & Haas, 2001).

Application of NIC to Research in Parish Nursing to Identify the Most Frequently Used and Core Interventions for the Ministry of Parish Nursing Practice

Use of the NIC 3rd Edition Survey
Method

In 2001, 2330 NIC 3rd Edition surveys (Center for Nursing Classification, 2000) were mailed as part of a larger survey instrument to parish nurses in the United States who had participated in the Basic Preparation for Parish Nurses as developed through the International Parish Nurse Resource Center. These respondents were required to be currently practicing as parish nurses. The respondent was asked to think of the number of times that they performed each of the 486 interventions listed in the survey. They were to then select one choice out of five choices ranging from "rarely, if at all" to "several times a day." The nurse respondents were also asked to identify which of the 486 interventions "are essential or core to the ministry of parish nursing practice." The definition used for core interventions for the purpose of this survey was "interventions that are essential and may not be the interventions used most frequently." This allowed for a distinction to be made between those interventions that are used most often by parish nurses and those core, or "essential," to the ministry of parish nursing practice. An additional question was added to the survey which asked "Are there any nursing interventions that you use in your parish nursing practice that are not included in this classification?" Space was allotted for 30 write-in responses. (Solari-Twadell, 2002, p. 67.)

Results

1161 (54%) useable surveys were returned. All states in the United States were represented except Alaska, Vermont, and Rhode Island (Solari-Twadell, 2002). Reporting indicates that parish nurses are practicing in these states;

however those nurses may not have met the requirements for the study and therefore were not included. This was an excellent response, given the length of the survey and the amount of the time it took to respond to the questions. This author will remain extremely grateful to all the parish nurses who took the time to participate in this research.

Each of the 486 interventions listed in the survey was used at least once. The use of some of the high-tech/invasive NICs raises concern regarding the responsibility and liability that parish nurses are assuming in their roles as parish nurses. Some of the respondents indicated that they are using NICs beyond the scope of the ministry of parish nursing practice (ANA, 1998). Whether these responses were errors, interventions used by parish nurses who may have been employed in other settings, or truly inappropriate activities for parish nurses is unclear (Solari-Twadell, 2002).

A table comparing the respondents from this research with respondents from other selected research in parish nursing is found in Appendix 3A. The research noted in Appendix 3A will not be reviewed as part of this chapter but is noted so that the reader can compare the research described in this chapter and some earlier parish nurse studies (McDermott & Burke, 1993; McDermott & Mullins, 1989; Kuhn, 1997; Lloyd & Solari-Twadell, 1994; Solari-Twadell, 2002).

Most Frequently Used Interventions Identified by Parish Nurse Respondents

The responses to the NIC 3rd Edition Survey were analyzed for frequency of the responses to the 486 interventions listed in the survey. The frequency of responses to each item were used to rank the interventions with the most frequently used interventions ranked as number one. The "several times a day" and "about once a day" responses were merged because their rankings were very similar and represented a like time frame. The several times a day/daily, weekly, and monthly responses were ranked (Appendixes 3B, 3D, and 3F) and then organized into the appropriate Domain and Class (Appendixes 3C, 3E, and 3G) as outlined by NIC (McCloskey & Bulechek, 2000). Appendix 3H combines all the frequently used interventions as identified in the several times a day/daily, weekly, and monthly tables into one table of 49 interventions.

These three sets of interventions—several times a day/daily, weekly, and monthly—listed interventions in six out of the seven NIC domains. No interventions were listed in the top 30 most frequently used interventions for any time frame in the Physiologic Complex Domain. Most of the interventions selected as being frequently used by parish nurses are from the Behavioral Domain, Coping Assistance, Patient Education, Communication Enhancement or Cognitive Therapy Classes. The weekly and monthly rankings, which also listed interventions in the Physiologic Basic Domain, included interventions in the Activity Management and Nutrition Support Classes. Other NIC classes represented in these sets of results are Risk Management in the Safety Domain, Life Span Care in the Family Domain, Health System Mediation and Information in the Health System Domain, and Community Health Promotion in the Community Domain. This reflects the scope of the parish nurse role (ANA, 1998).

Interventions found to be employed most frequently on a several times a day/daily and weekly basis are Active Listening, Presence, Spiritual Support, Emotional Support, Spiritual Growth Facilitation, Humor and Hope Instillation, and Health Education. Use of these interventions on a several times a day/daily and weekly basis is consistent with the notion of spiritual care being the hallmark of the ministry of parish nursing practice. The interventions identified as being used most frequently on a monthly basis—such as Health System Guidance, Teaching Disease Process, Caregiver Support, Grief Work Facilitation, Program Development, and Health Screening—are important to the ministry of parish nursing practice. However, these interventions as reported are not as frequently used by parish nurses and not as closely related to spiritual care.

These three sets of frequently used nursing interventions expand the current understanding and explicitly describe the complexity of the parish nurse role. Uses of a standardized language to describe what parish nurses do make the work of parish nurses intelligible to other nurses, policymakers, clergy, and possible funders. These findings will also be instrumental in future revisions of the parish nurse standardized core curriculum.

Core Interventions Identified by Parish Nurse Respondents

The 30 essential or core interventions (Appendixes 3I and 3J) identified by the respondents also did not include any interventions from the Physiologic Complex Domain of NIC. Similar to the most frequently used interventions most were in the Behavioral Domain, Coping Assistance Class. Again Active Listening, Spiritual Support, Emotional Support, Presence, and Spiritual Growth Facilitation rank high, as well as Health Education reflecting the significance of spiritual care to the ministry of parish nursing practice. NIC interventions identified as nonessential to parish nurses are noted in Appendix 3K.

In further analyzing this data, a correlation between the three sets of frequently used interventions and the essential interventions demonstrated that the set of frequently used monthly and weekly interventions were highly correlated with the set of essential interventions. This finding suggests that parish nurses frequently are doing what they believe is essential to their ministry of parish nursing practice. This finding contrasts research that was done by Hackbarth, Haas, Kavanagh & Vlasses (1995), which used a similar research method with ambulatory care nurses. Their findings revealed that ambulatory care nurses' most frequent tasks seldom were those they identified as most important to their role. Parish nurses' ability to execute activities felt to be essential to their role might explain their satisfaction in the ministry of parish nursing practice.

Parish nurse respondents listed additional interventions not listed in the NIC 3rd Edition Survey. Prayer was one intervention most often listed by the respondents as not listed in the 486 interventions. Prayer, however, is listed as an activity under the intervention of Spiritual Support in NIC. Because of the wide use of prayer as an intervention, it may require further study and needs to be included as a separate NIC. This work of designating and clarifying prayer as an intervention is important not only for parish nursing but also for nursing as a whole.

The outcomes of this research have profound implications for the way that the ministry of parish nursing practice is understood. For the first time, the parish nurse role, which was speculated as being more complex than the seven functions intimated, can be understood more fully.

Perhaps it would be more accurate to describe the functions of the parish nurse role as follows:

- Care that supports physical funtioning
- Care that supports psychological functioning and facilitates lifestyle change, with particular emphasis on coping assistance and spiritual care
- Care that supports protection against harm
- Care that supports the family unit
- Care that supports effective use of the health system
- Care that supports the health of the congregation and community

These descriptions mimic the definitions of the Domains found in NIC and provide a clearer, more comprehensive image of the functions of the parish nurse's role than the seven functions (integrator of faith and health, health educator, personal health counselor, referral agent, liaison with congregational and community resources, developer of support groups, trainer of volunteers and health

advocate). In addition, if the classes and activities that correspond with these NIC Domains are used as reference, there will be no doubt as to the meaning of these descriptions because the NIC system is based on years of nursing research.

Altering the naming for what parish nurses do may be a difficult, but this change is one that represents the maturation of the ministry of parish nursing practice and indicates progress to understanding more clearly the complexity of the role. This is fitting for a nursing service that is congregation-based, has evolved over 20 years, and is building the continued understanding of this nursing role on a broad base of research. Consequently, the preparation for the role can now be revised to address the specific work parish nurses do. In addition, those thinking about becoming a parish nurse or having a parish nurse in their congregations will have a much clearer idea of what the role encompasses.

The results of this research have significant implications for curriculum revisions for the basic parish nurse curriculum. This topic will be discussed in Chapter 11.

REFERENCES

American Nurses Association. (1998). *Scope and standards of parish nursing practice.* (9806st). Washington, DC: Author.

Androwich, I.M. & Haas, S.A. (2001). Ambulatory care nursing: Challenges for the 21st century. In McCloskey Dochterman, J & Grace, H.K. *Current issues in nursing.* 6th Ed. St Louis: Mosby.

Center for Nursing Research. (2000). *NIC 3rd edition, use survey.* Iowa City, Iowa: Author.

Hackbarth, D.D., Haas, S.A., Kavanagh, J.A., Vlasses, F. (1995). Dimensions of the staff nurse role in ambulatory care: Part I—Methodology and analysis of data on current staff nurse practice. *Nursing Economics,* 13(2): 89-98.

Holstrom, S. (1999). Perspectives on a suburban parish nursing practice. In P.A. Solari-Twadell & M.A. McDermott (Eds.). *Parish nursing: promoting whole person health within faith communities* (pp. 67-73). Thousand Oaks, CA: Sage.

Iowa Intervention Project Research Team (1996). *Core interventions by specialty.* Iowa City, Iowa: Author.

Journal of Christian Nursing. (1989). Parish nursing's pioneer: An interview. Author. Winter: 26-28

Kuhn, J. (1997). A profile of parish nurses. *Journal of Christian Nursing* (14)1: 26-28.

Lloyd, R. & Solari-Twadell, A. (1994). *Organizational framework, functions and educational preparation of nurses: National survey 1991 and 1994.* Ethics and Values: A Framework for Parish Nursing Practice. Proceedings of the Eighth Annual Westberg Symposium, Park Ridge, IL: The International Parish Nurse Resource Center.

McCloskey, J.C. & Bulechek, G.M. (2000). *Nursing interventions classification (NIC): Iowa intervention project.* 3rd Ed. St Louis: Mosby.

McDermott, M.A. & Mullins, E. (1989). Profile of a young movement. *Journal of Christian Nursing.* Winter: 29-30.

McDermott, M.A. & Burke, J. (1993). When the population is a congregation: The emerging role of the parish nurse. *Journal of Community Health Nursing* 10(3): 170-190.

Solari-Twadell, P.A. (2002). The differentiation of the ministry of parish nursing practice within congregations. *Dissertation Abstracts International* 63(06): 569A. UMI No. 3056442.

Westberg, G. (1986). The role of the congregations in preventive medicine. *Journal of Religion and Health* 26(3): 193-197.

Westberg, G. (1988). Parishes, nurses, and health care. *Lutheran Partners.* November/December.

A Comparison of Selected Parish Nursing Studies

Study	McDermott & Mullins, 1989	McDermott & Burke, 1993	Kuhn, 1997	Lloyd & Solari-Twadell, 1994	Solari-Twadell, 2002
Number of Participants	n=37	n=109	n=48	n=509	n=1161
Age	26 above 40 years	75 age 35-54 years Range 25-65	73% above 50 years	49-51 years old	Average age 55 years
Gender	M=1 F=36	M=1 F=108	M=1 F=47	M=2 F=507	M=13 F=1033*
Marital Status	M=33 W=2 D=2	All married, widowed, or divorced	Not reported	Not reported	M=964 W=65* D=72 S=58
Educational Preparation	BSN=17 MSN=9	Half had no BSN	Diploma=63% Associate's Degree=13% BSN=13% BA=2% MSN=4%	LPN=2% Diploma=40% Associate's Degree=7% BSN=21% BS nonnursing=11% MA=18% PhD=1%	Diploma=24% Associate's Degree=14% BSN=32% BS nonnursing=7% MSN=12% MA nonnursing=7% PhD=1%
Title	Parish Nurse=29 Min of Health=8	Not Reported	Parish Nurse=58%	Not Reported	Parish Nurse=98%
Compensation	Paid=25 Unpaid=12	Paid=63 Unpaid=46	Paid=25% Unpaid=71%	Paid=40% Unpaid=60%	Paid=32% Unpaid=68%
Denomination	Lutheran=17 Roman Catholic=7 United Methodist=6 Presbyterian=3 Nondenominational=4	Lutheran=36 Roman Catholic=29 United Methodist=21 Other=9	Not reported	Lutheran=45% Roman Catholic=30% United Methodist=21% Presbyterian=14% Baptist=9% Episcopalian=8% UCC=11% Other=10%	Lutheran=25% Roman Catholic=23% United Methodist=16% Baptist=6% Episcopalian=5% Presbyterian=7% UCC=4% Jewish=2% Mennonite=5% Nondenominational=5% Other=9%
Member of Professional Organization	ANA=6 Other=12 Non=19	ANA=21 HMA=53 Other=37	Not reported	Not reported	ANA=17% FOC=16% HMA=13% Other=26%
Evaluation	Yes=20 No=11 Too soon=6	109 some form of evaluation	Yes=50% No=25%	Not reported	Yes=35% No=65%
Geographic Location	Not Reported	Urban=48 Suburban=84 Rural=33	Not reported	Not reported	Town=47% City=42% Metro Area=11%

From Solari-Twadell, P.A. (2002). The differentiation of the ministry of parish nursing practice within congregations. *Dissertation Abstracts International, 63(06)*, 569A. UMI No. 3056442.

*Some respondents did not report age. Some respondents did not report marital status.

APPENDIX 3B

Nursing Interventions Selected by Parish Nurse as Used Several Times a Day/Daily or About Once a Day by Rank Order (n = 1161)

(THE NUMBER LISTED AFTER EACH INTERVENTION IS THE CODE NUMBER FOR THAT INTERVENTION.)

Intervention	Rank	Domain	Class
Active Listening (4920)	1 (n=479)	3. Behavioral	Q. Communication Enhancement
Presence (5340)	2 (n=349)	3. Behavioral	R. Coping Assistance
Touch (5460)	3 (n=300)	3. Behavioral	R. Coping Assistance
Spiritual Support (5420)	4 (n=289)	3. Behavioral	R. Coping Assistance
Emotional Support (5270)	5 (n=285)	3. Behavioral	R. Coping Assistance
Health Education (5510) C	6 (n=260)	3. Behavioral	S. Patient Education
Spiritual Growth Facilitation (5426)	7 (n=257)	3. Behavioral	R. Coping Assistance
Documentation (7920)	8 (n=236)	6. Health System	b. Information Exchange
Humor (5320)	9 (n=201)	3. Behavioral	R. Coping Assistance
Hope Instillation (5310)	10 (n=185)	3. Behavioral	R. Coping Assistance
Learning Facilitation (5520) S	11 (n=177)	3. Behavioral	P. Cognitive Therapy
Telephone Consultation (8180)	12 (n=175)	6. Health System	b. Information Management
Counseling (5240)	13 (n=173)	3. Behavioral	R. Coping Assistance
Decision-Making Support (5250) Y	14 (n=153)	3. Behavioral	R. Coping Assistance
Self-Esteem Enhancement (5400)	15 (n=137)	3. Behavioral	R. Coping Assistance
Support System Enhancement (5440)	16 (n=136)	3. Behavioral	R. Coping Assistance
Telephone Follow-up (8190)	17 (n=132)	6. Health System	b. Information Management
Religious Ritual Enhancement (5424)	18 (n=128)	3. Behavioral	R. Coping Assistance
Teaching Disease Process (5602)	19 (n=127)	3. Behavioral	S. Patient Education
Learning Readiness Enhancement (5540) S	20 (n=119)	3. Behavioral	P. Cognitive Therapy
Self-Awareness Enhancement (5390)	21 (n=118)	3. Behavioral	R. Coping Assistance
Truth Telling (5470)	22 (n=117)	3. Behavioral	R. Coping Assistance
Values Clarification (5480)	23 (n=107)	3. Behavioral	R. Coping Assistance
Teaching: Individual (5606)	24 (n=100)	3. Behavioral	S. Patient Education
Consultation (7910)	25 (n=98)	6. Health system	b. Information Management
Health Screening (6529) D	26.5 (n=96)	4. Safety	V. Risk Management
Coping Enhancement (5230)	26.5 (n=96)	3. Behavioral	R. Coping Assistance
Caregiver Support (7040)	28 (n=94)	5. Family	X. Life Span Care
Program development (8700)	29 (n=92)	7. Community	c. Community Health Promotion
Vital Signs Monitoring (6680)	30 (n=91)	4. Safety	V. Risk Management

From Solari-Twadell, P.A. (2002). The differentiation of the ministry of parish nursing practice within congregations. *Dissertation Abstracts International, 63(06)*, 569A. UMI No. 3056442.

Nursing Interventions Selected by Parish Nurse Respondents as Used Several Times a Day or About Once a Day by Domain and Class (n=1161)

(THE NUMBER LISTED AFTER EACH INTERVENTION IS THE CODE NUMBER FOR THAT INTERVENTION.)

Domain	Class	Intervention	Rank
1. Physiologic Basic: *Care that supports physical functioning.*	None	None	None
2. Physiological Complex: *Care that supports homeostatic regulation.*	None	None	None
3. Behavioral: *Care that supports psychosocial functioning and facilitates lifestyle change.*	P. Cognitive Therapy	Learning Facilitation (5520) S	11 (n=177)
		Learning Readiness Enhancement (5540) S	20 (n=119)
	Q. Communication Enhancement	Active Listening (4920)	1 (n=479)
	R. Coping Assistance	Presence (5340)	2 (n=349)
		Touch (5460)	3 (n=300)
		Spiritual Support (5420)	4 (n=289)
		Emotional Support (5270)	5 (n=285)
		Spiritual growth Facilitation (5426)	7 (n=257)
		Humor (5320)	9 (n=201)
		Hope Instillation (5310)	10 (n=185)
		Counseling (5240)	13 (n=173)
		Decision-Making Support (5250) Y	14 (n=153)
		Self Esteem Enhancement (5400)	15 (n=137)
		Support System Enhancement (5440)	16 (n=136)
		Religious Ritual Enhancement (5424)	18 (n=128)
		Self-Awareness Enhancement (5390)	21 (n=118)
		Truth Telling (5470)	22 (n=117)
		Values Clarification (5480)	23 (n=107)
		Coping Enhancement (5230)	26.5 (n=96)
	S. Patient Education	Health Education (5510) c	6 (n=260)
		Teaching Disease Process (5602)	19 (n=127)
		Teaching Individual (5606)	24 (n=100)
4. Safety: *Care that supports protection against harm.*	V. Risk Management	Health Screening (6520) d	26.5 (n=96)
		Vital Signs Monitoring (6680)	30 (n=91)
5. Family: *Care that supports the family unit.*	X. Life Span Care	Caregiver Support (7040)	28 (n=94)
6. Health System: *Care that supports effective use of the healthcare system.*	b. Information Management	Documentation (7920)	8 (n=236)
		Telephone Consultation (8180)	12 (n=175)
		Telephone Follow-up (8190)	17 (n=132)
		Consultation (7910)	25 (n=98)
7. Community: *Care that supports the health of the community.*	c. Community Health Promotion	Program Development (8700)	29 (n=92)

From Solari-Twadell, P.A. (2002). The differentiation of the ministry of parish nursing practice within congregations. *Dissertation Abstracts International, 63(06)*, 569A. UMI No. 3056442.

APPENDIX 3D

Nursing Interventions Selected by Parish Nurse Respondents as Used Weekly by Rank Order (n = 1161)

(THE NUMBER LISTED AFTER EACH INTERVENTION IS THE CODE NUMBER FOR THAT INTERVENTION.)

Intervention	Rank	Domain	Class
Emotional Support (5270)	1 (n=379)	3. Behavioral	R. Coping Assistance
Spiritual Support (5420)	2 (n=363)	3. Behavioral	R. Coping assistance
Presence (5340)	3 (n=341)	3. Behavioral	R. Coping Assistance
Spiritual Growth Facilitation (5426)	4 (n=330)	3. Behavioral	R. Coping Assistance
Health Education (5510) S	5.5 (n=316)	3. Behavioral	S. Patient Education
		7. Community	c. Community Health Promotion
Active Listening (4920)	5.5 (n=316)	3. Behavioral	R. Coping Assistance
Decision-Making Support (5250)	7 (n=310)	3. Behavioral	R. Coping Assistance
Teaching: Disease Process (5602)	8 (n=307)	3. Behavioral	S. Patient Education
Energy Management (0180)	9.5 (n=292)	1. Physiologic Basic	A. Activity and Exercise Management
Hope Instillation (5310)	9.5 (n=292)	3. Behavioral	R. Coping Assistance
Touch (5460)	11 (n=289)	3. Behavioral	R. Coping Assistance
Counseling (5240)	12 (n=272)	3. Behavioral	R. Coping Assistance
Support System Enhancement (5440)	13 (n=270)	3. Behavioral	R. Coping Assistance
Coping Enhancement (5230)	14 (n=269)	3. Behavioral	R. Coping Assistance
Humor (5320)	15 (n=258)	3. Behavioral	R. Coping Assistance
Religious Ritual Enhancement (5424)	16 (n=246)	3. Behavioral	R .Coping Assistance
Caregiver Support (7040)	17 (n=245)	5. Family	X. Life Span Care
Telephone Consultation (8180)	18 (n=241)	6. Health System	b. Information Management
Documentation (7920)	19 (n=228)	6. Health System	b. Information Management
Grief Work Facilitation (5290)	20.5 (n=224)	3. Behavioral	R. Coping Assistance
Self-Esteem Enhancement (5400)	20.5 (n=224)	3. Behavioral	R. Coping Assistance
Learning Facilitation (5520) S	22 (n=212)	3. Behavioral	P. Cognitive Therapy
Consultation (7910)	23 (n=211)	6. Health System	b. Information Management
Nutrition Counseling (5246)	24 (n=209)	1. Physiologic Basic	D. Nutrition Support
Self-Awareness Enhancement (5390)	25 (n=208)	3. Behavioral	R. Coping Assistance
Health System Guidance (7400)	26 (n=205)	6. Health System	Y. Health System Mediation
Family Support (7140)	27 (n=197)	5. Family	X. Life Span Care
Forgiveness Facilitation (5280)	28 (n=199)	3. Behavioral	R. Coping Assistance
Support Group (5430)	29 (n=198)	3. Behavioral	R. Coping Assistance
Teaching Individual (5606)	30 (n=190)	3. Behavioral	S. Patient Education

From Solari-Twadell, P.A. (2002). The differentiation of the ministry of parish nursing practice within congregations. *Dissertation Abstracts International, 63(06),* 569A. UMI No. 3056442.

Nursing Interventions Selected by Parish Nurse Respondents as Used Weekly by Domain and Class (n = 1161)

(THE NUMBER LISTED AFTER EACH INTERVENTION IS THE CODE NUMBER FOR THAT INTERVENTION.)

Domain	Class	Intervention	Rank
1. Physiologic Basic: *Care that supports physical functioning.*	A. Activity and Exercise Management	Energy Management (0180)	9.5 (n = 292)
	D. Nutrition Support	Nutrition Counseling (5246)	24 (n = 209)
2. Physiologic Complex: *Care that supports homeostatic regulation.*	None	None	None
3. Behavioral: *Care that supports psychosocial functioning and facilitates lifestyle change.*	P. Cognitive Therapy	Learning Facilitation (5520) S	22 (n = 212)
	Q. Communication Enhancement	Active Listening (4920)	6 (n = 316)
	R. Coping Assistance	Emotional Support (5270)	1 (n = 379)
		Spiritual Support (5420)	2 (n = 363)
		Presence (5340)	3 (n = 341)
		Spiritual Growth Facilitation (5426)	4 (n = 330)
		Decision-Making Support (5250)	7 (n = 310)
		Hope Instillation (5310)	9.5 (n = 292)
		Touch (5460)	11 (n = 289)
		Counseling (5240)	12 (n = 272)
		Support System Enhancement (5440)	13 (n = 270)
		Coping Enhancement (5230)	14 (n = 269)
		Humor (5320)	15 (n = 258)
		Religious Ritual Enhancement (5424)	16 (n = 246)
		Grief Work Facilitation (5290)	20.5 (n = 224)
		Self-Esteem Enhancement (5400)	20.5 (n = 224)
		Self-Awareness Enhancement (5390)	25 (n = 208)
		Forgiveness Facilitation (5280)	28 (n = 199)
		Support Group (5430)	29 (n = 198)
	S. Patient Education	Health Education	5 (n = 317)
		Teaching Disease Process (5602)	8 (n = 307)
		Teaching Individual (5606)	30 (n = 190)
4. Safety: *Care that supports protection against harm.*			None
5. Family: *Care that supports the family unit.*	X. Life Span Care	Caregiver Support (7040)	17 (n = 245)
		Family Support (7140)	27 (n = 197)
6. Health System: *Care that supports effective use of the healthcare system.*	Y. Health System Mediation	Health System Guidance (7400)	26 (n = 205)
	b. Information Management	Telephone Consultation (8180)	18 (n = 241)
		Documentation (7920)	19 (n = 228)
		Consultation (7910)	23 (n = 211)
7. Community: *Care that supports the health of the community.*			5 (n = 316)

From Solari-Twadell, P.A. (2002). The differentiation of the ministry of parish nursing practice within congregations. *Dissertation Abstracts International, 63(06),* 569A. UMI No. 3056442.

APPENDIX 3F

Nursing Interventions Selected by Parish Nurse Respondents as Used Monthly by Rank Order (n = 1161)

(THE NUMBER LISTED AFTER EACH INTERVENTION IS THE CODE NUMBER FOR THAT INTERVENTION.)

Intervention	Rank	Domain	Class
Health System Guidance (7400)	1 (n=459)	6. Health System	Y. Health System Mediation
Teaching Disease Process (5602)	2.5 (n=447)	3. Behavioral	S. Patient Education
Caregiver Support (7040)	2.5 (n=447)	5. Family	X. Life Span Care
Grief Work Facilitation (5294)	4 (n=443)	3. Behavioral	R. Coping Assistance
Program Development (8700)	5 (n=442)	7. Community	c. Community Health Promotion
Health Screening (6520) d	6 (n=430)	4. Safety	V. Risk Management
Consultation (7910)	7 (n=430)	6. Health System	b. Information Management
Dying Care (5260)	8 (n=428)	3. Behavioral	R. Coping Assistance
Health Education (5510)	9 (n=426)	3. Behavioral	S. Patient Education
Teaching: Prescribed Medication (5616)	10 (n=424)	3. Behavioral	S. Patient Education
Nutritional Counseling (5246)	11 (n=405)	1. Physiologic Basic	D. Nutrition Support
Teaching: Procedure/Treatment (5618)	12 (n=404)	3. Behavioral	S. Patient Education
Support System Enhancement (5440)	13 (n=398)	3. Behavioral	R. Coping Assistance
Family Support (7140)	14 (n=395)	5. Family	X. Life Span Care
Family Involvement Promotion (7110)	15 (n=393)	5. Family	X. Life Span Care
Decision-Making Support (5250) Y	16 (n=389)	3. Behavioral	R. Coping Assistance
Anticipatory Guidance (5210) Z	17 (n=387)	3. Behavioral	R. Coping Assistance
Teaching Prescribed Diet (5614) D	18 (n=383)	3. Behavioral	S. Patient Education
Coping Enhancement (5230)	19 (n=374)	3. Behavioral	R. Coping Assistance
Referral (8100)	20 (n=370)	6. Health System	b. Information Management
Environmental Management Safety (6486)	21 (n=369)	4. Safety	V. Risk Management
Family Integrity Promotion (7100)	22 (n=364)	5. Family	X. Life Span Care
Support Group (5430)	23 (n=361)	3. Behavioral	R. Coping Assistance
Hope Instillation (5310)	24 (n=359)	3. Behavioral	R. Coping Assistance
Teaching Individual (5606)	25.5 (n=358)	3. Behavioral	S. Patient Education
Fall Prevention (6490)	25.5 (n=358)	4. Safety	V. Risk Management
Forgiveness Facilitation (5280)	27.5 (n=353)	3. Behavioral	R. Coping Assistance
Weight Reduction Assistance (1280)	27.5 (n=353)	1. Physiologic Basic	D. Nutrition Support
Self-Esteem Enhancement (5400)	29 (n=351)	3. Behavioral	R. Coping Assistance
Health Care Information Exchange (7960)	30 (n=347)	6. Health System	b. Information Management

From Solari-Twadell, P.A. (2002). The differentiation of the ministry of parish nursing practice within congregations. *Dissertation Abstracts International, 63(06),* 569A. UMI No. 3056442.

Nursing Interventions Selected by Parish Nurse Respondents as Used Monthly by Domain and Class (n = 1161)

(THE NUMBER LISTED AFTER EACH INTERVENTION IS THE CODE NUMBER FOR THAT INTERVENTION.)

Domain	Class	Intervention	Rank
1. Physiologic Basic: *Care that supports physical functioning.*	D. Nutritional support	Nutritional Counseling (5246)	11 (n = 405)
		Weight Reduction Assistance (1280)	27.5 (n = 353)
2. Physiologic Complex: *Care that supports homeostatic regulation.*	None	None	None
3. Behavioral: *Care that supports psychosocial functioning and facilitates lifestyle change.*	R. Coping Assistance	Grief Work Facilitation (5294)	4 (n = 443)
		Dying Care (5260)	8 (n = 428)
		Support System Enhancement (5440)	13 (n = 398)
		Decision-Making Support (5250) Y	16 (n = 389)
		Anticipatory Guidance (5210) Z	17 (n = 387)
		Coping Enhancement (5230)	19 (n = 374)
		Support Group (5430)	23 (n = 361)
		Hope Instillation (5310)	24 (n = 359)
		Forgiveness Facilitation (5280)	27.5 (n = 353)
		Self-Esteem Enhancement (5400)	29 (n = 351)
	S. Patient Education	Teaching Disease Process (5602)	2.5 (n = 447)
		Health Education (5510) C	9 (n = 426)
		Teaching: Prescribed Medication (5616) H	10 (n = 424)
		Teaching Procedure/Treatment (5618)	12 (n = 404)
		Teaching Prescribed Diet (5614) D	18 (n = 383)
		Teaching: Individual (5606)	25.5 (n = 358)
4. Safety: *Care that supports protection against harm.*	V. Risk Management	Environmental Management: Safety (6486)	21 (n = 369)
		Fall Prevention (6490)	25.5 (n = 358)
		Health Screening (6520) d	6.5 (n = 430)
5. Family: *Care that supports the family unit.*	X. Life Span Care	Caregiver Support (7040)	2.5 (n = 447)
		Family Support (7140)	14 (n = 395)
		Family Involvement Promotion (7110)	15 (n = 393)
		Family Integrity Promotion (7100)	22 (n = 364)
6. Health system: *Care that supports effective use of the healthcare system.*	Y. Health System Mediation	Health System Guidance (7400)	1 (n = 459)
	b. Information Management	Consultation (7910)	7.5 (n = 430)
		Referral (8100)	20 (n = 370)
		Health Care Information Exchange (7960)	30 (n = 347)
7. Community: *Care that supports the health of the community.*	c. Community Health Promotion	Program Development (8700)	5.5 (n = 442)

From Solari-Twadell, P.A. (2002). The differentiation of the ministry of parish nursing practice within congregations. *Dissertation Abstracts International, 63(06),* 569A. UMI No. 3056442.

APPENDIX 3H

Combined Set of Interventions Derived from Nursing Interventions Selected as the Top 30 Interventions Used Several Times a Day/Daily, Weekly, and Monthly

(THE NUMBER LISTED AFTER EACH INTERVENTION IS THE CODE NUMBER FOR THAT INTERVENTION.)

Intervention	Daily	Weekly	Monthly
1. Learning Facilitation (5520) S	n=177	n=212	
2. Learning Readiness Enhancement (5540)	n=119		
3. Active Listening (4920)	n=479	n=316	
4. Presence (5340)	n=349	n=341	
5. Touch (5460)	n=300	n=289	
6. Spiritual Support (5429)	n=289	n=363	
7. Emotional Support (5270)	n=285	n=379	
8. Spiritual Growth Facilitation (5426)	n=257	n=330	
9. Humor (5320)	n=201	n=258	
10. Hope Instillation (5310)	n=185	n=292	n=359
11. Counseling (5240)	n=173	n=272	
12. Decision-Making Support (5250)	n=153	n=310	n=389
13. Self-Esteem Enhancement (5400)	n=137	n=224	n=351
14. Support System Enhancement (5440)	n=136	n=270	n=398
15. Religious Ritual Enhancement (5424)	n=128	n=246	
16. Self-Awareness Enhancement (5390)	n=118	n=208	
17. Truth Telling	n=117		
18. Values Clarification (5480)	n=107		
19. Coping Enhancement (5230)	n=96	n=269	n=374
20. Health Education (5510)	n=260	n=317	n=426
21. Teaching Disease Process (5602)	n=127	n=307	n=447
22. Teaching Individual (5606)	n=100	n=190	n=358
23. Health Screening (6520) d	n=96		n=430
24. Vital Signs Monitoring (6680)	n=91		
25. Caregiver Support (7040)	n=94	n=245	n=447
26. Documentation (7920)	n=236	n=228	
27. Telephone Consultation (8180)	n=175	n=241	
28. Telephone Follow-up (8190)	n=132		
29. Consultation (7910)	n=98	n=211	n=430
30. Program Development (8700)	n=92		n=442
31. Energy Management (0180)		n=292	
32. Nutrition Counseling (5246)		n=209	n=405

From Solari-Twadell, P.A. (2002). The differentiation of the ministry of parish nursing practice within congregations. *Dissertation Abstracts International, 63(06)*, 569A. UMI No. 3056442.

Continued

Combined Set of Interventions Derived from Nursing Interventions Selected as the Top 30 Interventions Used Several Times a Day/Daily, Weekly, and Monthly—cont'd

(THE NUMBER LISTED AFTER EACH INTERVENTION IS THE CODE NUMBER FOR THAT INTERVENTION.)

Intervention	Daily	Weekly	Monthly
33. Grief Work Facilitation (5290)		n=224	n=443
34. Forgiveness Facilitation (5280)		n=199	n=353
35. Support Group (5430)		n=198	n=361
36. Family Support (7140)		n=197	n=395
37. Health System Guidance (7400)		n=205	n=459
38. Weight Reduction Assistance (1280)			n=353
39. Dying Care (5260)			n=428
40. Anticipatory Guidance (5210)			n=387
41. Teaching Prescribed Medication (5616)			n=424
42. Teaching Procedure Treatment (5618)			n=404
43. Teaching Prescribed Diet (5614)			n=383
44. Environmental Management: Safety (6486)			n=369
45. Fall Prevention (6490)			n=358
46. Family Integrity Promotion (7100)			n=364
47. Family Involvement Promotion (7110)			n=393
48. Referral (8100)			n=370
49. Health Care Information Exchange (7960)			n=347

From Solari-Twadell, P.A. (2002). The differentiation of the ministry of parish nursing practice within congregations. *Dissertation Abstracts International, 63(06),* 569A. UMI No. 3056442.

APPENDIX 3I

Nursing Interventions Written-in by Parish Nurse Respondents as Essential or Core to the Ministry of Parish Nursing Practice by Rank Order (n=977)

(THE NUMBER LISTED AFTER EACH INTERVENTION IS THE CODE NUMBER FOR THAT INTERVENTION.)

Intervention	Rank	Domain	Class
Health Education (5510) c	1 (n=695)	3. Behavioral	S. Patient Education
Active Listening (4920)	2 (n=631)	3. Behavioral	Q. Communication Enhancement
Spiritual Support (5420)	3 (n=588)	3. Behavioral	R. Coping Assistance
Emotional Support (5270)	4 (n=523)	3. Behavioral	R. Coping Assistance
Presence (5340)	5 (n=502)	3. Behavioral	R. Coping Assistance
Spiritual Growth Facilitation (5426)	6 (n=479)	3. Behavioral	R. Coping Assistance
Caregiver Support (7040)	7 (n=396)	5. Family	X. Life Span Care
Grief Work Facilitation (5290)	8 (n=391)	3. Behavioral	R. Coping Assistance
Hope Instillation (5310)	9 (n=381)	3. Behavioral	R. Coping Assistance
Coping Enhancement (5230)	10.5 (n=358)	3. Behavioral	R. Coping Assistance
Counseling (5240)	10.5 (n=358)	3. Behavioral	R. Coping Assistance
Decision-Making Support (5250)	12 (n=340)	3. Behavioral	R. Coping Assistance
Forgiveness Facilitation (5280)	13 (n=338)	3. Behavioral	R. Coping Assistance
Health System Guidance (7400)	15.5 (n=303)	6. Health System	Y. Health System Mediation
Touch (5460)	15.5 (n=303)	3. Behavioral	R. Coping Assistance
Support System Enhancement (5440)	16 (n=294)	3. Behavioral	R. Coping Assistance
Humor (5320)	17 (n=290)	3. Behavioral	R. Coping Assistance
Dying Care (5260)	18 (n=277)	3. Behavioral	R. Coping Assistance
Health Screening (6520) d	19 (n=255)	4. Safety	V. Risk Management
Religious Ritual Enhancement (5424)	20 (n=250)	3. Behavioral	R. Coping Assistance
Consultation (7910)	21 (n=244)	6. Health System	Y. Health System Mediation
Support Group (5430)	22 (n=230)	3. Behavioral	R. Coping Assistance
Teaching Disease Process (5602)	23.5 (n=222)	3. Behavioral	S. Patient Education
Program Development (8700)	23.5 (n=222)	7. Community	c. Community Health Promotion
Referral (8100)	25.5 (n=212)	6. Health System	b. Information Management
Anticipatory Guidance (5210)	25.5 (n=212)	3. Behavioral	R. Coping Assistance
Telephone Consultation (8180)	27 (n=206)	6. Health System	b. Information Management
Documentation (7920)	28 (n=202)	6. Health System	b. Information Management
Family Support (7142)	29 (n=201)	5. Family	X. Life Span Care
Exercise Promotion (0201)	30 (n=200)	1. Physiologic Basic	A. Activity and Exercise Management

From Solari-Twadell, P.A. (2002). The differentiation of the ministry of parish nursing practice within congregations. *Dissertation Abstracts International, 63(06)*, 569A. UMI No. 3056442.

Nursing Interventions Written-in by Parish Nurse Respondents as Essential or Core to the Ministry of Parish Nursing Practice by Domain and Class (n = 977)

(THE NUMBER LISTED AFTER EACH INTERVENTION IS THE CODE NUMBER FOR THAT INTERVENTION.)

Domain	Class	Intervention	Rank
1. Physiologic Basic: *Care that supports physical functioning.*	A. Activity and Exercise Management	Exercise Promotion (0201)	30 (n = 200)
2. Physiologic Complex: *Care that supports homeostatic regulation.*	None	None	None
3. Behavioral: *Care that supports psychosocial functioning and facilitates lifestyle change.*	Q. Communication Enhancement	Active Listening (4920)	2 (n = 631)
	R. Coping Assistance	Spiritual Support (5420)	3 (n = 588)
		Emotional Support (5270)	4 (n = 523)
		Presence (5340)	5 (n = 502)
		Spiritual Growth Facilitation (5426)	6 (n = 479)
		Grief Work Facilitation (5290)	8 (n = 391)
		Hope Instillation (5310)	9 (n = 381)
		Coping Enhancement (5230)	10 (n = 358)
		Counseling (5240)	11 (n = 358)
		Decision-Making Support (5250)	12 (n = 340)
		Forgiveness Facilitation (5280)	13 (n = 338)
		Touch (5460)	15 (n = 303)
		Support System Enhancement (5440)	16 (n = 294)
		Humor (5320)	17 (n = 290)
		Dying Care (5260)	18 (n = 277)
		Religious Ritual Enhancement (5424)	20 (n = 250)
		Support Group (5430)	22 (n = 230)
		Anticipatory Guidance (5210) Z	26 (n = 212)
	S. Patient Education	Health Education (5510) c	1 (n = 695)
		Teaching Disease Process (5602)	23 (n = 222)
4. Safety: *Care that supports protection against harm.*	V. Risk Management	Health Screening (6520) d	19 (n = 255)
5. Family: *Care that supports the family unit.*	X. Life Span Care	Caregiver Support (7040)	7 (n = 396)
		Family Support (7142)	29 (n = 201)
6. Health System: *Care that supports effective use of the healthcare system.*	Y. Health system Mediation	Health System Guidance (7400)	14 (n = 303)
	b. Information Management	Consultation (7910)	21 (n = 244)
		Referral (8100)	25 (n = 212)
		Telephone Consultation (8180)	27 (n = 206)
		Documentation (7920)	28 (n = 202)
7. Community: *Care that supports the health of the community.*	c. Community Health Promotion	Program Development (8700)	24 (n = 222)

From Solari-Twadell, P.A. (2002). The differentiation of the ministry of parish nursing practice within congregations. *Dissertation Abstracts International, 63(06),* 569A. UMI No. 3056442.

APPENDIX 3K

Interventions Not Considered Essential to the Ministry of Parish Nursing Practice

(THE NUMBER LISTED AFTER EACH INTERVENTION IS THE CODE NUMBER FOR THAT INTERVENTION.)

Domain	Class	Intervention
1. Physiologic Basic: *Care that supports physical functioning.*	B. Elimination Management	Bowel Incontinence Encopresis (0412) Z
		Bowel Irrigation (0420)
	E. Physical Comfort Promotion	Acupressure (1320)
		Transcutaneous Electrical Nerve Stimulation (TENS) (1540)
2. Physiologic Complex: *Care that supports homeostatic regulation.*	G. Electrolyte and Acid Base Management	Acid Base Management: Metabolic Acidosis (1911)
		Acid Base Management: Metabolic Alkalosis (1912)
		Electrolyte Management: Hypercalcemia (2001)
		Electrolyte Management: Hypermagnesemia (2003)
		Electrolyte Management: Hypomagnesia (2008)
		Electrolyte Management:Hypophosphatemia (2010)
		Hemofiltration Therapy (2110)
		Hemodialysis Therapy (2100)
		Peritoneal Dialysis (2150)
	H. Drug Management	Conscious Sedation (2260)
		Medication Administration: Ear (2308)
		Medication Administration: Enteral (2301)
		Medication Administration: Epidural (2309)
		Medication Administration: Eye (2310)
		Medication Administration: Interpleural (2302)
		Medication Administration: Intradermal (2312)
		Medication Administration: Intraosseous (2303)
		Medication Administration: Intravenous (2314)
		Medication Administration: Rectal (2315)
		Medication Administration: Vaginal (2318)
		Medication Administration: Ventricular Reservoir (2307)
	I. Neurological Management	Cerebral Edema Management (2540)
		Cerebral Profusion Promotion (2550)
		Dysreflexia Management (2560)
		Intracranial Pressure (ICP)
		Monitoring (2590)
		Positioning Neurological (0844)
		Tube Care: Ventriculostomy/Lumbar Drain (1878)
		Unilateral Neglect Management (2760)

From Solari-Twadell, P.A. (2002). The differentiation of the ministry of parish nursing practice within congregations. *Dissertation Abstracts International, 63(06),* 569A. UMI No. 3056442.

Continued

Interventions Not Considered Essential to the Ministry of Parish Nursing Practice—cont'd

(THE NUMBER LISTED AFTER EACH INTERVENTION IS THE CODE NUMBER FOR THAT INTERVENTION.)

Domain	Class	Intervention
	J. Perioperative Care	Autotransfusion (2860) N
		Positioning (Intraoperative (0842)
		Postanesthesia Care (2870)
		Surgical Assistance (2900)
		Surgical Precautions (2920)
	K. Respiratory Management	Artificial Airway Management (3180)
		Chest Physiotherapy (3230)
		Cough Enhancement (3250)
		Endotracheal Extubation (3270)
		Mechanical Ventilation (3300)
		Mechanical Ventilation Weaning (3310)
		Tube Care: Chest (1872)
	L. Skin Wound Management	Leech Therapy (3460)
		Suturing (3620)
		Wound Care: Closed Drainage (3662)
		Wound Irrigation (3680)
	M. Thermoregulation	Hypothermia Treatment (3800)
		Malignant Hyperthermia Precautions (3840) U
		Temperature Regulation: Intraoperative (3902) J
	N. Tissue Perfusion Management	Bleeding Reduction: Antepartum Uterus (4021) U
		Bleeding Reduction: Gastrointestinal (4022)
		Bleeding Reduction Postpartum Uterus (4026) W
		Bleeding Reduction: Wound (4028)
		Blood Products Administration: (4030)
		Hemodynamic Regulation (4150)
		Invasive Hemodynamic Monitoring: (4210)
		Phlebotomy: Arterial Blood Sample (4232) G
		Phlebotomy: Blood Unit Acquisition (4234)
		Shock Management: Vasogenic (4256)
		Venous Access Devices (VAD)
		Maintenance (2440) H

From Solari-Twadell, P.A. (2002). The differentiation of the ministry of parish nursing practice within congregations. *Dissertation Abstracts International, 63(06)*, 569A. UMI No. 3056442.

Interventions Not Considered Essential to the Ministry of Parish Nursing Practice—cont'd

(THE NUMBER LISTED AFTER EACH INTERVENTION IS THE CODE NUMBER FOR THAT INTERVENTION.)

Domain	Class	Intervention
5. Family: *Interventions to assist in raising children.*	Z. Childbearing Care	Intrapartal Care (6830) Intrapartal Care: High-Risk Delivery (6834)
6. Health System: *Care that supports effective use of the healthcare delivery system.*	A. Health System Management	Bedside Laboratory Testing (7610) Controlled Substance Checking (7620) Emergency Cart Checking (7660) Specimen Management (7820)

Spiritual Formation for the Ministry of Parish Nursing Practice

4

Elizabeth Johnston Taylor

The Significance of Spiritual Formation to the Ministry of Parish Nursing Practice

Parish nurse Jane is listening empathically to the spiritual concerns of a homebound, 87-year-old, female congregant who prefers to be called Doris. Having begun to trust Jane, Doris begins to share her concerns:

> You know, I've been a Christian all my life. Sang in the choir 'til I retired. Attended faithfully every Sunday and contributed to the church fund regularly. My daughter even served as a missionary. I never doubted God—no, never. And even when church members stopped coming to visit me after I couldn't attend any longer, I still kept the faith. Yeah, I held on tight! But they don't come anymore. And I can't go out anymore. [Long pause.] But Jane, [tears well up] don't you ever wonder? I mean, when you get close to death like I am, you start wondering. Wondering if it did any good. Wondering if I've been good enough. You can't help but wonder these things.

Doris infers an unraveling "faith." When the religious community's presence becomes nominal, she also questions whether God is present. As death comes closer, she encounters an intrusion of doubt about her sense of worth and salvation. The rigid internal structure that prevented her from doubting now seems to be crumbling as she experiences what may be the most challenging time of her life.

How will parish nurse Jane respond? Will her fears about personal religious doubts compound Doris'? Or will her experience of embracing doubt (recognizing it as a requisite to faith) give her comfort as she allows Doris to explore her doubts further? How will parish nurse Jane's experience of God influence how she responds? Has God been mostly present to Jane during times when she put forth effort to connect with God or with others, as God was for Doris? Or has Jane also recognized God's presence when she did nothing, thought nothing, and even felt nothing? How will Jane's sense of self-worth affect her response? If Jane, unlike Doris, understands that faith is not limited to faithfulness to a religious institution, how will that affect her response?

These questions begin to uncover how deeply the parish nurse's personal spirituality determines responses to clients' expressions of spirituality. Parish nurses are only as comfortable with a client's spiritual pain as they are with their own. Not only do parish nurses' personal spiritual journeys influence their ability to hear and assess others' spiritual needs, but they also affect the nursing therapeutics they provide. Spiritual therapeutics, furthermore, are most effectively offered, taught, or practiced by a parish nurse who has personal experience with them.

Because personal spirituality affects parish nurses' ability to provide spiritual care (part of whole person nursing care), this chapter is devoted to exploring the formation of mature and healthy spirituality. After asking what spiritual formation is, the chapter reviews various theories about the process of spiritual formation. Next, various individual and collective approaches to spiritual formation will be described. The chapter concludes with suggestions for how parish nurse clinicians, educators, and coordinators can apply this theory and knowledge.

What Is Spiritual Formation?

Definitions

Within the discipline of nursing, spirituality is viewed as an integrating force that prompts one to make meaning and connect with self, others, nature, and God—or the Sacred Source, transcendent or ultimate Other, Life Force, or however "God" is defined by the individual (Taylor, 2002). "Formation" means organizing, structuring, making up, molding, devising; it indicates human work, methods, manipulation, and intention (Lewis, 1978). Putting the two terms together could suggest that one's interior life can be methodically organized and manipulated so as to produce certain outcomes. For example, the processes of meaning making or transcending self could be achieved if a certain method or practice were instituted. Although this may be true in a sense, it is also untrue and misleading.

Theological definitions for spiritual formation recognize that although practices can be pursued that facilitate spiritual development, there also is a divine contribution in the process that is graciously gifted to individuals. A review of varying Christian theological definitions for spiritual formation identifies it further. Spiritual formation is the following:

- "Progressive patterning of a person's inner and outer life according to the image of Christ through intentional means of spiritual growth" (Lawrenz, 2000, p. 15)
- "Discern[ing] patterns of God's presence within human life and ... respond[ing] in an increasingly open way to this presence" (Whitehead & Whitehead, 1992, p. 36)
- "Our cooperation with the Spirit's action over our lifetime ... noticing and responding to God's direction in our lives ... determining how best to respond to God" (Conn, 1999, p. 88)

- "The cultivation and acquisition of the values and perceptions of reality that are consistent with the will of God" (Leonard, 1990)
- "Learning to understand and to tell stories that will teach us how to recognize God's activity in our own ordinary week" (Wallace, 1999, p. 48)

These definitions accept that spiritual formation does involve intentionality in our response to the divine. This intentionality is applied to not only becoming more alert for God but also to being responsive to God.

Understanding what spiritual formation is *not* is another way of appreciating what it *is*. Conn (1999) stated: "People easily misunderstand spiritual formation to mean some attempt to find a secret guarantee of salvation. Or, worse, some see it as subtle manipulation of persons, an attempt to form them to an ideology rather than assist them to listen for their own 'still small voice of God'" (pp. 86-87).

Outcomes of Spiritual Formation

An assumption underlying any discussion of spiritual formation is that it is God who takes the initiative in relating to humans (Leonard, 1990). Spirituality allows humans to respond to God, in all aspects of living. The ability or quality with which persons are aware and responsive to God directly relates to their degree of authenticity (Bloom, 1970). Spiritual formation therefore is also about becoming authentic—peeling off the layers of our facades to reveal who and whose we are. This authenticity then contributes to the quality of relationships one has with self, others, and God. Thus spiritual and human formation are entangled processes (Conn, 1999).

Spiritual formation can also be understood by describing what are its psycho-social-spiritual outcomes. Steele (1990) identified five characteristics of maturing spirituality:

- Self-objectification (i.e., reflecting on experience and seeing it in a larger perspective, having a spirituality that integrates all facets of life, living responsibly and with self-discipline, and being stabilized by a faith that withstands the stressors of life)
- Self-criticism (i.e., assessing self honestly, being playful and able to laugh at oneself, accepting the complexity of life and living

with its ambiguities, being flexible and not given to "spiritual imperialism")

- Self-transcendence (i.e., being other-centered, hospitable, reconciliatory, and generous towards life and others, showing others preference)
- Self-in-community (i.e., participating in a community recognizing that it helps—by providing support *and* challenge—to develop spiritual identity, gifts, and purpose)
- Self-in-process (i.e., recognizing personal development is a process)

Conn (1999) proposed three F's as indicators of authentic spiritual formation:

- Fidelity to loving relationships
- Spiritual Freedom
- Fruitfulness in ministry to others

One does not pursue spiritual formation for the sake of achieving outcomes identified here; rather, our purpose is "to glorify God, and to enjoy him [sic] forever," as the Westminster Shorter Catechism states (Steele, 1990). These outcomes, however, can serve as indicators to validate and encourage those who journey the path of spiritual formation. These outcomes can also function as indicators of spiritual well being for parish nurse clinicians, educators, and coordinators as they provide spiritual care.

A Caveat About Christian Influence

Given the pervasive influence of Christian tradition and practice within the literature discussing spiritual formation, a caveat is appropriate. Although parish nursing was birthed within Christianity and although today the large majority of parish nurses are Christians delivering care to Christian parishioners, parish nurses from other religious traditions of the world also provide congregation-based nursing care. As the opening vignette illustrates, all parish nurses will be more effective if they engage in spiritual formation. Although some of Christians' underlying assumptions about spiritual formation are irreconcilable with other world religions, some fundamentals about the existence of God and spiritual disciplines that increase God-awareness or intentionality of response are consonant with most religious experience (e.g., fasting, service, prayer, devotional reading). Knowing how Christians pursue spiritual formation can still help those from other tradi-

tions to become more knowledgeable about the process and can stimulate ideas about spiritual practices that can be adapted to fit within their tradition.

The Context of Spiritual Formation

Theories of Spiritual Development

Theologians and psychologists have explored the question of how individuals mature spiritually. Selected theories will be briefly presented here so as to illustrate not only a range of thinking about spiritual development, but also the possible contributors to it.

To begin, consider Princeton theologian Charry's (2002) statement:

> "I come from a tradition that says we need teachers and we need to study all our life long in order to grow into the wisdom of God. It recognizes that we are capable of learning different things at different ages. A seven-month-old cannot learn to walk, but a 12-month old can. A 12-month-old cannot be toilet-trained, but a 36-month-old can. My tradition says that we are not able to learn the wisdom of God until we are 40 years old.
>
> This comforts me, although I have passed the deadline. It tells me that partaking of the wisdom of God for which I long does not come easily. I must be prepared for it. Spiritual maturity takes a long time" (p. 21).

In seeming contradiction, Talbert (2000) suggested that "it is children who hold the key to correct spiritual formation" (p. 21). Citing Jesus Christ's admonition to become as little children and a Wordsworth poem (i.e., "Heaven lies about us in our infancy! Shades begin to close upon the growing boy..."), Talbert described how young children are closer to God than adults. Charry and Talbert are probably both correct. But how do individuals develop spiritually?

The most prominent theory about spiritual development is that of the theologian Fowler (1981), whose team of researchers interviewed over 400 individuals (ages 3 to 84 years) while deriving the theory. Fowler identified seven sequential, hierarchical stages of faith development, which are summarized in Table 4-1.

Subsequently, Streib (2001) examined Fowler's theory and argued that religious development is better described by a typology of five religious styles.

TABLE 4-1   Fowler's Stages of Faith Development

Label for Stage	Age Range	Description
Undifferentiated Faith	0-3 years	Neonates and toddlers are acquiring the fundamental spiritual qualities of trust, mutuality, courage, hope, and love. The transition to the next stage of faith begins when the child's language and thought start to converge, allowing for the use of symbolism. These spiritual qualities can be undermined rather than developed (e.g., when a parent abuses a baby).
Intuitive-Projective Faith	3-7 years	A fantasy-filled, imitative phase when a child can be highly influenced by examples, moods, actions, and religious stories of the visible faith. Children relate intuitively to the ultimate conditions of existence through stories and images, the fusion of facts and feelings. Make-believe or mental magical concoctions are what is reality. For a child in this stage of faith, for example, Santa Claus is real and God may be viewed literally as a big, smiling (or frowning) granddaddy in the sky (depending on the stories the important adults in the child's life tell).
Mythic-Literal Faith	School age to 12 years, or even into adulthood	Are attempting to sort out what is fantasy from what is fact, by demanding proofs or demonstrations of reality. Stories become a critically important means for children this age to find meaning and to give organization to experience. It is a task of these children to learn not only the stories but also the beliefs and practices of their religion. They accept stories and beliefs literally rather than with abstract meanings.
Synthetic-Conventional Faith	Adolescence to teen years but possibly into adulthood	Experience of the world is now beyond the family unit (e.g., school, media). Spiritual beliefs must provide a helpful understanding of this extended environment. Individuals generally conform to the beliefs of those around them because they have yet not reflected or studied these beliefs objectively. Thus beliefs and values of teens are often held tacitly. For example, an adolescent raised by observant Jews will likely continue to observe the Jewish practices of parents and accept parents' beliefs.
Individuative-Reflective Faith	Young adulthood but possibly into later adulthood	Development of a self-identity and worldview that is differentiated from those of others. The individual forms independent commitments, lifestyle, beliefs, and attitudes (e.g., the child who obediently attended mom's Roman Catholic mass every Sunday will now examine independently what religious practices and beliefs to accept). Also develops personal meaning for symbols. (e.g., the young adult who was taught as a child not to place anything on top of holy scriptures because of their sacredness, now understands that this is not religious edict but rather an authority's attempt to teach respect for an object that informs the reader about what is sacred.)
Conjunctive Faith	Mid-adulthood (or later)	Newfound appreciation for one's past; increased value for one's inner voice; and more awareness of myths, prejudices, and images that exist because of one's social background (e.g., may practice prayer in way that allows listening to the deeper self, instead of petitionary praying). An individual in this stage of spiritual development attempts to unify opposites in mind and experience and remains open and flexible to others' truths. (e.g., instead of trying to dissuade or avoid another with differing spiritual beliefs, a person in this stage would embrace persons of other faith traditions, recognizing that in their faith may be new understanding.)
Universalizing Faith	Usually mid- to late adulthood	Believe and live out a sense that they are part of a greater, nonexclusive, community. These persons work to unshackle social, political, economic, or ideological burdens in society. They fully love life, yet simultaneously hold it loosely. Martin Luther King, Mahatma Gandhi, and Mother Teresa are persons who illustrate this stage.

From Kozier B., Erb G., Berman A., & Snyder S.J. (Eds.) (2004). *Fundamentals of nursing: concepts, process, and practice* (7th ed). Upper Saddler River, NJ: Prentice Hall.

Streib posits that these styles can overlap at points during one's life. Each style suggests a spiritual theme, which when observed over a lifetime, reveals a pattern. The "subjective religious style," for example, begins in infancy and involves the search for basic trust. As children age, they develop new God representations (i.e., God is not only like a parent figure). This theme of seeking trust and new God representations will continue throughout a life.

Spiritual director O'Hare (2004) also proposed a paradigm for spiritual growth (or, "opening to love") that also involves overlapping phases. Not only does the relationship to God evolve, but how one sees the self in relation to others also changes. The characteristics of these three phases are the following:

- Phase I—"Certainty," as evidenced by "deference to a higher authority and the sense of certainty one experiences in following a well-defined system of rules" (p. 28). Although this phase begins during adolescence it can last a lifetime. Poorly self-aware, these persons need approval from others and security from established rules and facts. They may not be aware of their truest feelings about God, think of God as a judge or other strong authority, and have difficulty accepting that God's love for them is beyond their comprehension. (This describes Doris in this chapter's opening illustration.)

- Phase II—"Searching," as often triggered by a personal crisis that challenges one's sense of security. It is characterized by searching that results from a tension between exploring one's own identity and finding others' approval. That tension results in questioning of previously held values, beliefs, motives, and expectations. It is not unusual to wonder if God is there, if God loves unconditionally, and if prayer is meaningless. Layers of the "false self" are lost in this process of asking "who am I?" and "who is God?" This purgative phase, however, begins to bring illumination as the "true self" is found and one realizes that God is amidst the inner confusion. (Doris may be just entering this phase.)

- Phase III—"Intimacy" is typified by: increased self-awareness and loving acceptance of self; appreciation for inner complexities, paradox, and questions; and greater honesty and openness in relationships with self, others, and God. One feels beloved by God and increasingly trusting in God—even though one may have discarded images and language for God. Though possibly experienced as a void, God is; and this mystical experience of the reality of God is lived deeply.

O'Hara's insights about spiritual formation loosely parallel medieval Christian descriptions of spiritual formation as evolving from phases of awakening, purgation, illumination, and union (Mulholland, 1993). They are helpful because they understand not only institutional but also mystical aspects of religiosity.

Whitehead and Whitehead (1992) build on Erikson's theory of adult development to describe spiritual development. They posit that ideal Christian maturity is "not located at some specific point on the developmental spectrum ... but will be discovered at each stage of adult growth, in appropriate response to the challenges of that stage" (p. 40). An adult confronts three essential tasks: to be able to love in a committed way special person/s (intimacy); to generate in a creative and responsible manner (generativity); and to find meaning in life (integrity). In contrast to these positive impulses, adults realistically are balancing their negative counterparts of isolation, self-concern, resentment, and doubt. Balancing these opposing impulses in a manner that is congruent with one's values and commitments is what contributes to spiritual health.

Although they do not focus on spiritual formation directly, several social-psychological theories describe how suffering can contribute to spiritual growth (Violanti, Paton, & Dunning, 2000). Because parish nurses typically witness much suffering, considering how this influences spiritual formation is important not only for themselves but also for their parishioners. These theories postulate that a life crisis or transition initiates a process of cognitive appraisal and use of coping strategies to achieve spiritual growth or transformation. Not all persons respond to such a challenge with such a positive outcome. Whereas some simply survive by functioning at a lower level and others recover to a similar level of function as before the crisis, others are transformed by it and thrive at a higher level of functioning. This transformation is characterized by changes in perception of self (e.g., feeling stronger, better, more confident, and experienced), changes in relationships with others (e.g., closer to family, increased sensitivity towards others who suffer, and deeper relationships), and changes in spiritual or philosophical orientation (e.g., reevaluation of priorities, more perspective and appreciation for life, and strengthened spirituality).

Tedeschi and Calhoun (1995), for example, are psychologists who offered a detailed theory identifying principles in the process of posttraumatic growth. They identified the initial response to transformational trauma as one of being overwhelmed. Survivors of trauma experience their distress as unmanageable. Their cognitive schemas are no longer comprehensible, and their attempts to control the trauma fail. This contributes to a response involving rumination about how to revise their assumptions about life and cope emotionally. Growth begins when the victim starts to accept unchangeable aspects of the situation, sets realistic goals, and gains new understanding about the trauma. As emotional distress eases, the situation appears more manageable, and cognitive schemas are revised. Particularly creative people engage in a more advanced type of reflective rumination, open to ideas and creative wisdom. Personality characteristics such as optimism, extraversion, and social support influence the entire posttraumatic growth process and its outcomes. Psychotherapist Barrett (1999) illustrated this theory with her extremely insightful personal account of how suffering brought forth spiritual transformation. Barrett observed that it is when persons are forced by suffering to draw inward because of their sense of forsakenness, that they also recognize the limits of being human and move to a greater awareness of God. (Thus Doris' spiritual distress could be reframed as a gift.)

Psychologists Oman and Thoresen (2003) extend Bandura's social cognitive theory to support "spiritual modeling" as a significant part of spiritual and religious growth. Spiritual modeling refers to the process by which an individual grows spiritually by "imitating the life or conduct of one or more spiritual exemplars" (p. 150). These theorists identify how in diverse world religions, spiritual formation has often occurred when religious mentors (e.g., gurus, spiritual directors) provided instruction formally or informally, directly or indirectly (e.g., through written records or oral traditions documenting the spiritual

exemplar's wisdom). Christians, for example, grow spiritually from reading about Jesus' life in the Gospels, reading biographies about spiritual giants such as Martin Luther or Joni Erickson Tada, and observing or interacting with contemporary spiritual role models.

Typologies of Personality and Spirituality

Among the numerous theories of personality, a couple offer typologies for the various personalities found among humans. Many clergy and spiritual mentors have found these typologies helpful for explaining spiritual formation. These include the Enneagram (Riso, 1987) and the Myers-Briggs (Myers & Myers, 1980) typologies of personality. Long (1992) labeled the Myers-Briggs typology and others like it "modern astrologies." Although completing the Myers-Briggs Type Indicator (MBTI) instrument can be a tool for initiating self-discovery, Long complained that this typology is used in church settings in an "uncritical, theologically naïve, rigid, and overly confident manner" (p. 293). Various factors in contemporary society steal away persons' ability to appreciate their unique identities. They crave to be known, by themselves and others. These "modern astrologies" provide a quick answer and may even determine one's future approaches to spiritual life when readily embraced. Given this concern, parish nurses need to cautiously use such tools to initiate self-discovery and discussion about spiritual formation for themselves or others.

The Myers-Briggs typology builds on four axes, which when combined in various ways produce 16 categories to describe personality (Stiefel, 1992). The axes, each with ends that are opposite, include: extraversion vs. introversion (i.e., how one focuses energy towards the world); sensing vs. intuition (i.e., how one takes in information); thinking vs. feeling (i.e., whether one reasons evaluatively or relationally); and judging and perceiving (i.e., whether one makes decisions that are outcome- or process-oriented). Thus a person could be an ESTJ (extraverted, sensing, thinking, judging) or any of the other 15 categories created by combining the dominant side of each of these four axes. The opposite ends of each of these axes are further described in Table 4-2, with thoughts about how they could influence spiritual formation.

Typologies for categorizing spiritualities also exist (e.g., Lawrenz, 2000; Ware, 1995). Ware's typology

---

TABLE 4-2   Myers-Briggs Types with Implications for Spiritual Formation

Type	Description	Implications (Examples)
Extraversion	Places and receives energy from people, events, places, things, and ideas put into practice. (May describe 75% of Americans.)	Receives most spiritual insights from interaction with others and events (e.g., interactive worship experience); hears the self/Self when verbally speaking (e.g., talking to a friend, colloquial prayers).
Intraversion	Places and receives energy from the inner life and may even find outer world irritating. Thinks much before acting and may choose not to act. (May describe 25% of Americans.)	May experience God as imminent (vs. transcendent) more; given to meditational approaches to prayer and apophatic practices; prefer nondemonstrative, noninteractive worship.
Sensing	Rely mostly on information acquired via the physical senses (e.g., visual, kinesthic); detail-oriented, working one-step-at-a-time; uncomfortable with ambiguity and are factually minded; oriented towards here-and-now. (Likely describes majority of Americans.)	Systematically study scriptural passages before jumping to conclusions; appreciate worship and prayer that incorporate sensory stimuli (e.g., incense, music, audiovisual presentations).
Intuition	Relies on preconscience-generated information (e.g., intuition, hunches, "sixth sense"); are unable to explain how they know something, and insights come expectedly; are global, futuristic, possibility thinkers. (May describe 25% of Americans.)	Predisposed to apply intuition and imagination to study; love to brainstorm about what could be known about God (vs. what is already accepted); appreciate the mysteries of God.
Thinking	Make decisions by using logic, determining right vs. wrong, what works—not whether it will hurt a relationship; like maintaining order and create it when it does not exist. (Possibly describes half of Americans, although tends to be more present among men.)	Tend to be uncomfortable with emotional expression during prayer and worship; enjoy scriptural study that is systematic and precise.
Feeling	Make decisions by considering values, emotions, relationships (e.g., What is merciful? How do I feel about it? Who will be helped or hurt?); usually more comfortable with people than abstractions.	Need religious instruction to not just cover theology but how that theology can contribute to healthy relationships; may tend to seek warm emotional feelings during prayer, as they may be thought to validate God's presence.
Judging	Closure-oriented decision making; oriented by a thinking or feeling function; dislike making a decision and is relieved once it is over; attempts to keep order in life and may expect this of others.	May tend to view their religious decisions as final, not open to further exploration; preferred predictable, ordered worship services.
Perceiving	Process-oriented decision-making; oriented by a sensing or intuitive function; enjoy gathering information for a decision and then afterwards wonder if they omitted something from the process; tolerate disorder and uncertainty.	Appreciate spontaneity and curiosity in worship services and personal devotions.

From Jones, W.P. (1991). Myers-Briggs Type Indicator: A psychological tool for approaching theology and spirituality. *Weavings, 6*(3): 32-43 and Stiefel, R.E. (1992). Preaching to all the people: The use of Jungian typology and the Myers-Briggs Type Indicator in the teaching of preaching and in the preparation of sermons. *Anglican Theological Review, 74*: 175-207.

---

is well described and is accompanied by a 12-item tool that can assess an individual's or group's (e.g., congregation's) dominant spiritual type. Both Ware and Lawrenz built their typologies on the work of Holmes who proposed two axes, which create four spiritual types. The horizontal axis hold at opposing ends the apophatic and kataphatic approaches to encountering God. (Apophatic is defined by Ware as understanding God nonconcretely—as mystery—whereas kataphatic means viewing God as knowable and revealed.) The vertical axes hold contrasting ways of knowing: the speculative (or rational thinking or intellectual) vs. the affective (or feeling) way. The spiritual types that these intersecting axes create are identified in Table 4-3. An individual or group typically tends toward a certain spiritual type, and each type of spirituality benefits from different forms of spiritual nurture. The optimal spirituality, however, is one that balances these four types. If, however, persons are entrenched in one type, the imbalance contributes to an unhealthy spirituality. Like understanding

personality types, knowing one's own spiritual types can help people to appreciate why their spiritualities and spiritual nurture needs are different. It can also help persons to plan spiritual nurture for themselves that is matched to their type and will help them to mature in a balanced way.

Smith (1993) identified institutionalized religious "movements" that have emerged in response

---

TABLE 4-3   Spiritual Types

Speculative

Speculative/Apophatic—A Kingdom Spirituality

Description: *active visionaries who are very focused on an ideal*
Aim: *to obey God*
What they do: *crusade against injustice, seek to transform society; theology and prayer equals action, service; often make personal sacrifices*
Preferred forms of nurture: *that which does not stifle, but enhances self-understanding; pursuing social justice with action*
When found in excess: *encratism, or moralistic single-mindedness that prevents them from appreciating others' perspectives*
Growing edge: *knowing that God is in control (not them) and that they do not have to be "driven" to be faithful*

Speculative/Kataphatic—A Head Spirituality

Description: *intellectual spirituality that prefers what it can sense and vividly imagine*
Aim: *to pursue God as truth*
What they do: *these persons codify beliefs, do theological reflection, get things done that build up religious structure*
Preferred forms of nurture: *word-based prayer, study groups, intellectual sermons, corporate worship—seek God through words*
When found in excess: *overintellectualization of spiritual life, void of feeling*
Growing edge: *to develop the interior connection with God*

(Apophatic) *(Kataphatic)*

Affective/Apophatic—A Mystic Spirituality

Description: *focus on hearing vs. speaking to God; seek to hear the inner voice more*
Aim: *to pursue God as love; union with the Holy*
What they do: *write inspirational literature; push further the spiritual frontiers*
Preferred forms of nurture: *live ascetic lives; solitude; contemplative practices and meditation; often leave institutional religion; read mystical and Eastern religious material*
When found in excess: *quietism, or the withdrawal from others and reality; breeds spiritual passivity*
Growing edge: *to incorporate interaction with others as part of spiritual discipline or lose guilt about wanting silent, "unproductive" retreats*

Affective/Kataphatic—A Heart Spirituality

Description: *affective, charismatic spirituality combined with theology that emphasizes scripture and anthropomorphic God*
Aim: *to pursue God as holy*
What they do: *evangelism, share experiences*
Preferred forms of nurture: *witnessing, testimonials, music in worship; loosely structured spiritual disciplines, extemporaneous prayer; relating personal stories to Biblical stories*
When found in excess: *pietism or devaluing nonemotional spiritual experiences of others*
Growing edge: *risk new experience of God, be open to diverse expressions of faith*

Affective

From Ware C. (1995). *Discover your spiritual type: A guide to individual and congregational growth.* Bethesda, MD: Alban Institute.

to various societal spiritual needs. That is, the social justice religions evolved to emphasize compassion for others (e.g., Franciscan order); the evangelical movement resulted from a need for more scriptural study and evangelism (e.g., Lutheranism); the contemplative movements have resulted from a need for greater devotion to God (e.g., ancient desert ammas and abbas); the holiness movement was birthed by a need for supporting virtue in all of life (e.g., Methodism); and the charismatic movement came from a hunger for the Holy Spirit's empowerment (e.g., Pentecostalism). Understanding the gifts each movement offers allows individuals to identify spiritual practices that will be comfortable given their religious tradition and consider practices that will stretch their spiritual muscles because of their linkage with a different movement.

Nurturing Spirituality

How can one form a more mature spirituality? That is, how can one become more intentionally alert and responsive to God? Numerous approaches to spiritual formation have been practiced by Christians and other religious seekers over the past millennia. An overview of spiritual practices and disciplines will be presented.

Spiritual Disciplines

Just as an athlete exerts tremendous discipline to earn an Olympic medal, an individual needs discipline to mature spiritually and, to use a Pauline metaphor, "win the race" of faith. Spiritual growth does not happen all by itself (Willard, 1991). Spiritual disciplines are "a means of receiving His [sic] grace … [and] allow us to place ourselves before God so that He can transform us … bless us" (Foster, 1978, p. 6). Foster acknowledged that the only requisite to practicing a spiritual discipline is to have a longing or thirsting for God. This longing along with the discipline transforms persons internally only because of the free gift of God's grace. Practicing a spiritual discipline is not about earning forgiveness, salvation, or God's love. It is not about proudly proving or controlling ourselves out of fear. Rather, it is about allowing ourselves to be controlled and internally changed by God (Foster; Willard).

Numerous spiritual disciplines have been identified (Foster, 1978; Mulholland, 1993; Willard, 1991). Traditional disciplines of abstinence include: solitude; silence; fasting; frugality or simplicity; chastity (appropriate, loving abstention from sex); secrecy (regarding our own good qualities and deeds); and sacrifice. Disciplines of engagement include: study, worship, celebration, service, prayer and meditation, fellowship, receiving guidance, confession, and submission. Box 4-1 provides examples of these spiritual disciplines. Willard observed that people grow spiritually not by practicing disciplines that are easy and enjoyable for them but by practicing those which are challenging—as this is what stretches and tones spiritual muscles.

Note also that many of these disciplines involve spirit, mind, and *body*. This is because the body functions as a "gatekeeper and instrumental means" for spiritual formation (Cox, 2002, p. 281). As Willard (1991) noted, one does not want "a headful of vital truths about God and a body unable to fend off sin" (p. 152).

Rule of Life

Another aid to spiritual formation is the "rule of life" or spiritual maintenance schedule (Alexander, 1999). A rule of life is what an individual creates for "a specific daily pattern for maintaining spiritual awareness" (Ware, 1997, p. 76). For millennia, Jews, Muslims, Christians, and others have organized their days around morning and evening prayers. When creating a life rule, one should consider how he or she plans to not only pray but also study and serve others. The life rule one creates answers the question "How can work, study, community, and prayer be done with my time, and in my time?" (Ware, 1997, p. 78). A life rule for a parish nurse might include 15 minutes of Bible reading and 15 minutes of various types of prayer every morning upon waking and every evening before sleep, weekly meeting with a small group, Sabbath-keeping, monthly meeting with a spiritual director, volunteering as a nurse for the homeless one day per month, or an annual three-day retreat of solitude. As with the disciplines, the life rule is to facilitate encountering God, not experience guilt for failing.

BOX 4-1 Examples of Spiritual Disciplines

CELEBRATION

- Throw a party when your prodigal family member returns "home."
- Whistle a song of gratitude while you walk in the woods.
- Bake a favorite treat to commemorate a project completed with God's grace.
- Keep a weekly Sabbath to celebrate the work and blessings of the week.

CHASTITY

- Abstain from reading popular magazines or novels that focus on sexuality.
- If in agreement with your spouse, refrain from intercourse while prayerfully considering your life's direction.

CONFESSION

- Discuss with a trustworthy friend aspects of your "false self" that you are discovering. Or, explore with a spiritual director your "shadow self."
- Provide restitution to someone you have hurt (e.g., face-to-face "I'm sorry, how can I ease the hurt I've caused?").

FASTING

- Observe a 24-hour fast; drink lots of water and have juice if necessary. Use the time usually spent preparing and eating food in Bible study (see Foster, 1978, for details on how to physically fast).
- Abstain from television for a month; use the extra time for family or intercessory prayer.

FELLOWSHIP

- Participate in a small group whose purpose is spiritual formation. Meet weekly or monthly for 1 to 2 hours. (See Ware, 1997, or Smith, 1993, for guidance and suggested discussion topics.)
- Weekly participate in a local congregation. Make a point of befriending newcomers and oldtimers.

FRUGALITY/SIMPLICITY

- Examine your motives for each purchase you make. Are they necessary? Use the saved money to support those who are living in poverty.
- Eat only that which you need for proper nutrition, and avoid overindulgence.

GUIDANCE

- Gather spiritual friends together to pray for you when you face a major decision. Seek their impressions of what is right for you.
- Visit a spiritual director monthly.

MEDITATION

- Pray without language for ten minutes every morning.
- Find an object in the natural world on which to focus. Consider how it reflects God's character.

PRAYER

- Take a walk and pray for each person you pass. Or, pray for each person present every time you enter a room.
- Write prayers in a journal.
- Consciously experience God in selected actions you perform (e.g., exercise, sexual intercourse, meal preparations, getting dressed, toileting).

SACRIFICE

- Give the income that is unspent at the end of each month to charity.
- Forego something you think is necessary (e.g., stop drinking anything but water, sell your television; discontinue your news magazine subscriptions).

SECRECY

- Shovel your neighbors' snowy driveway without informing them.
- Put money on a worthy student's school account anonymously.

SERVICE

- Vote. Or donate blood. Volunteer. Write letters to editors or your political representative stating your views of matters of social injustice.
- Help others in ways that train you away from possessiveness, envy, arrogance, and resentment.
- Help your "competition" at work or in a social circle to meet a goal.

SILENCE

- Awaken in the middle of the night for half an hour of silence. Do not expect anything, but know God is there.
- Listen to a friend for 20 minutes without speaking. (You may want to explain your discipline in a sentence before doing so!)

BOX 4-1   Examples of Spiritual Disciplines—cont'd

SOLITUDE

- Go on a silent retreat annually (perhaps camping or at a retreat center).
- Walk alone for 45 minutes every day, praying and reflecting on your relationships.

STUDY

- Write out a Bible text on a notecard and place it on your bathroom mirror or car dash. Repeated reading of the card will allow easy memorization of the text as well as analyses.
- Keep notes in a journal about what you are learning from your daily Bible reading.
- Choose a spiritual question (e.g., How can a loving God allow suffering?) and research it using scriptural and theological sources. (The library at the closest seminary will be helpful).

SUBMISSION

- Identify an experienced and godly person for whom submission is a mutual value and to whom you can be transparent and humble and receive guidance from him or her (e.g., a spiritual director).

WORSHIP

- Meditate on the hymn "Holy, Holy, Holy;" focus for 15 minutes each day on the greatness/worthiness of God.
- During meals, driving, telephone calls, or any part of living, intentionally recognize the goodness of God in you.

Based on data from Foster, R.J. (1978). *Celebration of discipline: The path to spiritual growth.* San Francisco: Harper & Row; Smith, J.B. (1993). *A spiritual formation workbook: Small group resources for nurturing Christian growth.* San Francisco: HarperSanFrancisco; and Willard, D. (1991). *The spirit of the disciplines.* San Francisco: HarperSanFrancisco.

Spiritual Direction

Spiritual directors are mentors who assist others to develop spiritually. Spiritual directors are "holy listeners" and "soul friends" who may be laypersons or clergy. Ideally, the spiritual director should be trained specifically in spiritual direction. Whereas some directors (or their employers) will request pay, others offer their direction as a gift to the client. Although a director and directee do not need to share the same religious orientation, directees must be comfortable relating intimate matters of the soul and be open to learning from the director. Thus a director who is of the same gender and from a similar religious tradition is sometimes recommended (Leech, 1992).

Spiritual direction sessions should be devoted to the directee's spiritual life and experience of God. A refrain addressed to directees during a session is often something like "How has God been present [e.g., in this relationship, during this crisis]?" A spiritual director can not only encourage and comfort but also challenge one to strive for increased spiritual awareness and discipline. For individuals desiring spiritual discipline, regular visits (e.g., every 4 to 6 weeks) with a spiritual mentor are recommended. Times of crisis may provoke more frequent meetings.

Theological Reflection

A method for study and growth called "theological reflection" has been welcomed in the Christian community during the past decade because it values personal experience as well as theology to determine action (Killen & deBeer, 2002; Whitehead & Whitehead, 1992). Killen and deBeer structured this process to include the following:

Focusing on some aspect of experience by writing, speaking, or reading it (i.e., personal experience such as distressing memory, conversation, or other life situation; culture, such as that expressed in a painting, essay, news story; or religious tradition or experience such as a Bible passage, theological text, or story about a devout person; or a position, such as an attitude or belief).

Describing that experience with depth and reflecting (i.e., considering what image/s emerge) on what the "heart of the matter" is in that experience or text.

Exploring the heart of the matter alongside the wisdom of the religious tradition. First imposing a question such as "What does my image indicate about my role in realizing God's love in the world?" or "How does my experience reflect longing for God?" Then allowing images, text, story from your religious heritage (e.g., scripture, theology, or folklore) to also emerge to your consciousness. Review this passage (or whatever you remembered) and ask of it the same question you asked of your experience in step two.

Compare the answers you arrived at in steps 2 and 3. Consider the similarities, contrasts, and themes. What strikes you? What is the conversation between your life experience and religious heritage?

Finally, ask if in the conversation between personal experience and theology you were called to any action.

This process of theological reflection requires time, honesty with self, deep introspection, and openness to whatever images are received. It is almost essential to write down these images (e.g., the experiences and the questions and answers that come in response).

Journal Writing

Another practice that supports spiritual formation is the keeping of a spiritual journal or diary (Klug, 1982). Whether one uses a looseleaf notebook, computer, fancy diary, or scratch papers that get placed in a special box, the act of writing one's response to life provides many benefits. These benefits include growth in self-understanding, increased awareness of daily life, guidance for decision-making, perspective that makes sense of life, increased creativity and self-expression, clarity of beliefs, and problem resolution. A spiritual journal should be a private place where one can freely (without worrying about the technicalities of writing) express thoughts, feelings, questions, joys, and failures. In a journal, one can reflect on world events, personal interactions, dreams, readings, and so forth. Ideally, this journal can also contain photos, sketches, idea maps, quotes, or meaningful clippings. This process of expressing the inner self is essentially prayer; the process of "harvesting" or

evaluating themes and growth within the journal over a period of time is also spiritually formative.

Small Groups

A necessary ingredient for spiritual formation is community. Many theologians advocate participation in a small group of believers who share similar religious orientations. The goals of such groups are to provide knowledge about spiritual formation, mutual encouragement, and accountability. Directions for forming and facilitating such groups exist (e.g., SmallGroupMinistry.net; Smith, 1993; Ware, 1997). A group facilitator must remember that members will not want to be told how to think, feel, or believe, but people do like to be told what to do and how to do it (May, 1982). Box 4-2 summarizes approaches to facilitating a small spiritual formation group.

Other Spiritual Practices

Numerous other practices for nurturing the spirit, many which overlap or illustrate the ones presented, have been identified (Alexander, 1999; Brussat & Brussat, 2000). These include instituting spiritual reading, Sabbath rest, simple or vegetarian dieting, quilting, yoga, art, weeping, marriage, creating altars, and so forth. Modern, spiritually thoughtful authors have also described "everyday" spiritual practices that allow one to hear and respond to God continually through the vicissitudes of life (e.g., exercise, parenting, cooking, and gardening). As Brother Lawrence of the Resurrection wrote long ago, "practicing the presence of God" can even occur while washing dishes (Delaney, 1977).

Another Caveat: Cognitive Defenses

Although the human spirit longs for fulfillment in God, human nature also has a shadowy nature. That is, individuals use cognitive defense mechanisms for remaining distant and disengaged from God (May, 1982). These defenses include the following:

- Repression (parts of spiritual experience or insight [e.g., extremely sensual religious experience] is pushed into unconsciousness)
- Denial (e.g., "God does not exist")

BOX 4-2   Small Spiritual Formation Group "How To's"

Convene meeting of potential members, for inquiry—not to ask for commitment to the group.
Determine group membership. Should have 6 to 10 members who share similar religious beliefs.
At first meeting, discuss and mutually agree on purpose, time (including frequency), and place for meetings. Establish trust by agreeing to pursue spiritual practices that are consonant with group's religious beliefs. Members need also to commit to active participation for specified time period (e.g., one year), praying for each other between meetings, and maintaining confidentiality.
Format for meetings can include quieting time, prayer, study, sharing, benediction. Previously agreed time for ending should be respected. Study guides, exercises, and reflective questions for discussion are available (e.g., Smith, 1993; www.SmallGroupMinistry.net).
At intervals during and at the end of the agreed-on time period (e.g., quarterly and at the end of the year), allow time for evaluation. Encourage members to evaluate the effectiveness of both the process and content of the meetings. Renegotiate as appropriate.

Compiled from Ware, C. (1997). *Connecting to God: Nurturing spirituality through small groups.* Bethesda, MD: Alban Institute.

- Projection (aspect of spirituality is denied in self and seen disparagingly in others; e.g., "I don't get warm fuzzies from God, and people who do are irrational about who God is")
- Rationalization (intellectual explanations are derived to devalue or misinterpret threatening insights or experiences)
- Intellectualization (talking about spirituality extensively while avoiding personal spiritual experience)
- Isolation (focusing on intellectual insights and repressing emotional aspects of spiritual experience)
- Displacement (substituting a longing for God with a nonthreatening activity [e.g., seeking meaning by striving professionally for peer's respect]).

Another type of resistance, observed by Conn (1999), is that some resist human assistance with their spiritual formation, believing that God alone does the formation—that is, these people believe that God does not use persons to assist others with spiritual formation. By becoming self-aware of such resistances towards God, one can consider why defenses are needed. This honesty can assist persons in overcoming these barriers to experiencing God more fully.

Implications for the Parish Nurse

Several implications for parish nurse practice can be derived from this theoretical and practical literature about spiritual formation. Implications for parish nurse clinicians, educators, and coordinators are summarized here.

Clinicians

Parish nurse clinicians can apply the knowledge about spiritual development to themselves and to their clients. Recognizing different phases (or types) helps the nurse to plan phase-appropriate care. For example, planning care for an adult who is experiencing a phase that includes questioning previously held religious beliefs should receive spiritual care that allows this purgation. (Remember Doris?) Defending the client's earlier beliefs may be comforting to the nurse but would not be helpful to the client. This literature also contains numerous ideas for congregational spiritual formation that the parish nurse can promote. Examples include having congregants organized into small groups for theological reflection, teaching various spiritual disciplines (and the health implications of observing them), or assisting members to understand their spiritual type and the implications for balanced spiritual growth. Underlying all these applications for parishioners, however, is the essential need for parish nurses to institute spiritual disciplines in their own lives if they are to be effective spiritual care providers.

Educators

Parish nurse educators must recognize that although they should teach methods for spiritual formation, any spiritual growth is a gracious gift of God. It is during parish nurse educational programs that nurses should be encouraged (if not mandated) to design a rule of life, find a spiritual director, complete self-assessments such as the Myers-Briggs Type Indicator and Ware's (1995) Spiritual Wheel, and reflect on which spiritual disciplines will tone their weakest spiritual muscles best. Examples of assignments that would be instructive include the following:

- Write a paper that describes your spiritual development. Include how the religion of your childhood influences you as well as spiritual milestones and what spiritual disciplines or practices you have used and why.
- Choose one of the traditional spiritual disciplines. Describe it and how it could be implemented in contemporary life. Explain what spiritual types might tend to use it most and which types need it most. Suggest how you will use it personally and professionally.
- Identify process and content for a small group devoted to spiritual formation. Practice leading such a group.

In light of the social modeling theory, it is important that the educator not only conveys knowledge but can also be a role model in seeking spiritual formation.

Coordinators

The manager who supervises parish nurses can also learn from this literature. Spiritual formation cannot occur in isolation; the coordinator must ensure support for parish nurse spiritual formation. The coordinator, for example, can encourage the nurse to participate in a small group and visit a spiritual director regularly. Although staff meetings are not the time to conduct a small group, the coordinator can allow time for some discussion related to spiritual formation. A question like "What spiritual practices have you found to be helpful lately?" or "How are you matching up with your congregation as far as spiritual type?" could produce much to inform the coordinator. Such open-ended, nonthreatening questions will likely also serve as prompts for the clinicians' reflection. When tensions arise between nurses and their congregations, the coordinator may find having the nurse complete Wares' Spiritual Wheel tool or the MBTI may be helpful in gaining perspective on the problem. Tensions often arise because of differences in personality or spiritual types.

Conclusion

Mulholland (1993) described the aim of spiritual formation as becoming what God wants us to be—in relationship with God and with others. The outcome of spiritual formation, by its very nature, is love towards others. The parish nurse has an "inside track" for spiritual formation. Not only can spiritual formation occur during parish nurse "work," but it also results in such "work." Parish nurses therefore must reflect on their spiritual formation and seek to nurture it.

REFERENCES

Alexander, S.W. (Ed.). (1999). *Everyday spiritual practice: Simple pathways for enriching your life.* Boston: Skinner House Books.

Barrett, D.A. (1999). Suffering and the process of transformation. *Journal of Pastoral Care,* 53: 461-472.

Bloom, A. (1970). *Beginning to pray.* New York: Paulist Press.

Brother Lawrence of the Resurrection (Translated by J.J. Delaney). (1977). *The practice of the presence of God.* Garden City, NY: Doubleday.

Brussat, F., & Brussat, M.A. (2000). *Spiritual Rx: Prescriptions for living a meaningful life.* New York: Hyperion.

Charry, E. (2002). Growing into the wisdom of God. *Christian Century,* 119(4): 21-22.

Conn, J.W. (1999). Spiritual formation. *Theology Today.* 56(1): 86-97.

Cox, D. (2002). The physical body in spiritual formation: What God has joined together let no one put asunder. *Journal of Psychology and Christianity,* 21: 281-291.

Foster, R.J. (1978). *Celebration of discipline: The path to spiritual growth.* San Francisco: Harper & Row.

Fowler, J.W. (1981). *Stages of faith development: The psychology of human development and the quest for meaning.* San Francisco: Harper & Row.

Hall, T.A. (1997). Gender differences: Implications for spiritual formation and community life. *Journal of Psychology and Christianity,* 16: 222-232.

Jones, W.P. (1991). Myers-Briggs Type Indicator: A psychological tool for approaching theology and spirituality. *Weavings*, 6(3): 32-43.

Killen, P.O., & de Beer, J. (2002). *The art of theological reflection.* New York: Crossroad.

Klug, R. (1982). *How to keep a spiritual journal.* Nashville: Thomas Nelson.

Kozier, B., Erb, G., Berman, A., & Snyder, S.J. (Eds.). (2004). Spirituality (pp. 1001-1011). *Fundamentals of Nursing: Concepts, Process, and Practice* (7th ed.). Upper Saddle River, NJ: Prentice Hall.

Lawrenz, M. (2000). *The dynamic of spiritual formation.* Grand Rapids, MI: Baker Book House.

Leech, K. (1992). Soul friend: *An invitation to spiritual direction.* San Francisco: HarperSanFrancisco.

Leonard, B.J. (Ed.). (1990). *Becoming Christian: Dimensions of spiritual formation.* Louisville, KY: Westminster/John Knox Press.

Lewis, N. (Ed.). (1978). *The new Roget's thesaurus in dictionary form.* New York: Putnam's.

Long, T.G. (1992). Myers-Briggs and other modern astrologies, *Theology Today*, 49: 291-295.

May, G.G. (1982). *Care of mind/Care of spirit: Psychiatric dimensions of spiritual direction.* San Francisco: Harper & Row.

Mulholland, M.R. (1993). Invitation to a journey: A road map for spiritual formation. Downers Grove, IL: InterVarsity.

Myers, I.B., & Myers, P.B. (1980). *Gifts differing.* Palo Alto, CA: Consulting Psychologists Press.

O'Hare, B. (2004). Opening to love: A paradigm for growth in relationship with God. *Presence: An International Journal of Spiritual Direction*, 10(2): 27-36.

Oman, D., & Thoresen, C.E. (2003). Spiritual modeling: A key to spiritual and religious growth? *International Journal for the Psychology of Religion*, 13(3): 149-165.

Riso, D.R. (1987). *Personality types: Using the enneagram for self-discovery.* Boston: Houghton Mifflin.

SmallGroupMinistry.net Retrieved May, 2004, from www.smallgroupministry.net

Smith, J.B. (1993). *A spiritual formation workbook: Small group resources for nurturing Christian growth.* San Francisco: HarperSanFrancisco.

Steele, L.L. (1990). *On the way: A practical theology of Christian formation.* Grand Rapids, MI: Baker Book House.

Stiefel, R.E. (1992). Preaching to all the people: The use of Jungian typology and the Myers-Briggs Type Indicator in the teaching of preaching and in the preparation of sermons. *Anglican Theological Review*, 74: 175-207.

Streib, H. (2001). Faith development theory revisited: The religious styles perspective. *International Journal for the Psychology of Religion*, 11(3): 143-158.

Talbert, B.W. (2000). Partners with listening hearts: Some thought on Christian formation in families. *Journal of Family Ministry*, 14(1): 20-29.

Taylor, E.J. (2002). *Spiritual care: Nursing theory, research, and practice.* Upper Saddle River, NJ: Prentice Hall.

Taylor, E.J. (2003). Spirituality (pp. 1001-1011). In B. Kozier, G. Erb, A. Berman, & S.J. Snyder. (Eds.). *Fundamentals of Nursing: Concepts, Process, and Practice* (7th ed.). Upper Saddle River, NJ: Prentice Hall.

Tedeschi, R.G., & Calhoun, L.G. (1995). *Trauma and transformation: Growing in the aftermath of suffering.* Thousand Oaks, CA: Sage.

Violanti, J., Paton, D., & Dunning, C. (Eds.). (2000). *Posttraumatic stress interventions.* Springfield, IL: Charles C. Thomas.

Wallace, C.M. (1999). Storytelling, doctrine, and spiritual formation. *Anglican Theological Review*, 81(1): 39-60.

Ware, C. (1995). *Discover your spiritual type: A guide to individual and congregational growth.* Bethesda, MD: Alban Institute.

Ware, C. (1997). *Connecting to God: Nurturing spirituality through small groups.* Bethesda, MD: Alban Institute.

Whitehead, E.E., & Whitehead, J.D. (1992). *Christian life patterns: The psychological challenges and religious invitations of adult life.* New York: Crossroad.

Willard, D. (1991). *The spirit of the disciplines.* San Francisco: HarperSanFrancisco.

Nurturing the Self

Mary Ann McDermott

5

"Please remember to place the oxygen mask on your self before attempting to help others in an emergency," instructs the flight attendant on each and every flight we take. How many have ever had to implement this imperative in the air? How many have reflected on the universal truth of this teaching in our personal lives on the ground as well?

I am always exhilarated by the arrival of the Westberg program announcement. I scan the various titles of the workshops and paper presentations. I am often delighted to find a keynoter who will speak and nurture my soul. I am quite certain the majority of the remainder of the symposium presentations will inspire me with ideas for enhancing the practice of parish nursing. I am disappointed, however, to discover that only a precious few will continue to speak to my own self-care, not unlike most nursing conferences. The literature, my own personal experience, and my work with other nurses, including parish nurses, is replete with examples of the little value placed by many of us on this dimension of our lives.

A Rationale for Self-Care

How would you describe yourself and other parish nurses you know? *Conscientious, hardworking, devoted,* and *always giving* are a few words that come immediately to my mind. *Exhausted, disheartened* and *spent* are also descriptors. Women always seem to have something else to do for someone else. We often feel guilty about taking time for our selves. For whatever reason, many of us are unable to give ourselves permission to have a moment's peace. A number of nurses that I have interviewed over the years have told me they were attracted to parish nursing because it gave them a chance to practice congruent with their personal values and ideals. This role provides many of us the opportunity to practice the way we were taught in our nursing education programs to care for the whole person. How many of us were also well taught in the nursing program to care for our selves, to nurture our own spirits?

It is widely agreed that the particular caregiver personality of many nurses, combined with increasingly frustrating professional conditions, lends itself to stress and potential burnout. The "caregiver personality" has been attributed to a variety of causes including the ways in which women are socialized, religious beliefs, and dysfunctional families. In examining work and personal satisfaction, Seligman (2002) states that nurses are among workers who experience high stress and a low decision latitude (referring to the number of choices one has or believes one has on the job) and thus are more prone to coronary disease and depression than in a number of other professions (p. 179). Kahn and Saulo (1993) put it this way: "Those who choose the helping professions often have an easier time giving to others than giving to themselves. In fact, many professional helpers do not know how to care for themselves" (p. 3). We tend to sweep our thoughts about self-care under the rug. We are not ready or willing to attend to ourselves. When we ignore ourselves for too long we become exhausted, weakened, disheartened—thus opening ourselves to diseases of the mind, body, and spirit.

I do not think nurses who practice in the church setting are exempt from the above description. The church milieu may even compound the self-expectation of being there solely for others. In congregations, the 80/20 principle is possibly even more prevalent than in the society at large. When volunteers are needed for a project, 80 percent of the work is done by 20 percent of the congregation. You are doubtless one of the 20 percent!

Both in our personal and professional lives we are busy all the time … for all time! We are over informed: too many books, too many newspapers, too many magazine subscriptions, too many cell phone calls, too many pagers and faxes. We are "plugged in" all the time, courtesy of computers with modems. We can even be wireless all over the world if we can find "hot spots"! E-mail has become the electronic fast-food intravenous drip. A recent Intel advertisement appearing in the *Wall Street Journal* (June 23, 2004) recommends increasing productivity with the words "stop wishing they would do two things at once and let them" (p. B2). To achieve performance gains of up to 25% we are urged to purchase their Hyper-Threading Technology. Gleick's (1999) discussion of hurry sickness points out that the human race has always been time and task obsessed. Now, however, he observes that because of the rapid heartbeat of technology, we can squeeze more and more of everything into the allotted time span.

The desk chair is full; the deck chair is empty. In the split-second timing of our lives, we are on fast forward. In "doing it all," are we "having it all"? The pause button is jammed. As much as we feel our heads are in two places, we are binary: we cannot do something and nothing at the same time—even if Intel believes differently! The ability to work anywhere enables us to work everywhere. We are constantly checking in, never checking out! We are never out of touch—except with ourselves. With the Olympics in Athens in 2004, I could not help but think there ought to have been an endurance event: "The Everydayathon." We could all probably have made it at least to the qualifying round. Look at the obituary page of

the newspaper. They appear almost as posthumous resumes with their list of the accomplishments of the deceased. There are no hallelujahs for idleness, for time spent with family, for afternoons given over to long dreamy walks, for a day at the beach or for having the "time of their life!" Fassel (1990), Helldorfer (1995), and Walker (2001) point out the distinction between the American Protestant work ethic and workaholism, between creative industriousness and out-of-control drivenness, between being involved and work-fixation. Following God's calling to work is about the value and purpose of work, about life and living. Workaholism and drivenness on the other hand, although perceived as clean addictions in our society, are really a substitute for life, and the work is never complete, never ending.

How do you respond when greeted: How are you? or how are you doing? "I'm so busy right now, really frazzled!" Some version of that refrain is quite often the mental response, even if the spoken response may be "just fine." Muller (1999) observes: "The busier we are, the more important we seem to ourselves and, we imagine, to others" (p. 2). We check in with our Palm Pilot calendars. To be unavailable to friends and family has become the model of the successful life. Multi-tasking is a highly valued skill today in business and healthcare; no longer an option for us, even in our personal lives. Many of us have allowed it to become a way of life. We even pride ourselves on this ability, and this "talent" is awarded high scores on work performance evaluations. Have you noticed how much you expect of yourself every single day? It would seem that we scarcely have time to organize our to-do lists even though most of us have attended a session or even an entire course on time management! We have out-stripped our creative stores. We have put our energies elsewhere. We need to replenish the stores, to nurture the self.

Who/Whose Do You Think You Are?

We have little evidence that hard work and no play, putting relationships on hold, foregoing pursuing a creative hobby, being sensible and frugal are actually qualities cherished by our Creator. Rather, abundant evidence suggests that God, who could have created the world in an instant, took some time. When satisfied, God rested and continues to seek cocreators among us to keep the process going! In "doing it all" and in our attempts at "having it all," we easily forget our divine origin. Our roots are not in soil rich enough for our needs. You know the feeling. In asking too much of yourself you let go of inner harmony, and devalue your own self-worth, not trusting God to do God's part. We need to blow gently on the divine spark dimmed by years of frenetic getting, going, and doing. Even the mythical Greek King of Corinth, Sisyphus, although condemned to roll a huge stone up the side of the mountain only to have it tumble down each time it neared the top, had to work for all time; he was not mandated to work all of the time!

Nurturing the self is a spacious way of living physically, psychologically, and spiritually. How do we find the time, create the space, and identify the activities to do this? Activities that change the pace, change the place, or change the nature of our experience of the ordinary in our lives assist us to rediscover ourselves: to redux, to return to health. Nurturing one's spirit, nurturing one's self requires attention. Often we give insufficient attention and appreciation to God's creation, ourselves. When we give ourselves the gift of attention, our consciousness blossoms. Attention is an act of love, an act of connection. Tending comes from the Latin *tendo,* meaning to bend, to lean in. When we tend to someone or something, we lean in a bit to do so. When we attend, give our attention, this process is even more accentuated, we lean in a lot. When we start to attend to ourselves, support for our acts of kindness to ourselves starts to appear. We "stumble" onto something: we "just happen" to see a flyer; we "overhear" a conversation. Books, conferences, and individuals who can serve as resources for our personal "restoration" project are somewhat miraculously there for us!

Last summer I sat on a beach attempting to read and was distracted and a tad disturbed by children playing nearby until I heard a scream of delight from a child of about six. "Look, look, look what I found!" He was summoning his playmate to see a Monarch butterfly who had lit on some milkweed to feed. He had been arrested by beauty. When was the last time you were stunned, experienced that much wonder and

delight, seized the opportunity to become more fully human, a more valuable member of society? I have begun to think consciously of these serendipitous moments as blessings, as truly being graced. The child's enthusiasm for his discovery was truly a manifestation of the Greek root of that word, *en Theo,* in God! Persons who know that life is a gift from God handle the world and themselves in a different way. They tend to themselves; they lean in and pay attention to God's world. They find the time, create the space, and engage in activities that nurture their souls.

Finding the Time to Nurture the Self

Gladys Taber said, "We need time to dream, time to remember and time to reach the infinite. Time to be" (Long, 2002, p. 89). I believe cycles and seasons for activity and dormancy exist; however, nurturing the self needs to be a daily practice, not on hold for the weekend or the summer vacation. It needs to be woven into "ordinary time," which is the longest season in church year liturgy. We need to develop a sense of the sacred and the holy in the particulars of each day. The phrase *work life balance* is often found in the self-care literature. I have often seen this expression used as an acceptable excuse for not becoming involved or for inactivity in an area outside the workplace. I think some may misinterpret the word balance to mean equal time. I also think of the balance beam or the teeter-totter/seesaw in the playground where balance is often rather precarious. Everyone seems to have a comfortable, natural sense of what is about right for a day for themselves. When our choices and our normal work and leisure patterns are in harmony with this natural rhythm, we are less vulnerable to the internal temptation to fall in love with being busy.

Some may be familiar with monasticism's Book of Hours. I learned in my Benedictine secondary school that the message of the canonical hours is to live daily with the real rhythms of the day, whether one chants or speaks the message. Monasticism makes it easy to pray the hours. Steindl-Rast and Lebell (1998) state, "The monastery is a place in which everything is arranged so that it is made easy to be here now" (p. 8). We probably do not have our lives arranged in quite that manner, to pray at eight appointed times in a 24-hour period.

As a realistic alternative, could we find time daily to nurture the self by pausing at periodic intervals? To pause is to hesitate, to cease for a time, a very temporary act. But often the world and we interpret this activity, or rather nonactivity, as idleness, laziness, loafing, wasting time, or being indolent. Time that is unstructured—downtime, wasted time, free time—is unproductive time and lacks purpose and profit. It makes many of us ill at ease. There is a certain voluptuousness in the most mundane comforting chores such as pulling weeds, writing letters, cleaning drawers, and untangling the necklaces in one's jewelry box that make them seem self-indulgent.

Coca-Cola used to have a marketing slogan: "The pause that refreshes!" When was the last time you paused and were refreshed? Pauses are meaningful in poetry and music. In haiku, silence and suggestion are as important as statement. Rilke in one of his poems asks us to imagine our lives as pieces of music, but to stop putting all of our attention on the notes. My favorite line: "I am the rest between two notes" (Whyte, 1994, p. 241) has been an inspiration to me over the last decade. I grew up in a neighborhood where the Angelus was played on church bells at noon, when the day, the sun, had reached its peak. On the academic lakeshore campus of Loyola University, Chicago, they have resurrected that practice. The Angelus has become a reminder to me to take the time to stop, to pause, even for a brief while and to respond, in the middle of the day, in the middle of everything, to be present and to nurture my self. What signals, what cues, what are the "best practices" you use to make time, even a few minutes, to nurture your soul? In *Receiving the Day: Christian Practices for Opening the Gift of Time,* Bass (2000) suggests, "Putting down an anchor or two amid the swells of each day is essential if we are to avoid the bobbing on its surface or being washed away by its demand" (p. 37). When you arrive home in the evening, consider greeting and treating yourself as a returning MIA, a refugee, a war veteran, a survivor, a guest in your own home, in your own body/God's home! Might that practice change the way you and I prepare and eat dinner, or spend the evening? "Finding time" and "making time" for nurturing the self will always be a challenge.

Creating the Space to Nurture the Self

Some years ago I had the opportunity to spend an afternoon at the Disney Institute in Orlando, Florida. I participated in a team-building process that I have replicated with some modifications in my work with parish nurse educators. The first activity in the process is to ask each member of a small group of five or six people to: Depict a place where you go to find renewal, relaxation, refreshment, and/or restoration. The word *depict* is used quite intentionally. Although there are art materials available (crayons, water colors, and colored paper), to allay the fears of those who "cannot draw" they are permitted to depict this place any way they wish. Most do draw, but a few write a paragraph or two. After 5 to 7 minutes the individuals within the groups are asked to share their depiction with the others in the small group. I then ask the larger group of 20 to 100 participants how many of them had a nature scene … how many had water in any form in their depiction, how many had mountains, a tree, flowers, a woods in their depictions … any animals present? By far a scene from nature is the setting depicted by most. As much as nature can be violent, chaotic, and random, it is also soothing, all embracing, and restorative. Ackerman (2001) suggests, "There is a way of sitting quietly and beholding nature which is a form of meditation or prayer, and like those healing acts it calms the spirit" (p. 6). Becknell (2001) asks us to live more deliberately and to be more attentive; his wonderful collection of nature writing and poetry is arranged around the seven virtues that can serve as beautiful prayerful meditations.

If the scene that has been depicted by a participant is indoors, it is often on a porch or close to a window doing a craft activity, playing or listening to a musical instrument, or reading. A church, a museum, or a library is occasionally mentioned and the description always conveys a feeling of spaciousness. There is always someone in every group, usually a young mother, who depicts herself in the bathtub with the door locked! In almost all of the above depictions, the individual is alone, occasionally with a spouse or close friend, but rarely with a group. It might be interesting for you to engage in this "depiction" exercise alone or with others. Where do you find renewal, relaxation, refreshment, and/or restoration? Do you picture yourself alone, with a significant other, or with a group? Is your restorative space/place indoors or out?

Over the course of the last two years I have worked with nurse managers and healthcare designers to look at the concept of restorative space in the workplace, but the concept is applicable at home as well. A growing body of research addresses specific dimensions of space that are restorative: sound (fountains, chimes); color (combination and integration of colors, interaction of color and light); light (lighting options, window treatments); privacy; furniture; plants (fragrance, arrangement, containers); music, artwork; and activities (creative or contemplative). Moore (1996) recommends inefficiency experts in the workplace who would value downtime for reflection, conversation, and beauty that is captivating and pleasuring.

We cannot always go to the water, the forest, or the mountains for renewal, but we can bring elements of those into our homes and workplaces. What would a nurturing restorative space look like in your life? Is it possible to have a clearly defined sense of place for nurturing your soul, your self? Might you consider marking out a special or even a sacred space/place with dimensions to fit only you? Rather than emphasizing the items or objects that might be used to fill this space (e.g., a fountain, stones, a plant, or an icon), most authorities would agree that the space should be relatively empty. The space between in Japanese flower arranging is called *ma*. I find that word quite intriguing when thinking about renewal. One of my former art teachers once suggested that this novice student see and draw the space between the objects in a still life I was attempting; the objects emerged. Emptiness is not always negative. It allows one room to act and concentrate, it forms and defines. It allows us to emerge.

All space is truly sacred; however, is the space that you are designing also the place where you have set aside to pray? If so, are there any special considerations that need to be taken into account? What do the phrases "seeking sanctuary, seeking refuge" mean to you? Moore (1996) and Whyte (1994) use the Greek word *tenemos*, which refers to the precinct of a god, goddess, or

another spirit that could have a beneficial effect on human life. Moore (1996) discusses sanctuary as a place of *tenemos* with an embracing perimeter that is set aside for breathing new life into our daily activities. He also deplores that real gateways and entrances and real thresholds that lead the soul in and out of such places no longer exist. What types of transition, physical or mental, might you make as you enter and exit your restorative space? In Europe, it is not unusual to tour a home of past royalty and visit their chapel that was built into their dwelling. Today you will find a body of literature focusing on the construction of small altars in the home. McMann (1998) has assembled a beautiful collection of home-altars and shrines on shelves, dresser tops, windowsills, and in the garden that supplies the reader with ideas for a lifetime.

Identifying Activities that Nurture the Self

Leisure Time

Leisure comes from the Latin *licere*, which means "to be permitted, allowed." The Zen pictographic for leisure is the moon captured among tree branches. What do we permit ourselves to do—or not to do—in our leisure? Gini (2003) recommends that in leisure we allow ourselves "to be free to pursue the unusual, the inexplicable, the irrelevant, the interesting, and the idiosyncratic" (p. 34). Both Gini (2003) and Rybczynski (1991) suggest that in our leisure we need to get absorbed in, focused on, something of interest outside ourselves. They recommend that we need to learn the differences between entertainment and recreation, laziness and leisure, rest and inertia, distraction and insight. Both point out that we often use these terms interchangeably. This inability to distinguish between them delimits and diminishes us. Immediately, however, we tend to ask ourselves, "if I am visibly nonproductive, how will my world and I measure my value?"

The meaning and history of leisure is well described by Rybczynski (1991) in his book: *Waiting for the Weekend*. The cover of this little treasure, a reproduction of Seurat's "Sunday

Afternoon on the Island of La Grande Jatte," immediately caught my eye in the bookstore several years ago. Since childhood trips to the Art Institute of Chicago with my Aunt Sally, that "work" has been my very favorite painting. Quite possibly this painting was a personal introduction to nurturing my self along with a volume on that same aunt's bookshelf that is now on mine: *A Guide to Civilized Loafing* by Overstreet (1934).

Basic Self-Care Activities

Norris (1998) points out that neglecting the elementary physical acts of self-care are signals of isolation from reality. Parish nurses would recognize these as early signs of depression. "Shampooing the hair, washing the body, brushing the teeth, drinking enough water, taking a daily vitamin, going for a walk, as simple as they seem, are acts of self respect" (p. 40). Walker (2001) points out that driven individuals frequently have poor health habits, do not exercise frequently, and are prone to eat junk food. All of these activities are basic, but look around you. Many of the nurses I know in the hospital do not ever stop to take some deep breaths during a crisis and rarely take a lunch break to either eat or take a walk outside. If they do eat, they often do so quickly at their desks. Kass, in his book *The Hungry Soul* (1999), states that "wolfing down food dishonors both the human effort to prepare and the lives of the plants and animals sacrificed on our behalf" (p. 10). One of the more famous imports from my favorite country of Italy is the "slow food" movement. Gini points out that this movement "is not just about flavor, freshness and nutritional value … It is a bonding and learning experience" (p. 160). We should also remember that all of the central religious rituals are meals. It was not the last meeting, but the last supper. What are your basic self-care habits, your dining rituals at home and at work? The joy of self-care practices are seamlessly merged into the joy of God's care for us … why not reflect that care in our care for ourselves?

Rarely—if ever—do nurses in the hospital enjoy the "lounge"/"break" room without bringing along some charting. Although bottled water and drinking fountains are often readily available and accessible on the hospital units, nurses admit they don't drink water during their shift because

that would mean numerous trips to the toilet … "And who has that kind of time!" Battaglia (1996) has a wonderful poem entitled "The Plight of Nursing." She begins "I am the Lady with the Lamp" and speaks of leaving some of herself behind and at the end of the shift; how she cannot account for all of herself. "I retrace my steps, in hopes of putting myself back together again" (p. 33). Most nurses for whom I have read this recognize themselves and agree that her "plight" is also theirs! It is clear that we need to address the basics of self-care. Are parish nurses different?

Beyond the Basics: Nurturing the Soul

I have not addressed in the following section several specific areas of nurturing the soul that are central integrative practices to the ministry of parish nursing. I refer you instead to other chapters in this book that have treated these in depth: Elizabeth Taylor's chapter on spiritual formation, Annette Langdon's chapter on prayer, and Carol Tippe's discussion of planning and implementing sabbatical time. Kundtz (1998) defines stopping as "doing nothing as much as possible for a definite period of time (one second to one month) for the purpose of becoming more fully awake and remembering who you are" (p. 14). I have recited many times a wonderful poem called "Lost" by an anonymous Native American that has been rendered beautifully into modern English by David Wagoner (Whyte 1994). Asked by a child, "What do I do when I am lost in the forest?," The elder responds, "Stand Still./ The trees ahead and bushes beside you are not lost./ **Wherever** you are / is called Here …" (p. 259). A sabbatical or retreat is a wonderful way to "stop" and to "stand still." Louden's (1997) descriptions of four ways to make a retreat—a long retreat, a mini retreat, a retreat with others, and retreats in the world—may be helpful in considering optimal time away to shift our attention toward listening to the Lord. Retreats can provide the periodic stillness and rest we desire until we can arrange for the longer sabbatical leave. We all need to "vacate" ourselves, no matter how important the work. As a reminder to myself, I reread at least once each summer Anne Morrow Lindbergh's (1965) *Gift from the Sea*. If you cannot arrange a formal retreat, read about hers!

I have also not given justice here to the classic and highly desirable spiritual practices of breathing, silence, meditation, and guided imagery; however an abundance of literature related to each of these is both available and accessible. Many articles and books on the rationale and techniques for journaling also exist, both as a self-care activity (Adams, 1990; Cameron, 1992) and as a deliberate spiritual practice (Kelsey, 1980; Klug, 1993). Cameron (1992) is quite famous for advocating a journaling technique she has labeled "Morning Pages." She believes this activity helps people to prioritize the day and render us present to the moments of the day. In her more recent book (2004), she has a list of journaling exercises. She challenges readers to try doing something they truly love, even if they do not feel they can do it perfectly. She also asks us how our kids or best friends would describe us? What would we do with an extra hour/day/week/month/year? Progoff's *At a Journal Workshop* is the spiritual journaling classic. Should you ever have the opportunity to enroll in one of the "authorized" workshops bearing his name, register! Although not yet a classic, a book I highly recommend is Peter Gilmour's *The Wisdom of Memoir: Reading and Writing Life's Sacred Texts* (1997). He tells us: "The product of creating memoir is an artistic combination of memory, reflection, and imagination, and this product manifests spirituality" (p. 13).

A great deal of current research stresses the importance of family and friends to self-care. For instance, the famed Harvard Nurses' Health Studies 1976 and 1989 (retrieved June 23, 2004 http://www.channing.harvard.edu/nhs/) found that the more friends women had, the less likely they were to develop physical impairments as they aged and the more likely they were to be leading a joyful life. Yet why is it so hard to find time to be with them? Josselson (1998) points out that when we get overly busy with work and family, the first thing we do is let go of our friendships.

Calendarizing Self-Nurturing Activities

A myriad of practices nurture the self. How does one identify the activities that are self-nurturing? They tend to be very individual and may vary throughout our lives. A number of people tried to convince me that shopping was a self-nurturing activity. They spoke about doing this in conjunction with a hobby or a special collection they prized. Some talked about "malling" as a fun activity with friends. Others spoke of shopping for and finding just the right outfit for a special occasion and the joy that resulted. Ford (2002) has published a volume of what she refers to as life lessons garnered from her shopping experience. Not for me! Not in the past or the present ... maybe in the future? The practices you select may even differ day-to-day depending on specific stressors that "come into play." You may already be very well acquainted with what "works" for you. I have some suggestions, certainly not all-inclusive, that I have found to be self-nurturing. I do believe all of the activities identified also nurture the soul but are less commonly referred to in that manner. I ask your indulgence!

What gives you energy rather than drains you? Some twenty-five years ago, my spiritual director suggested that I institute a Jungian practice of making a weekly appointment with myself. Placed in my calendar that appointment was to be honored above all others. I have tried over the years to honor that commitment. I am sure that there are those in my acquaintance who might refer to this as *"dolce far niente!"* ("How sweet it is to do nothing!") This is a fine Italian saying that refers to goofing off! I see it as essential time for self-nurturance.

Along this same line, Cameron (1992, 2004) suggests Artist Dates, scheduled weekly appointments with the self. These are solo festive outings and what might appear to outsiders as frivolous expeditions that enchant you. They can appear deceptively simple yet can be very powerful: a bike ride, a visit to a museum, a walk in the park, a journey to the zoo, or attending the theater for an afternoon matinee. These are weekly and may or may not require preplanning. I do believe they merit putting them into your calendar/Palm Pilot as important appointments with yourself.

Moving back to "Ordinary Time" (a term that is used to refer to a lengthy season in church liturgical time), I suggest you might try out some new activities on a daily basis that require little to no advance planning except the commitment to carry them out. Set up a week of 30-minute solitary sensory delights for yourself. *Monday*: In season or not, gather a bouquet of fresh flowers; slowly arrange them in a pretty container; notice the *ma*; smell them; feel their texture; sit back;

and bask in their beauty. *Tuesday*: plan a morning or afternoon tea party for yourself. Try a new flavor of noncaffeinated herbal tea; brew it in a beautiful (just for company) teapot and savor both the fragrance and the taste of the tea in a favorite teacup with your best silver spoon on a placemat that you have designed for a lover—yourself. *Wednesday*: Attend an afternoon compact disc concert, without interruption, of your favorite composer. Relish the Epicurean "stillness of the soul" and the "rest between two notes." *Thursday*: Take one of your coffee table art books and gaze at no more than five of the works that appeal to you and consider them in detail. *Friday*: "Easy does it" is an expression we often use, but seldom practice. It is surprisingly hard to take it easy. Imitate the Europeans and take a twenty-minute siesta, reposo, an afternoon nap! Both Long (2002) and Vienne (1998) urge us to create relaxation rituals, create a nap sanctuary a place where you can be undisturbed for 30 minutes. Napping, they suggest and I agree, should have the same status as daily exercise. Afterwards enjoy the sensation of feeling replenished. *Saturday*: Spa time! Many of us do not have the money to make regular, if any, trips to a luxury spa for manicures, pedicures, facials or body massage; however, we can create our own mini spa experience. Take out your best and most fragrant hand cream or lotion and give yourself a really good hand message. Feel the warmth of the one hand administering to the other. When finished, admire your hands and all that they do. Conclude by asking God's blessings on your hands. Next week, maybe you could give yourself a really fine foot massage! *Sunday*: Pull down a poetry book from the shelf and after looking at the table of contents and/or authors select two or three to read slowly aloud to yourself. Enjoy the sound of your own voice, the sound of the words, and their meaning to you on this particular day. When you have completed the "try-out" week, spend some time considering which, if any or all, of these simple activities you might incorporate in your self-care routine.

Using the Arts to Nourish the Self/the Soul

In 1995, Ann Solari-Twadell invited me—and I eagerly accepted—to present the keynote address for the annual Westberg Symposium on the topic of Ministering to Self and Others through the Arts (McDermott, 1995). At that time I was interested in how the arts could enhance our practice. I was convinced that they could teach us about many of the qualitative themes that parish nurses address—the quest for meaning, battles with uncertainty, denial of symptoms, endurance in the face of chronic suffering— to come to, if ever, the acceptance of the loss of a loved one. Several books related to the arts were published by nurses (Styles & Moccia, 1993; Chinn & Watson, 1994) around that time. The preparation for that presentation led to a decade plus interest in expanding on that idea.

I share in Appendix 5A the often-revised current edition of the "Arts Assessment Tool/Survey" from that program. I offer it as one way that you might explore the arts to nurture your own spirit. Consider this not as a teaching tool to enhance your practice, an assessment preliminary to intervening with others, but for your own self-nurturance, for the sheer delight that the arts can evoke. The arts often ask us to withdraw within ourselves to consider their full meaningfulness. The first new book celebrating the arts by nurses (Wendler, 2002) in a decade was a delight. We have the opportunity through the arts to increase our experience of awe and wonder. The tool here is limited to literature, music, art, and architecture. Certainly other arts to explore include—but certainly are not limited to—photography, dance, film, and video. Many arts and crafts projects and even scrapbooking could be included as well. You may already be engaged as either an appreciator or patroness of one or all of the arts. Quite possibly, although you do not earn your living in this manner, you are an artist in one or more of these. It is the making of art that makes an artist. You are an amateur, a beautiful word from the Latin *amare*— "to love"! Again, I urge you to use the tool first on your self as a clue to the arts that can nurture you. I assure you, however, the questions asked make great dinner conversation with family and friends.

Conclusion

The list of self-care activities is literally endless. So here and now, as a self-care measure, I give up! I request your forgiveness in my sins of omission. How might we increase the value given to self-care? How might we institutionalize this value as Henry and Henry (2004) have suggested in performance evaluations? I challenge the parish nurse coordinators reading this to include in the next revision of the Parish Nurse Performance Evaluation a category that is worth some significant percentage of the total, a review of a personalized plan for self-care that is developed and implemented by the parish nurse with set milestones and measurable outcomes.

The care, tending, and nurturing of one's self is a lifelong, challenging, demanding project. Take a deep breath; thank God; thank all those who give you the opportunity to care. Take care of yourself so that you can give from overflow, not from emptiness. Savor the benediction of play. Saunter over and make your "not to do" list. Nurture your soul. Give yourself the attention, care and compassion you are so willing to give others. Make God happy!

REFERENCES

Ackerman, D. (2001). *Cultivating delight: A natural history of my garden.* New York: HarperCollins.

Adams, K. (1990). *Journal to the self; Twenty-two paths to personal growth.* New York: Warner Books.

Bass, D.C. (2000). *Receiving the day: Christian practices for opening the gift of time.* San Francisco: Jossey-Bass.

Battaglia, C. (1996). *Murmurs.* Long Beach, NJ: Vista.

Becknell. T. (2001). *Of earth and sky: Spiritual lessons from nature.* Minneapolis: Augsburg.

Cameron, J. & Bryan, M. (1992). The artist's way: *A spiritual path to higher creativity.* New York: G.P. Putnam's Sons.

Cameron, J. (2004). *The sound of paper: Starting from scratch.* New York: Penguin.

Chinn, P. & Watson, J. (Eds.). (1994). *Art and aesthetics in nursing.* New York: National League for Nursing.

Fassel, D. (1990). *Working ourselves to death.* San Francisco: Harper.

Ford, A. (2002). *Retail therapy: Life lessons learned while shopping.* York Beach, ME: Conari Press.

Gilmour, P. (1997). *The wisdom of memoir: Reading and writing life's sacred texts.* Winona, MN: St. Mary's Press.

Gini, A. (2003). *The importance of being lazy: In praise of play, leisure, and vacations.* New York: Routledge.

Gleick, J. (1999). *Faster: The acceleration of just about everything.* New York: Pantheon.

Harvard Nurses' Study (1976, 1989). Retrieved June 23, 2004 from http://www.channing.harvard.edu/nhs/

Helldorfer, M.C. (1995). *The work trap: Rediscovering leisure, redefining work.* Mystic, CT: Twenty-Third Publications.

Henry, J. & L. (2004). Self-care begets holistic care. *Reflections on Nursing Leadership Sigma Theta Tau,* 30(1): 26-27.

Intel advertisement. *Wall Street Journal* (June 23, 2004). p. B2.

Josselson, R. (1998) *Best friends: The pleasures and perils of girls' and women's friendships.* New York: Three Rivers Press.

Kahn, S. & Saulo, M. (1993). *Healing yourself: A nurse's guide to self-care and renewal.* New York: Delmar Thomson Learning.

Kass, L.R. (1999). *The hungry soul.* Chicago: University of Chicago Press.

Kelsey, M. (1980). *Adventure inward: Christian growth through personal journal writing.* Minneapolis: Augsburg.

Klug, R. (1993). *How to keep a spiritual journal: A guide to journal keeping for inner growth and personal discovery.* Minneapolis: Augsburg.

Kundtz, D. (1998) *Stopping: How to be still when you have to keep going.* Berkeley, CA: Conari Press.

Lindbergh, A.M. (1965). *Gift from the sea.* New York: Vintage Books.

Long, J.M. (2002). *Permission to nap.* Naperville, IL: Sourcebooks. Inc.

Louden, J. (1997). *The woman's retreat book: A guide to restoring, rediscovering, reawakening your true self in a moment, an hour, a day, or a weekend.* San Francisco: HarperCollins.

McDermott, M.A. (1995). Parish nursing: Ministering through the arts. In *Proceedings of the ninth annual Westberg parish nurse symposium: Parish nursing ministering through the arts* (pp. 9-27). Northbrook, IL: National Parish Nurse Resource Center, Advocate Health Care.

Mc Mahon, J. (1998). Altars and icons: *Sacred spaces in everyday life.* San Francisco: Chronicle Books.

Moore, T. (1996). *The reenchantment of everyday life.* New York: Harper Collins.

Muller, W. (1999). *Sabbath: Restoring the sacred rhythm of rest.* New York: Bantam.

Norris, K. (1998). *The quotidian mysteries: Laundry, liturgy, and women's work.* New York: Paulist Press.

Overstreet, H.A. (1934). *A guide to civilized loafing.* New York: W.W. Norton.

Progoff, I. (1975). *At a journal workshop: The basic text and guide for using the intensive journal.* New York: Dialogue House.

Rybezynski, W. (1991). *Waiting for the weekend.* New York: Penguin.

Seligman, M. (2002). *Authentic happiness.* New York: Free Press.

Steindel-Rast, D. & Lebell, S. (1998). Music of silence: *A sacred journey through the hours of the days.* Berkeley, Ca: Seastone.

Styles, M. & Moccia, P. (1993). *On nursing: A literary celebration.* New York: National League for Nursing.

Vienne, V. (1998). *The art of doing nothing.* New York: Clarkson Potter.

Walker, S. (2001). *Driven no more: Finding contentment by letting go.* Minneapolis, MN: Augsburg.

Wendler, C. (Ed.) (2002). *The heart of nursing: Expressions of creative art in nursing.* Indianapolis: Sigma Theta Tau International.

Whyte, D. (1994). *The heart aroused: Poetry and the preservation of the soul in corporate America.* New York: Currency Doubleday.

Nurturing the Self Through the Arts:
A Reflection on Personal Well-Being
An Assessment Tool/Survey
Mary Ann McDermott, RN, EdD, FAAN

"The artist is the person who makes life more interesting or beautiful, more understandable or mysterious, or probably, in the best sense, more wonderful."
—George Bellow (1882-1925)

Literature

What is your taste in literary works?

What are your favorite books?

Are they in categories by type, by author, by theme?

Can you remember the first complete book you ever read and enjoyed?

Can you remember any of the illustrations from that book or other "early" books?

Have you ever studied Greek/Roman mythology?

What was the last book you read? The last novel you read?

Do you listen to books on tape/CD?

Do you go to the movies or rent the video of books that you like?

What is your favorite sacred text?

Do you have a favorite spiritual writer?

Do you ever take and keep notes from the books you read (best lines, quotes, and descriptions) or make journal entry reflections on your readings?

Have you ever read a book aloud to someone?

Have you ever authored your autobiography, a memoir... other than on a resume?

If someone were to write your biography, whom would you choose to author it? What would you suggest as the title? What are the ten chapter titles? What will be your input for the two illustrations per chapter (both subject matter and medium: photographs, watercolors etc.)?

Do you have a favorite poem?

Do you have a favorite poet?

Have you ever read poetry aloud with others?

Have you ever attended a poetry reading or a poetry slam?

Have you ever committed any poetry to memory? Can you still recite some poetry from memory?

How often do you go to the theater? Do you have a subscription?

What was the most moving play you ever attended?

Have you ever participated in reader's theatre?

Were you ever in a play? Why, and what memories of it do you have?

If a playwright of your choice were to write a play about some unique facet of your personal or professional life, what shape would it take: a melodrama, a musical, a comedy, a morality play? What would the play be entitled? How many acts would be required? Who would play the leading role, who might be in the cast of supporting players?

What author, playwright, and/or poet might you like to take to lunch?

Art

What are your favorite works of art? Are they in categories by genre, type, medium, artist, theme?

Do you have a favorite artist?

Do you have a favorite mosaic, fresco, and icon?

Do you frequent a local or regional art museum? Are you a member, a patron of the arts?

If you journal, do you ever make reflection entries on art?

Have you ever taken up art—enrolled in classes, invested in materials, shown it to anyone, exhibited anywhere?

Is there a work of sacred art that has been of special inspiration to you?

Is there an artist you would like to interview? Have you ever read his/her biography/autobiography or rented a video on his or her story?

Imagine you commissioned a great artist, your pick, to do your portrait. Will anyone else be in the portrait? What will the setting be? What will you wear? What posture or attitude would you choose? Would you be engaged in an activity? Should a favorite object or any appropriate symbols or inscriptions be included?

Another great artist, more into landscapes, has been commissioned by you to place you into your most favorite landscape. Using some of the detail above as well as considerations such as season, time of day or evening, the weather, give language to this picture.

Have you ever done a museum walk alone or with others of specific works at holiday and/or liturgical times (i.e., Advent/Christmas, Lent/Easter, Ordinary Time)?

Do you have a favorite sculpture?

Do you have a favorite sculptor?

What materials does that sculptor work with—stone, marble, metal?

Do you have any monument of which you are particularly fond?

Have you ever tried your hand at carving, sculpting, or ceramics?

Architecture

Do you have a favorite space or a restorative space? What are its characteristics?

Do you have a sacred space? How does it touch you? What are its qualities?

Have you ever considered an altar in your home?

Are there certain buildings that you find awesome and/or that you have a certain "feel" for?

Are there specific entrances of which you are fond?

Are you ever acutely aware of the adjacency (relationship) of one room/area to another?

Are you alert to the punctuations, pauses within a space?

What effect does the height of a structure or of a specific room have on you?

How do you respond to certain building materials/textures?

How does the space and the use of the space around a building influence your perception of the building?

How do the decorations/inscriptions/furnishings/contents of a building influence your perception of the building?

How do the color, light, and temperature of a structure influence you?

Are there some common characteristics shared by churches, museums, opera houses, concert halls and libraries? Do hospitals share any of these common characteristics?

Music

What is your favorite music? Is it categorized by form, type, instrument, composer, performer or by theme? Are there any reasons for your preferences?

Have you ever read a biography or autobiography of a favorite composer?

What music do you have in your collection?

What do you do when you listen to this music: sing/hum along, brood, exercise, listen, meditate?

How do you "tune in" and/or "tune out"?

Is there a work of sacred music that has been of special inspiration to you?

What is your favorite Christmas carol?

Have you ever conducted the music you listen to?

Have you neglected making music?

Do you/have you ever played an instrument, sung, been in an orchestra, been in a chorus/ choir? Do you ever "play it by ear" or strike a sympathetic chord?

Are you conscious of the pauses and rests within musical compositions?

Have you ever "been" the music you listen to?

Do you ever "whistle while you work"?

Do you have a special time and/or place for listening to music?

Do you/have you ever used making or listening to music for relieving stress, when you are feeling "out of tune," "out of harmony," or "out of rhythm"? Do you ever "sing the blues"?

Do you have a song that is "mine" and/or "ours"?

What factors, life events, contributed to your choices?

Can you remember "first music"?

Do you like to orchestrate or "re-orchestrate" things?

What musician would you like to meet and get to know better—one with whom you feel like you are "on the same wavelength"?

A famous composer of your choice has been commissioned to write and dedicate a composition to your memory. What type of composition will it be? What will it be entitled? For what instruments will it be written? Will there be lyrics? Where will the premiere be held? Who will perform? Who will be invited, and how will they respond?

Other Thoughts for Reflection Related to Potential Self-Nurturing Interventions

Have you ever thought about literature, poetry, drama, art, architecture, and music as prayerful—as prayer?

Is there any particular piece of literature, music, or art that came to your mind or spoke to your heart when you were experiencing difficult times in your life or perhaps maybe when you were feeling really good? Do you consider the arts as healing?

Is there one of these arts (literature, music, art, architecture) for which you feel a particular affinity at this point in your life?

Would you like to consider exploring one or all of these arts as a way you might promote health and healing and/or as a way of working through, having a better understanding, or coping with a particular issue/situation/crisis? If so, might you subscribe to a magazine, attend a conference or a workshop, or take a class related to this art?

Do you have the energy at this time to mobilize the resources to assist yourself in using this mode/these modes of nourishing your spirit, and/or do you have family and friends who will assist you?

Might there be a child—a niece/nephew or grandchild—who would find it fun to accompany you on a visit to an art museum, a gallery opening, a poetry reading, a concert, or an architectural tour of your town?

ENJOY!

Parish Nursing: A Collaborative Ministry

6

Kathleen Cleary Blanchfield
Reverend Edward McLaughlin

This chapter will address the need for collaboration in parish nurse ministry and illustrate various opportunities for collaboration at the congregational level and beyond. It focuses on the spiritual basis for collaboration in the many dimensions of parish nurse ministry. The authors, a parish nurse and a pastor, will share their experiences in fostering collaboration into the various facets of parish nurse ministry. The authors serve a congregation of 5000 Catholic families in a Midwestern suburban area. The professional nurse has been a parish nurse for 8 years, and the pastor has served for 18 years. The parish nurse is employed full-time and is affiliated with a large, church-sponsored healthcare system. Collaboration in our congregation is a necessity, not an option!

The Concept of Collaboration

The verb *collaborate* is derived from two Latin words: *com*, meaning "together," and *laborare*, meaning "to labor" (Webster, 1999). Webster's dictionary (1999) offers one definition for *collaborate* as "To work together, especially in a joint intellectual effort" (p. 219). The word *intellectual* is derived from a Latin word, *intellectus,* meaning "perception." *Intelligence* is defined as "the capacity for understanding knowledge, the ability to think abstractly or profoundly" (Webster, 1999, p. 576). The concept of collaboration is appropriately enriched when thought of as an intellectual effort. Collaboration in the ministry of parish

nursing practice does increase knowledge and understanding among participants and demands the ability to think abstractly and at times profoundly. Collaboration is a human interaction that takes place when individuals work together to promote joint efforts and effective goal attainment. Collaboration occurs when individuals work together in a manner that promotes collegiality, joint efforts, and effective goal attainment (Bausch, 1997; Pattillo, Chesley, Castles, & Sutter, 2002). Organizations can collaborate only because individuals participate and commit to it (Henneman, Lee & Cohen, 1995; Peters, 1992).

Articles in a wide variety of professional journals in healthcare discuss several common elements of collaboration. These common elements are communication, shared goal-setting, trust, and respect for each person's abilities (Hallas, Butz, & Gitterman, 2004; Knaus, Draper, Wagner, & Zimmerman, 1986; Pattillo et al, 2002; Sheer, 1996; Sohn, 2003). The concept of collaboration is a basic component in The Health Ministries' Association and American Nurses Association (ANA) *Scope and Standards of Parish Nursing Practice* (1998) and in the ANA's *Code of Ethics for Nurses with Interpretive Statements* (2001). The ANA *Code of Ethics for Nurses* (2001) states that "The nurse collaborates with other health professionals and the public in promoting community, national, and international efforts to meet health needs" (p. 4). Many articles in nursing journals describe nurses collaborating as team members in hospitals and ambulatory health settings. Additionally, the need for collaboration with physicians has been in the nursing literature for many years. An early research study by Knaus et al (1986) found that collaboration between physicians and nurses was a vital factor in achieving positive outcomes for patients in intensive care units. Pattillo et al (2002) describes how collaboration is the framework for their interagency model of community and parish nurse initiatives. The model emphasizes such elements as shared decision-making, shared vision, competence, and stewardship. They state, "The collaborative model ... provides evidence of good results when individuals bring together their gifts and talents to make their community something more than individuals can on their own" (p. 50).

Three Essential Elements of Collaboration in Ministry

Collaboration in ministry has three essential elements that need to be developed among the individuals involved. These elements are the three C's of collaboration: communication, connections, and cooperative goal-setting.

Communication

Communication takes place in many forms, such as meeting together, phone conversations, worshiping together, e-mail, retreats, letters, and congregational and community gatherings. Prayer and worship together are vital forms of communication and connection in the congregational setting.

Connections

Connections take the form of knowing each other and staying in contact with each other. Connections in collaborative relationships need to be actively developed and maintained. In a congregation, connections take place over many years of interacting as members of the specific congregation. Because parish nurse ministry is a shared ministry, many congregants can make a significant contribution and can use their connections to assist others. These connections among members can lay the vital groundwork for parish nurses to

invite members to share their unique gifts and talents. Previous connections can also be vital to preparing the way for meaningful collaboration with individuals and families in time of need or crisis.

Connections with individuals in community agencies and health facilities are needed to expand the initiatives and resources available to parish nurse ministry. When the parish nurse works collaboratively and shares the ministry with members of the congregation, vital connections to the community can be facilitated. For instance, a member of the congregation's health cabinet introduces the parish nurse to his neighbor, the director of the township health services agency. The connection is made; now the collaboration can begin over cooperative goal-setting and initiation of joint partnerships.

Cooperative Goal-Setting

Cooperative goal-setting requires time and attention be given to the individual needs and objectives of each person and or/agency. The "what's in this for me" factor must be discussed and acknowledged (Gunderson, 1997). When working with individuals or families in the congregation, one must identify the goals and outcomes for interaction with the parish nurse. Starting with this identification allows everyone to share expectations. This criterion is especially important with family members who can have very different goals and objectives both for themselves and for each other. For example, adult children often seek the aid and resources of the parish nurse in caring for/about the needs of their elderly parent. The elderly parent may not feel that he or she needs any help. The adult children may feel that the elderly parent not only needs help but also needs to relocate to another setting to receive care. The parish nurse is in a unique position to bring everyone together and to help them identify their basic concerns and goals for each other and for themselves. The parish nurse who knows about community resources and congregational services while also remaning sensitive to the emotional and spiritual issues involved during this difficult time can aid each of the individuals in this process.

Cooperative goal-setting between parish nurse ministry and other church ministries is vital to successful working relationships between ministries. This takes time and needs to be done with intent and specific goals being jointly developed. Unfortunately, this task is easily overlooked because of time constraints and the assumption that each ministry understands the needs and abilities of the other ministry.

When organizations are involved in interorganizational collaboration and goal-setting, the mission of each organization needs to be identified and respected. This is especially important when different religious organizations are involved. The tenets of the religious denomination may foster or limit certain health initiatives. Religious beliefs surrounding end of life issues, conception, abortion, organ transplantation, and a theory of just war are examples of the religious issues that need to be considered and respected during cooperative goal-setting.

When healthcare organizations fund parish nurse salaries a written contract between the organization and the church is necessary. This process of developing and signing a contract helps both parties to understand the expectations and responsibilities of each and to enter a partnership together. Cooperative goal-setting about the parish nurse ministry purpose, relationship, and primary responsibilities to the congregation needs to take place. Cooperative goal-setting about the health organization's needs and cooperative role also needs to take place. This is an ongoing effort on both the healthcare organization's part and on the church's part and needs to take place on a regular schedule. With any change in leadership in the church, healthcare organization, or parish nurse position, cooperative goal-setting needs to occur along with establishing connections and communication.

Collaboration for and with God

Caring for the spiritual needs of patients can be challenging in a fast-paced health system serving a religiously diverse population. Reverend Granger Westberg (1987), the founder of parish nursing, developed the role to address this need. Reverend Westberg's (1955) early experiences of working with nurses as a hospital chaplain taught him the value of working together to effectively identify when patients and family members need spiritual as well as emotional and physical care. He realized a great need to reach people with health and wellness information before they become hospitalized. His early experiences as a chaplain evolved into his visionary belief that whole person care could best take place in the congregational setting and that registered nurses were prepared to do this by working with the clergy and members of the congregation (Paterson, 1982; Westberg, 1987).

"Being a parish nurse is like working in the cathedral of healthcare" (Blanchfield, 2001, p.160). One unique characteristic of working in a congregational setting is the opportunity to invite others to share in carrying out the work of the Lord. This takes many forms, such as inviting members of the congregation, community agencies, and health organizations to participate in health initiatives based in the congregation. Parish nurse ministry provides abundant opportunities for members of the congregation and for health agencies to collaborate and make available needed whole person health initiatives that foster self-care and health and wellness.

The congregational setting for parish nurse ministry is a unique setting for professional nursing. Congregations have distinct missions and ministries. They also have several characteristics in common. Gunderson (1997) has written and spoken extensively on the characteristics of congregations. He has identified eight strengths of congregations that foster health ministry. These strengths are the following: to accompany, to convene, to connect, to tell stories, to give sanctuary, to bless, to pray, and to endure. He believes these strengths can improve the quality of life in congregations and communities. Gunderson (1997) views collaboration as the way that these strengths come alive in congregations. A vivid example of these strengths occurs in church sponsored support groups. The congregation literally accompanies, convenes, connects, fosters storytelling, gives sanctuary, blesses, prays, and endures with members in support groups, such as for those who are grieving, who are struggling with addictions, or who are caregivers.

Parish nurses can minister to the spiritual needs of individuals, which can make a significant difference in offering whole person care. Gunderson's (1997) strengths of congregations such as to accompany, to bless, to pray, and to endure are powerful ways to minister to individual's spiritual needs. Blanchfield (2002) writing about shame in the homebound explains how ministering to the spiritual needs of an isolated, medically needy elderly woman makes the difference between refusing needed care or accepting this care. The woman's isolation and refusal of medical care was lifted by prayer and collaboration with lay ministers who were willing to accompany, to pray, and to endure while supporting this elderly parishioner.

Isaiah 6:8 reads, "And I heard the voice of the Lord saying: Whom shall I send? And who shall go for us? And I said: Lo, Here am I. Send me." Collaboration in ministry starts with being open to what God is calling you to do. Many parish nurses will state that they truly feel called or directed to this ministry by God (McDermott & Mullins, 1989; O'Brien, 2003). Ruffing (2000), in her book *Spiritual Direction*, explains that as we become closer to God we can develop a sense of mutuality with God. When we place God in the center of our ministry, we are together. The Lord assures us in the very last words of Matthew's gospel that we are not alone as we struggle with this work of the Lord. "And behold, I am with you always, until the end of the age," reads Matthew 28:20.

The parish nurse needs to have time to pray and to discern what God is asking and the ability to be in tune with God's opportunities for interactions with others. Nouwen (2003), a theologian and author, challenges all in ministry to pray. He states the following:

> Very few ministers will deny that prayer is important. They will not even deny that prayer is the most important dimension of their lives. But the fact is that most ministers pray very little or not at all. They realize that they should not forget to pray, that they should take time to pray; and that prayer should be a priority in their lives. But all these "shoulds" do not have the power to carry them over the enormous obstacle of their activism. There is always one more phone call, one more book, and one more party. Together these form an insurmountable pile of activities (p. 67).

Obviously, we need to take time to focus, to pause, and to reflect as a believing person. We call this process prayer. Without prayer we can easily forget that we are doing God's work and that we need a lot of help.

Because spirituality is the core of parish nursing, placing God at the center of the ministry of parish nursing practice places every aspect of parish nursing as connected to God. Collaboration in parish nurse ministry evolves as an outcome of recognizing that God is entrusting the work of caring for each other to each of His followers. The parish nurse as a person involved in ministry needs to trust that God continues to speak to us and to call us. God calls to us in the people, situations and responsibilities of our life.

Collaboration with the Pastor and Staff

Initially, a parish nurse wanting to collaborate with the pastor, staff, and lay ministers can be perceived as burdening ministers who already have too much to do. When the idea of collaborating and sharing the work of ministry is suggested, suspicions can be raised about burdening each other. Why work together when there is already so much work to be done in each separate ministry? Additionally, when a nurse becomes a parish nurse, the desire to make a difference and the uniqueness of the parish nurse role can pressure a nurse to try to start this new ministry alone. It is easy to believe that working with others will come later when the new parish nurse understands his or her role and the needs of the congregation.

Because of their professional knowledge and experience as well as their position in ministry that demands a collaborative approach, parish nurses must realize their excellent opportunity to model collaboration in all their efforts. This ministry demands that people and resources be brought together to meet the health and wellness of the congregation. Consequently, the parish nurse needs to use his or her skills in teamwork and collaboration by inviting staff and lay leaders to join in working together. This effort can begin by attending staff meetings and actively showing interest and concern for staff members and the ministries they serve.

Two roadblocks should be carefully considered before collaborating. One is approaching our ministry as if we are alone and forgetting that this is God's work we are about. We do this not alone but with God's constant help, some of which is in the form of the people we work with or those whom God sends to us.

The other roadblock to collaboration is the temptation to focus on the regrets or failures and to beat ourselves up because of the things we haven't done or because of programs that were "not successful." Things are going to go wrong. Programs at times will fail. Not everything we attempt will be successful. God's mysterious plan for continuing His work and building His Kingdom depends on human beings continuing that work in a human and therefore, less than perfect, manner. Mother Teresa is a model for this with her challenge to each of us in ministry that God calls us to be faithful not successful.

Working with the leader of a congregation is essential. Communication, connections, and cooperative goal-setting take time and understanding of each person's role and vision for the congregation. Both pastor/leader and parish nurse need to establish how they will do this and why it is necessary for the success of achieving their goals. Solari-Twadell's dissertation research (2002) found that parish nurses attributed "the support of their pastor" as one of three major factors accounting for the success of their programs (p. 127).

Pastors need to accept the reality that they cannot accomplish the entire ministry of a parish by themselves. Acts 6:1-7 tells of the original disciples realizing that they cannot do everything alone. They needed to care for the widows' needs and to pray and preach. The disciples carefully chose others to respond to the needs of the widows. They explained that the congregation needed the widows to be cared for and also needed leaders who pray and preach. By asking others to help, the work of God spread and the number of disciples increased.

The pastor and nurse need to respect the competence of each other. Each must recognize that he or she has different gifts, roles, and talents. Realistic expectations need to be discussed, with neither of them expecting perfection of the other or in others with whom they will work. A written parish nurse job description that is jointly developed and agreed upon will facilitate this process.

The following items are a list of a few of the challenges for a pastor who is collaborating with a parish nurse:

- Effectively articulate the need for a parish nurse ministry to the congregation, to the

parish council, and to the finance committee.
- Actively support the parish nurse and her programs.
- Give honest, ongoing feedback.
- Facilitate and support her position on parish staff.
- Foster collaboration between the parish nurse and other staff.
- Pray for the nurse and for the parish nurse ministry.

The following are a few of the attributes and abilities a pastor finds essential in a parish nurse:
- Be a self-starter.
- Make himself or herself known to groups and parishioners.
- Be present at parish functions and worship services.
- Be available and patient with the process of beginning a new ministry.
- Network both within and outside of the congregation.
- Realize good things have been and are happening in the congregation.
- Listen, listen, listen.

Collaboration with Congregation Members

The roles of professional staff in congregations are to call, unite, empower, and support all the members of the body of Christ to use their gifts to continue the work of the Lord and to build His Kingdom. Therefore the parish nurse and the pastor need to invite skilled, competent parishioners to serve in parish nurse ministry. They are invited to use their expertise for the good of the congregation and the community. The pastor hopefully listens and is guided by the wisdom of the congregation and elicits their enthusiasm and help.

In the congregation the parish nurse can empower people of good will (e.g., Communion visitors to the homebound) to be alert to and to respond to needs of the sick, aged, or infirmed parishioners. The parish nurse is a source of wisdom, support, and reassurance concerning issues of health and disease to the pastor, other staff members, and parishioners.

In our congregation many people were invited to participate in either the nursing cabinet or the health cabinet to work with the parish nurse ministry. These cabinets multiply the ministers in parish nurse ministry. Initially, Reverend Granger Westberg (1987) recommended the idea of the health cabinet in parish nursing. He believed that just as every home has a medicine cabinet, congregations need health cabinets of health resources. We decided that because our parish is so large, both a health and nursing cabinet were needed. Reverend Westberg envisioned the health cabinet as a group of health professionals and leaders who could advocate for and work to gather the resources necessary for parish nurse ministry. The number of members for both cabinets is kept small to foster group cohesiveness. Each person brings unique skills and gifts to the ministry. Members are encouraged to make a commitment of two years service and then to discern whether they need to move on to other areas of ministry. This works well for us. People often are reluctant to become involved because leaving the ministry later on does not seem to be an option. As other health professionals hear of parish nurse ministry, they often volunteer to join. When one member discerns to leave, another person is given the opportunity to become a part of the nursing or health cabinet.

The Nursing Cabinet

At our parish the nursing cabinet comprises registered nurses who have a wide variety of skills and nursing expertise. Currently, the twelve members of our nursing cabinet are employed in various hospitals, ambulatory care centers, community and home health agencies, and schools of nursing. Each brings a unique gift to the ministry. They work with the parish nurse to develop programs and resources and serve as consultants to the parish nurse. Often one of the nurses specializes in an area that meets a specific need in the congregation. She then works with the parish nurse and the person or family to help guide them through the process of receiving necessary health resources.

Initially, the nursing cabinet met frequently to identify its role and to determine ongoing congregational needs for whole person health. As the ministry expanded over 8 years, various members moved on to other ministries, and new members were asked to join the parish nurse ministry

nursing cabinet. The number of meetings has been reduced, but the contact has increased between the parish nurse and the individual nursing cabinet members.

The nursing cabinet members collaborate with each other and with many other healthcare agencies. They draw from their contacts and experiences to bring programs, resources, health information, and referral sources for members of the congregation and community. Their collaborative approach has resulted in the following outcomes:

- Development of a Caregiver's Community Resource Book
- Development of a guide for reducing the cost of prescription drugs
- Development of a series of healthy eating programs and bulletin articles
- Development of weekly bulletin articles on a wide range of health issues
- Development, in partnership with the health cabinet, an annual Adult Health Fair and a Children's Health and Safety Fair
- Development of monthly health education programs
- Development of contacts with community agencies to facilitate referrals and identification of needs for additional health services

The Health Cabinet

The health cabinet comprises various health professionals (e.g., physicians, nutritionists, counselors, elected officials, paramedics, and congregational leaders). Both the health and nursing cabinet members collaborate with the parish nurse to bring resources to the parish nurse ministry. The health cabinet members work to support the parish nurse ministry by assessing and documenting what is needed and then helping to secure these resources. The health cabinet helped clarify the need for a full-time position when the parish nurse was working more than the initial, agreed-on 20 hours a week.

Health cabinet members can make introductions to local government departments, community agencies, health organizations, and businesses. This fosters the ongoing working relationships the parish nurse needs with vital community agencies. For example, by working with a paramedic on the health cabinet, the parish nurse can call on the fire department and paramedic division to help conduct ongoing community needs assessments and to assist individuals who do not understand how to use this expanding community service.

Listed here are a few of the outcomes of collaboration with the health cabinet and parish nurse:

- Development of brochures, bulletin articles, and speaking opportunities that explain the mission and offerings of parish nurse ministry to the congregation and the larger community
- Development of formal introductions and creation of contacts with various hospital systems, local governmental agencies, community agencies, and businesses
- Development of advocacy initiatives to secure needed services and to raise awareness of gaps in delivery of healthcare
- Development of health education programs using the knowledge and expertise of the various cabinet members, their colleagues, and/or their healthcare organization affiliations

Collaboration with Physicians

Parish nurse ministry provides a unique opportunity for collaboration between nurses and physicians. Physicians on the health cabinet are in a unique role to help foster whole person health of body, mind, and spirit. For example, one early proponent of the need for a parish nurse and a founding member of the health cabinet was an emergency department physician. He helped identify the need and lobbied for the parish financial resources to establish a parish nurse ministry. He was in an excellent position to provide witness to the need for health and wellness information and for services that would be grounded in the faith community. His years in the emergency department made him a firm believer in helping people stay well and in the need for whole person care. His experience with the needs and frustrations of families surrounding such issues as end-of-life care, suicide prevention, treatment for depression, care for the frail elderly, well-child health, and safety precautions convinced him of the need for parish nurse ministry.

This physician's leadership role subsequently became even stronger as both cabinets worked together to bring health and wellness programs and screenings to the parish and surrounding community. The cabinets struggled with the challenge to provide spiritual as well as physical and emotional health and wellness programs. With the physician's help and insight, we began to offer programs focusing on the spiritual aspect of health. We wanted to offer programs that would have a spiritual focus in the title, with spirituality integrated into the content and experience. We believed these programs were authentic offerings for the faith-based setting of the church. We decided to title them "Spiritual Strength" programs. We knew we had a need for these programs because public and nondenominational health systems and agencies are not equipped either by mission or expertise to provide these programs.

Our physician leader volunteered to coordinate our first offering, which was called "Spiritual Strength for Survivors of Suicide." After the success of this program, we developed and we continue to develop more "Spiritual Strength" programs, such as Spiritual Strength for Dealing with Addictions, Spiritual Strength for Dealing with Anger, Spiritual Strength for Depression, Spiritual Strength for Postpartum Depression, Spiritual Strength for Caregivers, and Spiritual Strength for Facing End-of-Life Issues. The nature of the "Spiritual Strength" programs called us to collaborate with other ministries and with other church-affiliated agencies to organize the necessary resources before and after the program. We needed the help of clergy so members of our congregation can ask the questions about what is morally acceptable to the Catholic church—for example, the following:

- What happens when a person takes his or her own life?
- Do addictions separate you from God?
- Can you morally sign a living will?

These programs can be emotionally draining for participants who are dealing with issues perceived as very private and that may have sometimes gone unanswered for years. Often a "disconnect" from the church occurs. Members of both cabinets work together to personally invite people who might be in need of these programs.

Cabinet members also work together to ensure a strong presence and a willing person to help someone who has chosen to attend.

We have asked parishioners who have previously attended to collaborate with us as we develop follow-up programs and initiatives. For instance, a mother of a child who committed suicide now works with the parish nurse and the grief minister to reach out to other families who are suffering the loss of a loved one by suicide. She helps parish nurse ministry refine our outreach to survivors of suicide. This mother works with us to invite and to accompany parishioners and members of the community to attend our spiritual strength programs for survivors of suicide. She also challenges us to become more actively involved in organ donor registration and awareness. One offering often leads to many other offerings and to more people becoming involved in the ministry of parish nursing. Collaboration promotes the expansion of ministry and helps us as we seek to serve God and reach out to others spiritually!

Collaboration with Existing Ministries

Collaboration among ministries avoids duplicating various ministries' efforts. Instead, ministries join together to share the load, to gather new ideas, and to recruit volunteers to work toward a common goal. This is especially true when a long-term need has been identified and no one ministry has been successful in meeting this need. One example occurred when youth, education, and parish nurse ministries wanted to invite a nationwide speaker to present a faith-based topic. None of them had the budget or ability to undertake this responsibility alone. When the various leaders of these ministries started working together to identify a common goal, the roadblocks were lifted. A speaker was identified that would appeal to both youths and adults. The topic "What it Means to be a Catholic Today" was selected. All the various responsibilities were defined and shared among the members of the three ministry groups. The necessary funds were gathered by combining budgets and identifying each ministry's ability to support this endeavor.

All ministries differ in purpose, numbers of volunteers, abilities, and leadership. These differences need to be recognized and discussed. If one

ministry has significantly fewer members, this needs to be taken into consideration when undertaking necessary jobs. Helping with sales of books may only take a few people, but greeting and hosting could take many more people. If it is not addressed, then responsibilities may be incorrectly assigned. A fundamental need with successful collaboration is to honestly recognize the gifts God has given each group and to work toward promoting use of these gifts, even if every job is not equal. In our situation it was decided that youths and adults would work together to introduce the speaker, to help sell tapes and books for the speaker, to do publicity, and to offer hospitality by greeting and serving refreshments. In some cases more youths were available to help, and in some cases more adults were available. Every detail was taken care of because direct communication and connections were in place throughout the event.

An unexpected benefit was the many parishioners who remarked about how inspiring it was to see youths and adults work together to provide for a major presenter and to take care of the hundreds of people who attended. Ironically, the speaker was very well received, but we heard more specific comments about how wonderful it was to have youths and adults working together on a program dealing with faith. These combined, collaborative efforts have led to several other joint sharing of large initiatives such as sponsoring a parish mission. The communication, connections, and ability to cooperatively set goals have been established. We have learned that there is synergy with collaborating together. We now have a successful history and a legacy we can build upon.

Here are a few lessons we have learned about collaborating with other ministries:

- Decide on a common goal.
- Do not duplicate each other's efforts.
- Respect each ministry's differences.
- Nurture and promote each ministry's unique gifts.
- Work toward recognizing and respecting the limitations of each ministry.
- Seek and plan for future efforts together to build upon what you have learned about collaborating together.
- In developing the ability to work together, address issues regarding budgeting, shared resources, combined efforts.

- Evaluate and review each ministry's needs and expectations.
- Share the evaluation of the event with all participants and use this to start your next effort to work together.
- Celebrate the outcome!

Collaboration with Individuals and Families

Parish nurse ministry provides a sacred mission for parish nurses to live out the scriptural call of Jesus to provide for each other (O' Brien, 2003). Because the focus of parish nursing is to provide others with knowledge and resources to care for their own health, the nurse needs to establish a collaborative relationship with individuals and families. Parish nurses do not care for "patients"; they care about the congregation and the health and wellness of the members of the congregation. The traditional health expert approach of caring for patients does not fit this ministry. The journey together begins when the parish nurse takes the time to meet with individuals and families to establish a collaborative relationship. Relationships in parish nursing are not episodic, these occur over years of interaction. Both members of the congregation and the parish nurse know a great deal about each other. Many joys and sorrows can be shared over life events and by coming together for worship.

Confidentiality is essential to the success of collaboration with individuals and families. The issues relating to confidentiality need to be discussed at the first meeting, especially when previous communication and connections have been informal. Now a change in the relationship and confidentiality becomes a topic that needs to be addressed. Here are a few issues that need to be discussed: Who else, including family members, does the individual want involved? Does the individual know that the parish nurse documents their meetings and interactions? How are these documents kept secure? Why is documentation necessary, especially if no other staff members keep records of interactions? The Health Ministry Association/ANA Scope and Standards of Parish Nursing Practice (1998) states, "The parish nurse collaborates with the client system, other health ministers, healthcare providers, and community

agencies in promoting client health" (p. 20). If confidentiality is broken, collaboration will cease. Before the parish nurse collaborates with anyone, permission must be granted by the individual or family involved.

Documentation can foster collaboration when the individual or family is involved in what is to be documented. This topic can be reviewed in future meetings and the information can support ongoing collaboration and evaluation. An example occurred when a young father who knew the parish nurse through their daughter's participation on the same sports teams happened to meet the parish nurse on his way to his child's basketball game. The nurse was on her way to the parish health fair. She invited him to stop in. He did and chose to have his blood pressure screened. His B/P was very high. Several additional readings were taken with the same results. He refused a referral for medical care and left for his daughter's game. That evening the parish nurse called him to inquire how he was. His wife answered and thanked her for getting her husband to seek needed treatment. The parish nurse did not know how to respond since she had no permission to discuss this with his wife. His wife seemed to understand this and went on to say her husband was at the hospital for treatment of this life-threatening, high-blood pressure. He had told his wife how the parish nurse persuaded him to have his blood pressure checked and to see his doctor immediately, which he did after his daughter's game was finished. The young father was happy to receive a call from the parish nurse. He truly felt the nurse saved his life. After the nurse received permission to discuss this with his wife, all of them met to plan follow-up health initiatives. The couple felt that this "chance encounter" with the nurse at the church was God's way of helping them to seriously evaluate their own health. They in turn told many members of the congregation and sent a letter stating their belief in the value of having the health fair at the church. They have given the parish nurse permission to tell their story to those who are reluctant to take the time for health screenings. Fortunately, the parish nurse's previous communication and connections with the family resulted in an invitation being offered and accepted for a blood pressure screening. The issue of confidentiality and the clarification of each person's role took time, yet the outcome was one in which the work of the Lord was real to each involved. The documentation of the man's original blood pressure, his visit to the hospital, and the subsequent lower readings support the collaborative efforts to improve his health and wellness.

Collaboration with Coordinators and Directors of Parish Nurse Ministry

Not every parish nurse has a coordinator or director of parish nurse ministry, but if he or she does, it provides another opportunity for collaboration. When a parish nurse is part of a formal structure for parish nurse ministry, someone in a leadership role can oversee the parish nurses affiliated with the sponsoring organization or hospital. Sometimes a formal employment arrangement is made; other times a cooperative arrangement is made.

Coordinators and directors have the advantage of seeing the big picture in parish nurse ministry. They understand the numerous demands for parish nurse services, and they can support the individual parish nurse, who can become overwhelmed by the many needs of the congregation. In turn, the parish nurse can offer the coordinator insight into the ongoing congregational needs and opportunities for other resources to be made available at the congregational level. Each needs the other and must work together to enhance the quality and growth of parish nurse ministry.

The old concepts of supervision and authoritarian leadership do not work well in parish nurse ministry. Christ Himself provides a model of servant leadership. When He wanted to tell his disciples how to care for others, He started by washing their feet. Nouwen, a respected theologian (1989) and Bausch, a pastor and author (1997), both assert that ministry and leadership need to work in collaborative ways that increase cooperative interaction and responsiveness to individuals' needs for growth, sharing their gifts, and feeling valued. Parish nurse coordinators can be excellent at this when they work collaboratively with parish nurses.

An example of the positive benefits of collaboration between a coordinator/director of parish nursing and a parish nurse occurred several years ago during a shortage of flu vaccine. Our parish nurse ministry was collaborating with the township health department to offer flu vaccine at the congregational health fair. All members of the congregation and community were to be invited. Unfortunately, a shortage of vaccine left the township without the hundreds of dosages necessary for the health fair. Consequently, many people who were at risk would not receive the flu vaccine because even their doctors could not get the vaccine. The elderly were particularly affected. A lack of transportation is often a major barrier to participation by seniors. In our congregation, however, rides had already been arranged.

As an employee of a large health system, parish nurse Blanchfield contacted her director. In turn the director communicated this great need and opportunity for an effective community health initiative to other system administrators. She sought their assistance and was successful in procuring a supply of hundreds of dosages of flu vaccine. The township was also able to obtain a limited amount of vaccine. At the last minute, enough vaccine was available to offer flu shots to everyone who had signed up. We were also able to accommodate those additional individuals who now felt they should participate because so much attention was being paid to getting this scarce vaccine! Through the collaboration of the parish nurse with the parish nurse ministry director, a congregational/community service was offered that could never have been accomplished by either party alone.

Here are a few lessons learned about collaborating with parish nurse coordinators/directors:

- Coordinators and directors of parish nurse ministry have a unique leadership role.
- Parish nurses and their coordinators need to make time for communication, connections, and cooperative goal-setting to ensure collaboration.
- Both have chosen to be on a journey together in parish nurse ministry.
- Faith-sharing and spiritual development are vital to ongoing interactions.
- Coordinators are well equipped to pose the hard questions about ministry and balance of the parish nurse role.
- Coordinators and parish nurses need to be sensitive to their own health and wellness needs as well as to those of others.
- Coordinators and parish nurses need to afford the same whole person care and

concern for each other that is offered in parish nurse ministry.

Collaboration with Other Parish Nurses

The synergy of working together is a reality when parish nurses across a health system or a geographical region collaborate on health initiatives. Working together affords an opportunity to share each nurse's unique gifts, talents, and knowledge. One nurse may be skilled in writing bulletin and newsletter articles. Many more people will benefit from these articles if they can be shared with other parish nurses for use in their bulletins and local newspapers. Another parish nurse may be skilled at presenting self-care or spiritual programs. By combining efforts and inviting several congregations to attend a program, a wider audience can be served. Helping each other with large initiatives such as health fairs can make the difference between success or a single parish nurse becoming overwhelmed by a large health event.

Speakers and organizations often will only become involved if several congregations are working together, especially if their resources are stretched and they fear if they do for one congregation they will have to do for all. When parish nurses work together to cosponsor one program, they can assure speakers and agencies they will have a broad audience.

Parish nurses know the delicate balance that each health initiative demands and can help each other stay focused and centered in the spiritual dimension of parish nurse ministry. Praying and reflecting together is a wonderful way to collaborate and to support each other.

Collaboration among parish nurses has resulted in some of the following initiatives:

- Developing shared retreats and prayer services
- Mentoring new parish nurses
- Creating an interdenominational walking program
- Participating in research to study documentation, outcomes, and dimensions of parish nurse ministry
- Jointly sponsoring programs on such topics as ethics, cardiovascular health, end-of-life issues and domestic violence
- Developing professional, continuing education programs
- Advocating for access to affordable healthcare
- Writing grants for congregational health initiatives
- Collaboratively authoring books and articles on parish nurse ministry

Collaboration with Schools of Nursing and Nursing Students

Parish nurse ministry and schools of nursing have a great deal to gain from working collaboratively. Schools of nursing need learning opportunities for students, and parish nurse ministry needs the stimulation, interest, and help that students offer. A learning experience with a parish nurse provides a vivid interaction in nursing with a focus upon fostering health and wellness for the congregation as a population/aggregate. Whole person interaction with individuals and families allows nursing students to grasp the importance of the spiritual dimension of health. The three C's of collaboration in ministry must be formally worked out before nursing students are placed with a parish nurse. Communication between the instructor and parish nurse needs to address the specific needs and expectations for this collaborative learning experience. Here are a few of the questions that need to be addressed:

- What are the course objectives for the student?
- What is the student's skill level?
- What are the required hours for the learning experience?
- Can the student accompany the parish nurse on home visits or would this be a violation of confidentiality?
- Can students be present on Sundays, and would they be comfortable participating in workshop services?
- Are there tenets of the faith about which students need to be sensitive and informed?

Many other specific details need to be collaboratively worked out. The parish nurse needs to be very clear about what would be an appropriate learning experience and what would be inappropriate. A written contract helps with formal communication of the needs and expectations of both the school and the congregation. The contract needs to cover such basics as the responsibility for the school, instructor, parish, and parish nurse. The following issues also need to be covered: confidentiality, liability, licensure, health status of students, and the terms of contract renegotiation and/or termination.

Basic nursing students have a need for specific clinical hours and for learning clinical skills, such as administrating medications and/or injections, that parish nurses cannot offer. Is this fact clearly understood by all concerned? Can the student vary the hours needed based upon the parish nurse's schedule? Are various Sunday and evening hours a possibility for the student?

Degree-completion and master's degree students already have clinical skills and experience. Most understand and value the need for a health and wellness focus in a congregational setting. Experienced professional nurses can bring a wealth of experience and insight into current healthcare practices. The collaborative interaction between student, teacher, and parish nurse preceptor can be a very rewarding experience. One master's degree student, a school nurse, collaborated with the parish nurse to identify learning needs for a program on bone health for mothers of school-age children. She then created a program and a learning evaluation tool on bone health for the congregation. When her learning experience was finished, she used the program for education of parents and children in her role as a school nurse.

Large endeavors such as congregation and community health fairs are excellent learning experiences for all levels of nursing students and for chaplain students, residents and interns, and other healthcare professional students.

Here are a few lessons about collaborating with schools of nursing and nursing students:

- Written objectives need to be developed by the student and discussed with the parish nurse.
- When an instructor leaves a school, the new instructor needs to meet with the parish nurse to ensure each understands the other's expectations.
- Parish nursing ministry is a relatively new specialty in nursing. Each ministry is so unique that misinterpretations can occur when faculty believe that parish nurse ministry is the same in all congregations or when home health nursing is confused with parish nursing.
- Students can be a source of profound insight and sharing of the need for a spiritual focus with health and wellness.

- A parish nursing learning experience can reinforce the student's desire to make a difference in others' lives and provide insight into the sacred nature of the practice of nursing.
- The spiritual nature of parish nursing is not for every student or instructor.
- Students can feel lost in a congregational setting if they are not oriented to parish nursing.
- Parish nurses need to set aside time to meet with the student on an ongoing basis.
- A written contract is necessary.
- Invite the instructor to attend a parish nurse initiative that has student involvement.
- Keep the instructor informed and ask for feedback.
- Parish nursing can be overwhelming for students who have no frame of reference for congregational life and ministry.

Collaboration with Community Agencies

The work of the Kingdom is not restricted to people of one denomination or one worldview. Rather, all people of good will who are trying to make the world a better place by reaching out to others with compassion are part of building the Kingdom. Congregations can and must look for ways to cooperate with and to foster and facilitate the good efforts that are present in our community and our world. No person or group has a corner on the market as we try to bring about the work of the Lord.

Community healthcare organizations and agencies provide an excellent opportunity for forming collaborative health initiatives. Parish nurse ministry provides community involvement for agencies that are charged with meeting community needs. Hospitals, ambulatory care facilities, and public health organizations can fulfill their mission to provide health services to the community. Congregations can fulfill their respective missions to serve others.

The organization's collaboration with parish nurse ministry fosters better understanding of the community's needs and provides an opportunity to enter the community at the congregational setting. Opening programs to members of the community and reaching out to the community benefit all parties. To form collaborative relationships with community agencies, one must do the basic groundwork to ensure the success of a collaborative relationship. The 3 C's of collaboration need to be addressed. Communication needs to be established, and meaningful connections among the key individuals and cooperative goal-setting must take place. This takes time, patience, honesty, and perseverance. This groundwork to build collaborative working relationships is necessary to avoid misunderstandings, mistakes, wasted efforts, and feelings of a burdensome workload.

An example is our parish nurse ministry's relationship with our township's health services. An elected official who served on the health cabinet introduced the director of the township health services and the parish nurse 7 years ago. The parish nurse was asked to present to the township governing board information about parish nurse ministry services and any identified community needs. As a result of the presentation, the director of the health services and the parish nurse began to meet regularly to form a working relationship.

Initially, two joint-sponsored major initiatives were developed: an adult health fair and a children's health fair. Because these fairs were very large in scope, a great deal of collaboration was needed. All the members of the health and nursing cabinets, along with the township health director, worked together to plan the events and to expand the resources by inviting other agencies to become involved.

The parish nurse's affiliation with a major healthcare system brought several needed screenings to the health fairs. Pediatric residents and their director were recruited to do well-children physicals; hospital laboratory director became involved; and cholesterol screenings were provided. The township health services director secured various agencies to perform hearing, vision, and dental screenings. When dentists were not available, the parish nurse invited a dentist who was a member of the parish to participate.

After several successful events the township director and the parish nurse partnered together to expand services and screenings. The police and fire departments were invited to participate. They helped to expand the children's health fair to a children's health and safety fair. The church parking lot was transformed into a safety education center complete with a fire safety house, car safety-seat checks, asthma information, nutrition, and

bike helmet distribution and fittings. A medical center helicopter landed and displayed emergency medical evacuation equipment.

After the fairs, follow-up evaluation meetings were held with the participating agencies and our cabinet members to decide what enhancements would be needed for future events. Written evaluations were sought from participants at both health fairs. A follow-up evaluation was mailed several months after the health fair to ask how participants have used the health information they received. People often report, for example, sharing their cholesterol screening findings with their doctors. As a result, a need was identified and subsequently met for more educational programs on diet and exercise to reduce cholesterol.

A spiritual emphasis is interwoven throughout the adult health fair. This emphasis starts with inviting many parishioners to volunteer and share their professional expertise or personal ability to offer a spirit of welcoming hospitality. An effort is made to have volunteer parishioners waiting to welcome and accompany hesitant people, harried parents, or people with disabilities to the screenings or needed services. Each adult is greeted and given a prayer card, which also offers a formal welcome to our adult health fair. Our events start with a gathering for the volunteers to pray together and to offer intentions for prayer as we begin this major health initiative. The prayer includes the fact that we are all gathered together to work toward fostering health and wellness for members of the congregation and the community. Staff members are involved with a spiritual health booth that offers care notes, prayer cards, and the opportunity to speak to parish clergy and ministry staff.

The outcome of the collaborative efforts of parish nurse ministry and the director of the township health services is that thousands of flu shots, immunizations, and well-children physical exams have been administered. Thousands of screenings have also been conducted (e.g., cholesterol, hemoglobin, osteoporosis, prostate cancer and PSA tests, skin cancer, dental, vision, hearing). Announcements of our joint events are placed in the local newspapers and in the church bulletin. Newsletters are mailed to everyone in the community to ensure that all are informed and invited. Educational follow-up programs are set up to follow these major screenings.

For instance, a series of nutrition programs ranging from cardiovascular health to food choices and faith practices have been developed in collaboration with the cabinet members and the township health services.

Communication and connections need to continue throughout the year to maintain an ongoing collaborative relationship. For example, initially the township health director and the parish nurse only worked on two annual events 6 months apart. When communication was only around these events, follow-up and additional opportunities rarely happened. Attendance at common events by both parties increased opportunities for communication and connection. Additional opportunities for collaboration naturally evolved. Speakers are shared, and information is coordinated between our offerings. When the township had an opportunity to buy cholesterol screening equipment, they did. The adult health fair evaluations have indicated a need for follow-up screenings and information. By working together the parish nurse and the township director were able to plan for future programs to address cholesterol issues and to incorporate the screening into the follow-up programs. With this ease of availability, more people were motivated to participate and to communicate with their doctors about their progress or lack of improvement.

Many benefits and risks are involved in collaborative relationships with community agencies and healthcare organizations. Listed here are a few of the benefits involved when congregations and community agencies collaborate:

- Synergy between the mission of the congregation and the mission of the agency can result in the joint effort being more effective than either can do alone.
- Both the congregation and the agency can reach more people by working together.
- Barriers that previously limited effective participation by members of the community can be reduced.
- The positive reputation of both organizations can bring added interest and status to the serious work being done together.
- Duplication of efforts can be reduced.
- Increased participation can be achieved.
- Relationships are established that can result in additional collaborative efforts.

Listed here are a few of the risks involved when congregations and community agencies collaborate:

- The collaborating parties may not reach agreement on shared goals.
- The missions of the agencies demand more than either party can give or are in opposition to each other.
- The needs of the collaborating agencies or parties dramatically change.
- A key person leaves the agency, and the next person does not have the time or the inclination for a collaborative relationship.
- A collaborative effort fails, and no one has a desire to try again.
- What started out as a collaborative effort becomes an unloading of the work of one agency on to the other agency or organization involved.

An example of some of these risks occurred when the parish nurse ministry was invited to work with a major health organization on a new community program to reach people at risk for a certain disease. The health and nursing cabinet members enthusiastically agreed to join this effort. All the contacts from the members of the cabinets helped bring many community leaders and health organizations to work collaboratively on this new program. The program was started in the parish and in numerous related sites. At first, the health organization members visited and enthusiastically met members of the community. The program was a great success that resulted in many people being reached and several being identified and referred for further workup and treatment. The parish nurse ministry received a commendation from the state for reaching out to the most people at risk in the state and for getting them to needed screening services. Then the key people from the health agency changed, and the new people were not interested in working collaboratively. They wanted the church and other community agencies to run their programs but had no time for meeting or for working with the large group of community leaders who had worked so hard to get this program started. Soon, calls were not returned, and contacts were not available. Communication stopped except for requests from the health organization that everyone work harder on their programs. This experience has been a valuable lesson in how to know when collaboration stops and when to refocus upon what parish nurse ministry can do. Lack of communication indicates a need to leave or renegotiate an interagency relationship that is draining and not reciprocal and to seek out other sources of help for community/congregation health initiatives.

Collaboration with Larger World Movements

Collaboration with larger world movements helps parish nurse ministry and members of the congregation follow Jesus' call for us to serve others and to spread the good news. These collaborative efforts with larger world movements take a great deal of time and energy. The pastor and cabinet members must understand the opportunity that is being offered to the parish nurse by becoming involved beyond the congregation. In reality the congregation supports the parish nurse's involvement. Therefore as many parishioners as possible need to be informed and invited to offer their support (i.e., prayer, time, talent, and funds) for this ministry beyond the congregation's boundaries.

An example of this type of collaboration is our opportunity to work with the Catholic Charities organization in our diocese when they sponsor health fairs that are reaching out to the entire community in need at indigent parishes. Our parish nurse ministry has been blessed to have successful health fairs for several years, and we have learned a great deal about this faith-based opportunity for health. When Catholic Charities began these summer health fairs, they discovered many needs but increasingly lacked dentists and nurses to staff the fairs. They found this especially difficult as the long summer wore on and health professionals started canceling on the Saturdays they had promised to help. Our parish nurse ministry volunteers knew what was involved and also knew they could not commit to six Saturdays during the summer. A compromise was reached by offering to staff one site and to help contact nursing schools to become involved. One of our parish dentists also volunteered to staff four of the health fairs. One of our diabetic educators volunteered to help procure equipment and education materials. We are now working to enlist other parish nurses from a wide variety of

denominations to commit a group to one Saturday to staff these health fairs. The health fairs have been distributed throughout the spring, summer, and fall so that more students from health professions schools can be involved. Our experience and the contacts that we have made are now being used and optimized in this large effort in the Chicago Metropolitan Area.

Another example of collaboration beyond the congregation and the immediate community is our opportunity to work with medical missions. Mission trips afford healthcare professionals the opportunity to serve others in need and to witness God's love by their actions and words. A physician on our health cabinet invited the parish nurse to join a medical mission group to serve Native American Indians on a reservation in the Southwest. The pastor gave his approval to this plan. Several other parishioners joined the mission trip. The parish nurse shared her experience in the bulletin and in a Lenten reflection booklet prepared for the parish. This generated much interest. The initial venture resulted in many positive comments from the parishioners and expressions of a desire to support these missions. We hope that more health professionals will participate in future mission trips and other parishioners can assist by collecting needed supplies and donations to support the mission. The congregation's initial question of "why do this?" developed into "how can more parishioners support and become involved in the medical missions?"

A final example of working collaboratively with larger world movements is our ministry's work with a large metropolitan community organization called United Power. This group's purpose is to help communities and congregations to organize together to improve their community. An example of this work is United Power's ecumenical work with Christian and Muslim congregations to work toward better access to affordable healthcare. Our parish became involved because of our recognition of this need. Our focus, however, changed after the terrorist attacks on the United States on September 11, 2001. We switched our efforts and focused upon building meaningful relationships between our Christian and Muslim congregations to counter suspicion and misunderstandings. Our parish hosted a meeting for members of our congregation to meet with several hundred members of a neighboring mosque. United Power was able to work with all of us as we planned for this meeting and worked on follow-up initiatives. Neither of our organizations/congregations could have done this alone.

Here are a few of the lessons we have learned from collaborating with larger world movements:

- Clearly explain to the congregation the reasons and benefits for working cooperatively with larger world movements.
- Be prepared for misunderstandings that can arise over the benefit of the congregation working outside their congregation.
- Be sensitive to teachable moments for illustrating the importance of being involved with larger movements.
- These collaborative efforts can and will lead to other unanticipated opportunities for working toward improving the world.

Conclusion

Collaboration is a vital dimension of parish nurse ministry. When parish nurses collaboratively work with others, they are actively carrying out the work of the Lord. Mark Link (1992), a noted Catholic theologian and author, shares a story that tells of Jesus' trust in others to carry out His work on earth:

Legend says that when Jesus returned to heaven, the Angel Gabriel asked Him if all people knew of his love for them. "Oh no!," said Jesus, "only a handful do." Gabriel was shocked and asked, "How will the rest learn?" Jesus said, "The handful will tell them." "But," said Gabriel, "what if they let you down? What if they meet opposition? What if they become discouraged? Don't you have a back-up plan?" "No," said Jesus, "I'm counting on them not to let me down." (p. 160).

This story captures the amazing truth that God's plan to continue the work of Jesus and to build His Kingdom relies on humans working together. The parish nurse's role and ministry is one concrete way the community is manifesting its concern and mercy for all of God's people. We are honored to share our experiences in collaboration as a vital dimension of parish nurse ministry. We will conclude with a closing prayer for the gift of collaboration.

Thank you, God, for creating us a people who are better together than alone. Thank you for giving us opportunities to use our talents and skills in ministering to others. May we always remember that wherever two or more are gathered in your name so too You are there also. Confident that You are with us, may we seek to collaborate with those You bring to us and may we work together in trust, faith, and honesty as we strive to do Your will. Amen.

REFERENCES

American Nurses Association. (2001). *Code of ethics for nurses with interpretive statements*. Washington, DC: Author.

Bausch, W. (1997). *The parish of the next millennium*. Mystic, CT: Twenty-Third Publications.

Blanchfield, K. (2001). Spiritual development as parish nurse: Reflections about striving to develop from novice to expert. *Proceedings of the Fifteenth Annual Westberg Symposium*. Park Ridge, IL: International Parish Nurse Resource Center.

Blanchfield, K. (2002). Homebound with shame: Caring for the spiritual, emotional and physical needs of an isolated elderly person. *Journal of Advocate Health Care*, 4(2): 37-40.

Gunderson, G. (1997). *Deeply woven roots*. Minneapolis: Fortress Press.

Hallas, D.M., Butz, A., & Gitterman, B. (2004). Attitudes and beliefs for effective pediatric nurse practitioner and physician collaboration. *Journal of Pediatric Health Care*, 18(2): 77-86.

Health Ministries Association/American Nurses Association. (1998). *Scope and standards of parish nursing practice*. Washington, DC: American Nurses Association.

Henneman, E., Lee, J., & Cohen, J. (1995). Collaboration: A concept analysis. *Journal of Advanced Nursing*, 21(1): 103-109.

Holy Bible. (New Catholic Edition). (1957). New York: Catholic Book Publishing.

Knaus, W,. Draper, E., Wagner, D., & Zimmerman, J. (1986). An evaluation of outcomes from intensive care in major medical centers. *Annals of Internal Medicine*, 104(3): 410-418.

Link, M. (1992). Vision 2000. Allen, TX: Tabor Publishing.

McDermott, M. & Mullins, E. (1989). Profile of a young movement. *Journal of Christian Nursing*, Winter: 29-30.

Nouwen, H. (1989). *In the name of Jesus: Reflections on Christian leadership*. New York: Crossroad.

Nouwen, H. (2003). *The way of the heart*. New York: Ballantine Books.

O' Brien, M.E. (2003). Parish nursing: Healthcare ministry within the church. Boston: Jones and Bartlett Publishers.

Paterson, W. (1982). *Granger Westberg verbatim: A vision for faith and health*. St. Louis: International Parish Nurse Resource Center.

Pattillo, M., Chesley, D., Castles, P., & Sutter, R. (2002). Faith community nursing: Parish nursing/health ministry collaboration model in Central Texas. *Family Community Health,* 25(3): 41-51.

Peters T. (1992). *Liberation Management*. New York: Knopf.

Ruffing, J. (2000). *Spiritual direction: Beyond the beginnings*. Mahwah, NJ: Paulist Press.

Solari-Twadell, P.A. (2002). The differentiation of the ministry of parish nursing practice within congregations. *Dissertation Abstracts International* 63(06): 569A. UMI No. 3056442.

Severynse, M. (Ed.). Webster. (1999). *Webster's II new college dictionary*. Boston: Houghton Mifflin.

Sheer, B. (1996). Reaching collaboration through empowerment: A developmental process. *Journal of Obstetric, Gynecologic, and Neonatal Nursing,* 25(6): 513-517.

Sohn, M. (2003). Public health law: The values of global collaboration. *Public Health and the Law in the 21st Century* (Supplement) 31(4): 30-32.

Solari-Twadell, P.A. (2002). The differentiation of the ministry of parish nursing practice within congregations. *Dissertation Abstracts International* 63(06): 569A. UMI No. 3056442.

Westberg, G. (1955). *Nurse, pastor, and patient*. Philadelphia: Fortress Press.

Westberg, G. (1987). *The parish nurse: How to start a parish nurse program in your church*. St Louis: International Parish Nurse Center.

The Public-Private Partnership: Expansion of the Ministry

7

Wendy Zimmerman

The impossible is possible when people align with you. When you do things with people, not against them, the amazing resources of the Higher Self within are mobilised.
—Gita Bellin (Hayward, 1984)

A central theme that reaches to the core of the ministry of parish nursing practice and health ministries is making connections: making the connections of mind, body, and spirit as the concepts of whole person health are embraced (Solari-Twadell & McDermott, 1999); making the connections between faith-based communities and our traditional healthcare delivery system to be responsive to the human needs in our midst (Patterson, 2003); and making the connections as directors and coordinators with institutions that sponsor parish nurse programs and with individuals and organizations that carry out the good work (Westberg & McNamara, 1987).

Inherent in making connections is the opportunity for the development of partnerships. Partnerships have certain elements. They include the following:

- A relationship that includes two or more parties.
- Each participant or participant group in the partnership must have trust in the other party.
- Partners share in the profits and losses in whatever proportion they have agreed upon.
- Partnerships begin when two or more individuals or groups determine the basis and parameters of the relationship.

- There is usually some sort of written agreement that includes the specifics of the relationship and the particular responsibilities of each partner (Clifford & Warner, 2001).

Partnerships offer ways of combining resources for meeting mutually beneficial goals as the United States' healthcare delivery system and world become increasingly more complex. The usual partners for parish nurse coordinators are faith communities, secular and religious healthcare systems, nurses, pastors, and physicians (Ludwig-Beymer & Sarran, 1999). A less typical partner—but one that deserves attention—is the public sector. A major portion of this chapter is devoted to exploring public resources found in federal, state, county and local governments. The scope of partnering opportunities continues to grow in this arena with the current healthcare climate and government trends.

Partnership Considerations: Opportunities and Realities

Parish nurse coordinators are in an ideal position to assess, plan, implement and evaluate program needs and ways to achieve positive outcomes.

Partnerships provide an opportunity to join with other entities that provide valuable services and resources that cannot be provided independently (SmithBattle, Diekemper, & Drake, 1999). Partnerships may be informal or formal. An informal partnership might be created through accessing health information or referral sources to disseminate to the parish nurses.

For example, the National Institutes of Health (NIH) sponsors an online resource called *Healthfinder®*. *Healthfinder®* publishes an annual calendar called *The National Health Observances Calendar*. This calendar lists the dates of a myriad of health observances, such as Breast Cancer Awareness Month and American Heart Month. It gives addresses, telephone numbers, and Internet links for further information and research. Through this resource a parish nurse may be encouraged to contact specific agencies or resources in the local community that will assist in developing programming for members of the congregation consistent with a particular health issue. This is a valuable resource for parish nurses and health ministers as they plan and disseminate health information through newsletter articles and bulletin board displays and as they identify potential partners in the community. Federal, state, and local entities provide endless opportunities for this informal partnering.

More formalized partnerships are possible when people and the agencies they represent come together. When combined in a well-organized and coordinated approach, formalized partnerships draw upon combined expertise and material resources. The result is a greater potential for meeting the needs of those that are served. For example, when a parish nurse plans a health fair for his or her congregation, the parish nurse may choose to offer only those services or screenings that can be provided by people within that congregation. These services might include blood pressure screenings by the parish nurse and immunization and safety information provided by a congregational member who is a pediatrician. A dentist that serves on the health cabinet may offer dental health and hygiene demonstrations, whereas a massage therapist could offer seated massages. Drawn from only internal, congregational resources, four health and wellness initiatives can be offered in this health fair scenario.

With the addition of more formalized partnerships, that same health fair can be transformed into a health initiative that provides significantly more comprehensive services. Joining forces with the local hospital, a health professional from the community outreach department may be able to assist with a stroke screening or nutritional counseling after an elevated blood pressure reading was assessed by the parish nurse. As needs are identified by the pediatrician, partnering with the local health department could provide an opportunity for a low-income, single mother to follow up with low-cost or free immunizations for her children. Having representation from the state-funded, local dental clinic would provide a referral resource for the dentist who identifies a needy adult who lacks dental insurance. Although the coordinator does not make the individual contacts to set up these expanded services, he or she can establish partnerships with the organizations that he or she represents and can facilitate the process for the parish nurse.

Before entering into partnerships or other relationships, such as coalitions whether formal or informal, one must be intentional regarding the nature of the relationship. If the relationship is intended to deliver a particular program, one must identify the needs that the program will create. Discussing and clearly identifying, with the intended partners, what each partner can and cannot offer, the possible resources and needs created by entering into this agreement, and the agenda or anticipated outcome are important. In addition, any knowledge of individual personalities and positions of influence is valuable information to have in advance.

Building relationships and ultimately partnerships takes time, with much of that time spent in meetings, on the telephone, or completing paperwork. Coordinators often face limited time and money resources, so the benefit obtained by building partnerships needs to outweigh the time and energy that would otherwise be spent on different program priorities.

Coordinators may consider tapping the expertise of those parish nurses who demonstrate strong collaborative, leadership, and communication skills. Capable parish nurses may serve as regional representatives on local or state coalitions, thus sharing the responsibility and demands required of initiating and maintaining partnership projects. The benefits are not only to the coordinator but also the parish nurse, who is offered an opportunity for further personal and professional growth.

Once partnerships are established through an initial successful health initiative, the doors are opened to future endeavors. Successful working relationships, professional connections, known personalities, and a track record of positive outcomes all contribute to a willingness to continue working together and undertake new ventures. As new projects arise, the pros and cons of each program must be evaluated individually. Be attentive to any changeover in staff or administration within the same partnering organizations. Individuals can make all the difference in the success or failure of a project, and a history of positive outcomes with one project does not always ensure repeated success.

Educating Potential Partners

For private, public, and faith-based partnerships to flourish, formally addressing the subtleties inherent in working with faith-based communities may be necessary (Pape, 2004). Being clear about the role of parish nurses and health ministers is vital. One should emphasize the focus on prevention and wellness rather than on hands-on care. Familiarity with the faith or denomination of the partnering congregation and their belief system must also be considered as related to the initiative (i.e., sexuality or end-of-life issues). Congregations usually expect that resources will be offered without cost, and outside agencies may be viewed with suspicion. Therefore trust is important (Castro et al, 1995). It is also important to stress the benefits of the anticipated services and to ensure the congregation's autonomy and integrity. Coordinators can often provide this education and screen out potential partnerships where parish nurses and congregations may be used solely as marketing agents or as research participants with little or no benefit to the congregation members.

Educating the Faith Community

Involving congregational representatives in the process of partnering is key to establishing a foundation for success (Lloyd & Ludwig-Beymer, 1999). Congregational input encourages ownership and investment into the overall project and facilitates communication and power-sharing on all levels. Key participants may need to be educated about the benefits of partnering, especially with public entities. Enough time must be allowed for the relationships to develop and to bring clarity to the mutual work of the parties involved. Coordinators who are pursuing program funding must include their parish nurses in the planning process to encourage success. A congregation must always be allowed the freedom to decline participation for practical, ethical, or legal reasons.

Written Agreements

Written agreements will be structured differently depending on the scope and nature of the partnership. Informal partnering and some formal partnering situations do not require written agreements. In these cases, personal communications and meeting minutes are enough to establish trust and provide a clear delineation of each stake-holder's responsibilities. For example, the partnering agencies used in the illustration of the parish nurse's health fair probably would not share a written agreement. Written agreements should be considered when the following apply:

- Any employment arrangement is involved.
- Liability considerations are inherent to the proposed project.
- Grants, payments, or any money will be changing hands.
- Specific responsibilities of each partner need to be stipulated and reinforced.
- Trust between partners is in the early phases of being established.

The most common partnership in which written agreements are seen is between institution-based parish nurse programs and faith communities.

When parish nurse or health ministry programs are institution-based (paid or unpaid), written agreements with faith communities are essential. The content of the agreement always depends upon the nature and sophistication of the partnership, and legal counsel is always recommended. Assistance with obtaining sample agreements or covenants for institution-based and congregation-based programs is available from the International Parish Nurse Resource Center and the Health Ministries Association or through networking with other parish nurse directors or coordinators.

Confidentiality

In partnerships in which confidential information will be collected or maintained, the details of protecting confidentiality must be addressed. This protection can be facilitated by coding client identity, obtaining consent for release of information when applicable, keeping records secure and locked, and clearly defining who will store and maintain records. Again, the specific nature of the partnership and the program endeavor will determine the extent of each of these needs. In situations in which a client's medical information and fee-for-service is involved, HIPAA (Health Insurance Portability and Accountability Act) regulations become the standard by which confidentiality decisions are made.

In partnering situations, one of the most common examples that parish nurses/health ministers encounter in regard to confidentiality regards ownership of congregants' health records. The following excerpt offers guidance on this topic:

> If the parish nurse is employed by a healthcare institution or the congregation, the institution that hires the parish nurse owns the health record and is responsible for the maintenance of the health record, regardless of whether the nurse is paid or unpaid. In a paid organizational framework, the institution—be it the church or the health institution—whose name appears on the parish nurse's paycheck owns the health record. Even though a church may provide some funding for the program, if the health system directly pays the nurse, the health system owns the record and is responsible for maintaining the record. Many churches view this arrangement as a benefit so that the health system maintains the responsibility and the liability for the health record and care provided. In an unpaid organizational framework, the contract between the church and the parish nurse should stipulate who owns the health record (Burkhart, 2000, p. 75).

This publication also provides excellent examples of policy statements and sample release forms to facilitate the professional handling of health records in a parish nurse/health ministry practice.

Expanding the Possibilities with Public Partners: An Overview of Public Resources

Our public health system is the means by which federal, state, and local agencies assess current health trends, develop policies, and ensure an effective healthcare delivery system for our population. Health initiatives are set at the federal level and implemented through the many departments of Health and Human Services (HHS). A program such as Healthy People—Health Communities is one example of a national health initiative that guides decision-making at the state and local levels. An overview of federal, state, and local health agencies is included in the following discussion in order to identify points of entry for new partnerships.

Federal Programs

The United States Department of Health and Human Services (HHS) is "the United States government's principal agency for protecting the health of all Americans and providing essential human services, especially for those who are least able to protect themselves ..." (US HHS, n.d.). The department oversees the operation of over 300 programs, administers more grant funding than all other federal agencies combined, and is the nation's largest health insurer. The secretary is the senior-most official of HHS and is appointed by the President of the United States and approved by the Senate.

The nation is divided into ten regions, with HHS offices and services available in each region. Knowing which region represents your area may afford you fuller access to information and regional services. The ten HHS regions are determined by population and can be found at the HHS website.

Many of the United States' public service agencies administered by HHS provide valuable health information and health-related services that enhance parish nurse practice and health ministry coordination. These agencies within HHS are constant and sustain many ongoing programs. New agency programs arise as indicated according to current health trends. Listed here are the agencies most frequently accessed with a brief summary of their range of services.

National Institutes of Health

National Institutes of Health (NIH) is a research-focused medical organization that supports thousands of research studies across the nation. NIH comprises 27 individual health centers; its main campus is in Bethesda, Maryland. In addition to clinical research, NIH offers extensive amounts of health information through *MEDLINEPlus®*, funding for research and fellowships, and information about prescription and over-the-counter drugs. Their Healthfinder® National Health Observances Calendar is an especially helpful resource for health ministry. NIH also provides access to information about complimentary and alternative medical therapies (NIH, n.d.).

Centers for Disease Control and Prevention (CDC)

Centers for Disease Control and Prevention (CDC) is our primary national resource for protecting public health and safety. Providing credible health information; controlling infectious diseases such as tuberculosis and HIV/AIDS; promoting child and adult immunizations; and actively working with national, state, and local agencies on matters of environmental exposures, pollution, and bio-terrorism are all functions of this agency. Their website offers a mailing list for regular updates on public health advisories such as influenza, West Nile virus, monkey pox, and SARS. The CDC is located in Atlanta, Georgia (CDC, n.d.).

Health Resources and Services Administration (HRSA)

Health Resources and Services Administration (HRSA) is principally a funding agency that serves to promote primary healthcare to the underserved and special-needs populations in rural and urban settings. Local primary care clinics funded by HRSA serve referral agencies that parish nurses can access for the underserved in their congregations (HRSA, n.d.).

Substance Abuse and Mental Health Services Administration (SAMHSA)

The focus of Substance Abuse and Mental Health Services (SAMHSA) is to provide services for people with or at risk for mental and substance-abuse disorders. SAMHSA partners on the state level by providing block-grant funding for local substance abuse and mental health services. It also provides materials for public information programs, data, and other information on best practices (SAMHSA, n.d.).

Food and Drug Administration

The Food and Drug Administration (FDA) ensures the safety of our food supply, prescription and over-the-counter medications, cosmetics, medical devices, and veterinary products. The FDA has been the leading force behind improved food labeling. It offers health professionals a place to report any serious problems they detect with drugs or medical devices. Reporting is done through *MedWatch*. Recalls are also posted regularly on their website (FDA, n.d.).

Administration for Children and Families (ACF)

Through partnerships with state and local services, the Administration for Children and Families (ACF) serves children and their families. Programs such as Head Start, family assistance (welfare), child care assistance, child abuse and domestic violence prevention, and adoption and foster care services are provided through ACF (ACF, n.d.).

Administration on Aging (AoA)

The Administration on Aging (AoA) provides services to the elderly to assist them in remaining independent. Services such as Meals-on-Wheels, adult day care and at-home care, legal assistance and transportation services are coordinated nationally and implemented at the state and local level (AoA, n.d.). A Kansas-based health ministry program has formally partnered with AoA to provide education to detect Medicare and Medicaid fraud (Wescott, 2004).

Other HHS Programs

Some programs that fall under HHS are not a permanent part of the organizational structure.

These programs are usually determined by the current administration and are under the direction of the Surgeon General. One example of this is the Office on Women's Health. This office offers valuable women's health education and prevention materials, screening tools and resource packets that would enhance what parish nurses might offer to their congregations (www.4women.gov). This office, however, is subject to political whims and may change with election of a new president.

Another example is the White House Office of Faith-Based and Community Initiatives (FBCI). Under the current administration of George W. Bush, faith-based organizations have been embraced in their ability to provide help and services to the needy (Federal Register, 2001). The areas that have been targeted include at-risk youth, ex-offenders, homeless and hungry, substance abusers, those with HIV/AIDS, and welfare-to-work families (White House Office of FBCI, n.d.).

State and Local Resources

The State Department of Health, or the State Department of Health and Mental Hygiene, (the title differs from state to state) is the agency that is responsible for the oversight of health-based initiatives at the state level. Each state determines its own budget, structure, and initiatives, but each department generally is responsible for regulating healthcare quality, access and cost, professional licensing and certification, policy development and enforcement, consultation, vital statistics, and the implementation of health initiatives determined at the federal level. Each state department of health is located in its respective state capital and can be reached by calling the state government offices or online.

Funding at the state level is determined, to an extent, by the federal government. Federal funds are appropriated to each state by need and population. The states also can apply for additional federal money through block grants and other discretionary grants. The states contribute to their own budgets through state taxes and, based on budget priorities, determine the amount that is allocated to health-related initiatives. So, from state to state, great disparities in the funds available for

health programming exist, and within states, urban areas tend to be better funded than rural areas are (Christoffel, 2004).

Public Health Departments

Public health departments are the most common means by which direct health services are delivered to the public. Public health departments can be administered at the county or local government level and the Chief Health Officer has the highest level of authority on the local level relating to public health issues.

At the federal level, major health programs are identified and usually are implemented at the state and local levels. This is a common point of formal partnership with parish nurse and health ministry programs. Some of the major health programs are breast and cervical cancer, school health, HIV/AIDS, immunizations, colo-rectal cancer, testicular cancer, substance abuse, family planning, heart disease, tobacco risk reduction and chronic diseases. Some examples of successful program partnerships at this level include the following:

- Parish nurses and health ministers in Texas partner with the Texas Department of Health (TDH) for networking and accessing expert resource support. The TDH staff gives educational presentations and provides resource and referral information. This has resulted in a more efficient and a further-reaching public health delivery system (Lafferty, 2004).
- A parish nurse from Wisconsin has developed a valuable service for nonEnglish speaking families by partnering with local and county agencies. Potluck suppers bring together a primarily Hispanic community on a quarterly basis. After dinner, a speaker is featured along with an interpreter. They present topics of nutrition, immunizations, programs for children and public school updates (Scott, 2004).
- The Ohio State Department of Health, with federal funds from NIH, is promoting a program called Know Your Numbers. In a collaborative effort, local hospitals, public health departments, and parish nurse/health ministry programs are providing health promotion information on blood pressure and cholesterol control, weight maintenance, and knowing the dosages of prescription medications (Pape, 2004).

Department of Social Services

The Department of Social Services (DSS) is a state agency, separate from the health department, that coordinates programs that assist parents and children. Many of the programs offer financial assistance, whereas others foster financial and social independence. DSS has county or local offices and is overseen by the Department of Human Resources of the federal government.

DSS provides many services, some of which are state specific. In general, the most common services provided by DSS include cash assistance, child care and child support services, food stamps, support for individuals with disabilities, coordination of foster care, and licensing for child care. DSS also oversees adult and child protective services and is the central location for reporting cases of elder or child abuse or neglect or cases of domestic violence. Parish nurses have forged formal and informal partnerships with DSS as they advocate, educate, and serve as case managers for parents and families in need.

Women, Infants and Children (WIC)

Women, Infants and Children (WIC) is another public service provider that targets the nutritional needs of pregnant, breastfeeding or postpartum women. Services are also provided for infants and children up to the age of five. Participants must meet income guidelines and state residency requirements and be deemed nutritionally at-risk. WIC provides checks or vouchers to purchase specific foods that supplement the participant's diets. WIC technically falls under the United States Department of Agriculture's Food and Nutrition Services Department. Local state offices partner informally with parish nurse programs to provide nutritional services and educational resources related to nutrition for eligible parishioners (WIC, 2004).

State Universities

State universities, specifically those with associated nursing programs or medical schools, have been active partners with parish nursing programs. The University of Maryland coordinated with a local parish nurse coordinator to design, implement, and maintain a website for parish nurses. This same university also provides continuing education opportunities for parish nurses to the western, more rural, parts of the state via teleconference presentations. Many nursing education programs match nursing students with parish nurses for community nursing and service learning experiences.

Public Sector Funding: Benefits, Caveats, and Guidelines

Federal, state, and local funding has been secured for parish nurse programs across the nation. Because the dollar amounts of grants are high, funds at the federal level are more difficult to obtain and require large organizations or extensive partnering networks to meet grant requirements. Coordinators often use grant writers for these larger initiatives. State and local funding is more accessible to smaller networks, thus enabling coordinators and parish nurses to obtain these grants independently. In either situation, attention must be given to the issue of separation of church and state.

First Amendment Considerations

Parish nurse programs that have been most successful in securing public funds have done so through targeting specific health initiatives. Public funds are not to support activities that are inherently religious. This refers to any activities that include religious worship, religious instruction, or proselytizing. Every effort must be made to separate the time and location of inherently religious activities from any government-funded services. The current administration has published *Guidance to Faith-Based and Community Organizations on Partnering with the Federal Government*, which can be found at the website for the White House Office for Faith-Based and Community Initiatives (2004).

First Amendment Litigation

The Office of Rural Health in Montana, located at Montana State University–Bozeman and funded by the Federal Office of Rural Health Policy, Health Resources, and Services Administration (HRSA), was awarded one of George W. Bush's initial faith-based awards through the Compassion Capital Fund (CCF) Program of 2002. The funding has provided support to primarily small, grassroots, faith-based and community-based organizations to expand their capacity of social and health service programs for the needy and underserved. Funds also support a parish nurse and health ministry basic preparation course conducted by the Parish Nurse Center at Carroll College in Helena, Montana. The 35-hour preparation course uses the standard core curriculum developed through the International Parish Nurse Resource Center, in consultation with the National League for Nursing (NLN) and the American Nurses Association (ANA) Credentialing Center. The Health Ministries Curriculum of the Health Ministries Association, Inc. is also included in the course content. Every effort has been made to keep the course faith-neutral, and all chapel services are optional for course participants.

A lawsuit was served in May, 2003, and filed in the U.S. District Court, District of Montana. The plaintiffs filing the suit included the Freedom from Religion Foundation and three of its members who reside in Montana. The codefendants named in the suit were representatives of the Montana Office of Rural Health, Montana State University Bozeman, and the Montana Faith-Health Cooperative. The major complaint of the lawsuit was an alleged violation of the establishment clause of the First Amendment to the U.S. Constitution. This clause provides that federally funded activities may not endorse or advance religion. The principal focus of the complaint appeared to be the federal funding of the parish nurse and health ministry basic preparation course.

The defendants did not feel they violated the terms of the federal cooperative agreement of the CCF award (Young, 2004); however, the plaintiffs contended that parish nursing is a religious activity, which constitutes endorsement and advancement of religion. The plaintiffs stated that public funding of programs with religious content has the effect of endorsing religion, in part because the religious component effectively becomes the government's own speech. Thus the establishment clause of the First Amendment is violated. The plaintiffs sought a federal court injunction to halt the Montana Office of Rural Health from funding parish nursing/health ministry preparation courses and from any involvement with the Montana Faith-Health Cooperative.

On October 26, 2004, the Magistrate of the federal District Court for the State of Montana ruled that the Office of Rural Health and Montana State University–Bozeman violated the Establishment Clause of the U.S. Constitution by providing direct and preferential funding to parish nursing and subsidizing and endorsing the activities of the Montana Faith Health Cooperative. The Magistrate ordered the director of the Office of Rural Health and Montana State University to terminate the funding of parish nursing programs and to discontinue any involvement with the Montana Faith Health Cooperative. The university chose not to appeal the Magistrate's decision and has complied with the order.

Success Stories

Public Health in Parish Nursing, Frederick, Maryland

Public Health in Parish Nursing Program (PHPN), based in Frederick, Maryland, is one example of a parish nurse program that operates strictly on public (state) funds. Based in the county health department, this parish nursing program supports 54 congregations with over 100 parish nurses (primarily unpaid) and a part-time coordinator at 24 hours a week. This program follows the core public health functions of assessment, policy development, and assurance as it has provided a creative approach to providing health and wellness services to the community (Kub & Groves, 2003).

The PHPN program supports parish nursing in the traditional ways of many institution-based parish nurse program. Monthly meetings are held for continuing education and networking. Individual support is provided to the parish nurse, clergy, and congregation in the process of beginning and maintaining active programming. An advisory board oversees program direction and supports the coordinator. The program also partners with Frederick Community College to provide the basic preparation course for beginning parish nurses.

Because this program receives public funds, the coordinator has been very careful about how spirituality is integrated into the program. As an employee of the state, the coordinator is not responsible for providing spiritual support to the parish nurses. That function is clearly and intentionally delegated to the sponsoring congregation and clergy representative/s. Parish nurses take the lead in providing devotional materials at networking meetings and support each other as they share methods of integrating faith and health in their practices. In this way, the program has been able to successfully operate within the parameters separating church and state (Rudy & Gunnerson, 2004).

The Witness Project

The Witness Project is a "culturally sensitive, community-based breast and cervical cancer education program through which cancer survivors and lay health advisors increase awareness, knowledge, screening, and early detection behaviors in the African-American population in an effort to reduce the mortality and morbidity from cancer" (Griffin, & Jones, 1998, p. 60). The program was originally established in 1990 with collaboration from the Arkansas Cancer Research Center, University of Arkansas for Medical Sciences, and the University of Arkansas.

The program engages volunteer African-American breast cancer survivors in the role of witness role models (WRMs). Other African-American women who are interested in supporting the project serve as lay health advisors (LHAs). Witness Project programs are most often presented in churches, but hospitals and other community sites are used as well. Small group presentation is the format for this program, which includes as many as 25 participants.

Sessions begin with several WRMs presenting their personal experiences with cancer. Early detection is stressed, and fears and concerns are discussed. The lay health advisors then follow up with practice sessions teaching self-breast exams with ethnic breast models. Large numbers of women who historically have been difficult to reach are receiving vital health information.

In 1997, the Director of the Parish Nurse Program in Moline, Illinois, heard about the program and presented it to her steering committee (Griffin & Jones, 1998). The idea was received enthusiastically, and program planning began. Funds were secured from the hospital auxiliary, and educational materials were obtained from the American Cancer Society and the county health department. Churches and community centers would host the presentations. Local physicians, the hospital, and the county health department would provide follow-up services.

During the first year of the project, May 1998 to April 1999, 56 African-American women were reached. Program activity increased over the next five subsequent years, and participants numbered over 800 (Robinson, 2004). This program has been successfully replicated in 28 sites across the nation with funding provided by local entities, the University of Arkansas for Medical Sciences, Centers for Disease Control and Prevention, and the Susan G. Komen Foundation. Further information about the Witness Project can be obtained from the University of Arkansas for Medical Sciences.

Conclusion

Partnerships create opportunities to join with other agencies and organizations to offer valuable services and resources that could not be provided independently. Inherent to partnerships are the elements of trust, clearly established responsibilities, a sharing of profits and losses, and written agreements as needed. Our public health system at the federal, state, and local level is expanding in its capacity to partner successfully with faith communities. This success has been clearly demonstrated in parish nurse and health ministry practice but depends on educating all stake-holders, respecting confidentiality, and being aware of the issues of separation of church and state.

REFERENCES

Administration for Children and Families. (n.d.). Home page. Retrieved May 17, 2004 from http://www.acf.gov

Administration on Aging (n.d.). About AoA. Retrieved May 17, 2004 from http://www.aoa.gov

Burkhart, L. (2000). Administration of parish nurse documentation applying NANDA, NIC, and NOC. Solari-Twadell, A. (Ed.). Park Ridge, IL: The International Parish Nurse Resource Center.

Castro, F.G., Elder, J., Coe, K., Tafoya-Barrazo, H.M., Morattu, S., Campbell, N., & Talavera, G. (1995). Mobilizing churches for health promotion in Latino communities: *Companeros en la salud. Journal of the National Cancer Institute Monographs,* 18: 127-135.

Centers for Disease Control (n.d.). About CDC. Retrieved May 17, 2004 from http://www.cdc.gov

Christoffel, W. (personal communication, May 14, 2004).

Clifford, D., & Warner, R. (2001). *The partnership book: How to write a partnership agreement* (6th ed.). Berkeley, CA: Nolo.

Federal Register. (2001). Executive Order 13198, Agency responsibilities with respect to faith-based and community initiatives. 66(21): 8495-8498.

Food and Drug Administration. (n.d.). Recalls, Market Withdrawals and Safety Alerts. Retrieved May 17, 2004 from http://www.fda.gov

Griffin, J.L., & Jones, S.A., (1998). Breast cancer awareness: Witnessing to save lives. *Twelfth Annual Westberg Parish Nurse Symposium Proceedings,* Park Ridge, IL: Advocate Health.

Hayward, S. (1984). *A guide for the advanced soul, a book of insight.* Boston: Little, Brown and Co.

Health Resources and Services Administration (n.d.). Home Page. Retrieved May 17, 2004 from http://www.hrsa.gov

Kub, J., & Groves, S., (2003). *Evaluation of the program: Public health in nursing.* Frederick County Health Department. Frederick, MD (Unpublished Report).

Lafferty, G. (2004). Questions of the quarter. *Parish nursing perspectives,* 3(2): 2.

Lloyd, R., & Ludwig-Beymer, P. (1999). Listening to faith communities: Collaboration with, those served. In P.A. Solari-Twadell & M.A. McDermott (Eds.). *Parish nursing: Promoting whole-person health within faith communities.* Thousand Oaks, CA: Sage.

Ludwig-Beymer, P., & Sarran, S. (1999). Parish nurse-physician partnerships: A continuum of care. In P.A. Solari-Twadell & M.A. McDermott (Eds.). *Parish nursing: Promoting whole-person health within faith communities.* Thousand Oaks, CA: Sage.

National Institute of Health (n.d.). About NIH. Retrieved May 17, 2004 from http://www.nih.gov

Pape, L. (personal communication, May 12, 2004).

Patterson, D.L. (2003). *The essential parish nurse.* Cleveland: The Pilgrim Press, pp. 96-97.

Robinson, C. (personal communication, September 7, 2004).

Rudy, J., & Gunnerson, A. (personal communication, April 1, 2004).

Scott, P., (2004). Featured parish nurse. *Parish Nursing Perspectives,* 3(2): 2.

SmithBattle, L., Diekemper, M., & Drake, M.A. (1999). Articulating the culture and tradition of community health nursing. *Public Health Nursing,* 16(3): 215-222.

Solari-Twadell, P.A., & McDermott, M.A. (1999). *Parish nursing: Promoting whole person health within faith communities.* Thousand Oaks: Sage.

Substance Abuse and Mental Health Services (n.d.). About SAMHSA. Retrieved May 17, 2004 from http://www.samhsa.gov

U.S. Department of Health and Human Services (n.d.). About HHS: What we do. Retrieved May 17, 2004 from http://www.hhs.gov

Westberg, G.E., & McNamara, J. (1987). *The parish nurse program: How to start a parish nurse program in your church,* Park Ridge, IL: International Parish Nurse Resource Center.

Westcott, J. (personal communication, May 21, 2004).

White House Office of Faith-Based and Community Initiatives. (n.d.). *Guidance to faith-based and community organizations on partnering with the federal government.* Retrieved May 17, 2004, from http://www.gov/government/fbci/guidance

Women, Infant and Children (WIC). (2004). Nutrition Program Facts. Retrieved on May 22, 2004 from http://fns.usda.gov/wic

Young, D. (personal communication, May 17, 2004).

The Growing Accountability in the Ministry of Parish Nursing Practice

Lisa Burkhart
Phyllis Ann Solari-Twadell

8

It is the year 2042. How have the talents of parish nursing been used over the past 50 years? In particular, what happened to "whole person accountability"? Has it been buried along with a myriad of other passing fads of the 20th Century? Or has it blossomed into a workable method of operating within healthcare and organized religion, empowering both healthcare providers and receivers? Thank you in advance for investing wisely.

—Reverend Granger Westberg (1992)

As professional registered nurses and members of a recognized nursing specialty, parish nurses are called to be accountable, upholding certain standards of practice. These professional standards are epistemologically grounded in philosophy, particularly Plato's *Republic* (trans. 1993). As discussed in the *Republic*, one of the defining ideals of being a professional is accountability. Accountability implies that professionals behave— not based on self-interest—but based on a higher set of values and ideals. These values and ideals include having authority to take on a role, maintaining responsibility to carry out that role, having the legal recognition to perform that role, and taking responsibility for liabilities inherent in the role and in making mistakes. Although Plato discussed accountability in an abstract ideal sense, parish nurses must apply accountability in their everyday lives as practicing professionals within a ministerial context. This includes identifying to whom and for what nurses are accountable.

Early References to Accountability and Parish Nursing

Sally Lundeen, RN, PhD, FAAN, (1992), the keynote speaker at the Sixth Annual Westberg Symposium, identified parish nurses as pioneers in nursing. Her recommendations regarding what all nursing pioneers are accountable for included the following: 1) the people and the communities served; 2) professional practice, and 3) the vision of healthcare reform. Greg Kirschner, MD, MPH, who was also a presenter on a panel at the same conference noted that parish nurses are also accountable for 1) whole person care; 2) the "unique deep trust which people place" in the parish nurse; and 3) ultimately to our creator (Kirschner, 1992). Anne Marie Djupe, RNC, MA (1992), then the Director of Parish Nursing Services for Lutheran General Health System, stated at the same conference that the parish nurse is accountable to the pastor of the congregation, pastoral staff, Health and Wellness Committee,

93

Church Council, congregation members, institutional administrators, themselves, and God.

McDermott (1999) explores the rationale for accountability, giving definitions and identifies elements of accountability that apply to parish nursing. She states, "There is an obvious relationship of accountability to procedures, to processes, to programs (such as quality control, quality assurance, continuous quality improvement, total quality management, evaluation) and to the new emphasis on healthcare outcomes" (McDermott, 1999, p. 228). More recently Van Loon and Carey (2002) note the mutual accountability parish nurses have with members of the ministerial team "for work being clearly defined, fairly delegated and appropriately shared" (p. 151). O'Brien (2003) discusses that parish nurses are accountable for documenting their activities "for the protection of the ministry, to provide an ongoing witness of the value and usefulness of the program and its impact on improving the quality of parishioners' lives" (p. 143). Parish nurses clearly are accountable to a number of people for many important reasons and purposes. This chapter is intended to explore the context of accountability and the nature of documentation for the ministry of parish nursing practice as it applies to today and the near future.

Context of Accountability for the Profession of Nursing

State law, institutions, and professional nursing organizations define accountability for nursing practice. Professional nursing standards have been developed through the American Nurses Association (ANA). These standards are published in the *Nursing Scope and Standards of Practice* (2004), the *Code of Ethics for Nurses* (2001), and *Nursing's Social Policy Statement* (2003). In 2004, the ANA revised the definition of nursing from "the diagnosis and treatment of human response" to the following:

> The protection, promotion, and optimization of health and abilities, prevention of illness and injury, alleviation of suffering through the diagnosis and treatment of human response, and advocacy in the care of individuals, families, communities, and populations.

The ANA also recognizes that nursing is both an "art" and a "science." The art of nursing refers to the elements of the dynamic relationship between nurse and patient/client, which include spirituality, healing, empathy, mutual respect, and compassion (ANA, 2004). The science of nursing pertains to critical thinking and the nursing process: assessment, diagnosis, outcomes identification, planning, implementation, and evaluation. This revised definition better captures the health promotion, disease prevention focus, and recognizes the spiritual dimension of the ministry of parish nursing practice better than previous definitions.

Nurses are also expected to meet an ethical standard as described in both the *Scope and Standards of Practice* (2004) and the ANA *Code of Ethics* (2001). The ANA *Scope and Standards of Practice* (2004) is organized in terms of the nursing process and lists measurable criteria in meeting those standards. Each standard incorporates not only what is to be performed but also each element that must be documented. These standards pertain to the ministry of parish nursing practice. Any parish nurse documentation system must capture the nursing process. The standards of practice developed through ANA also direct nurses to use recognized standardized nursing taxonomies when they are documenting. *Integration* (Burkhart, 2002), a documentation system developed specifically for parish nursing, incorporates the nursing process as well as standardized nursing taxonomies.

The ANA *Standards of Practice* (ANA, 2004) also includes standards of performance, which identifies nursing values. Professional nursing standards are ideals—that is, they call nurses to strive to maximize their practice. Nurses are to promote quality of care, apply current nursing knowledge, integrate research findings into their practice, use appropriate resources to improve practice, and continually evaluate one's own practice. Nurses are also called to be members of the professional nursing community by exemplifying collegiality and collaboration. Each standard includes measurable criteria per element.

Each state through established laws defines the minimum level of practice that constitutes professional nursing in the respective state nurse practice act. Parish nurses are encouraged to obtain a copy of their state nurse practice act through the state board of nursing. Healthcare common law also affects parish nursing practice, in particular, in maintaining patient confidentiality. Every nurse is to respect patient/client privacy by maintaining confidentiality. In response to these legal requirements, parish nurses should develop and comply with policies and procedures that are compatible with state laws.

Some federal laws may also have implications for nurses. For example, the Health Insurance Portability and Accountability Act of 1996 (HIPAA) applies to nursing and may have implications for parish nurses. As stated in the final regulation, as of April 2003, health plans, healthcare clearinghouses, and those healthcare providers who conduct certain financial and administrative transactions electronically must comply with the law (US Department of Health and Human Services, 2003). In general, HIPAA requires these healthcare providers and financiers to maintain patient confidentiality when transmitting patient data. Parish nurses who are affiliated with healthcare systems may need to seek further consultation through their related healthcare system regarding the application of this law to their practice. HIPAA does not affect parish nurses who are not affiliated with health systems and who do not file for insurance reimbursement electronically. However, regardless of whether the parish nurse is affected by HIPAA, parish nurses must maintain confidentiality and develop policies, procedures, or guidelines related to confidentiality.

Parish nurses must uphold denominational, congregational, and healthcare institutional standards. These standards are developed by the institution, be it the congregation and/or the health system, with input from parish nurses and are defined in terms of policies, procedures, or guidelines (see Chapter 22). Development of these policies, procedures, or guidelines can be particularly challenging because parish nurses may be the bridge to multiple institutions that are very different.

Accountability calls for adherence to laws, professional standards, and code of ethics no matter what the setting or reporting relationships. Professional nursing practice is not contingent on reimbursement. Whether a nurse is paid or unpaid in his or her nursing practice, accountability is expected to be honored.

Parish Nursing's Call to Be Accountable

Parish nurses, as a community of nursing professionals invested in a congregation-based health ministry, are called to live out professional mandates. The community of parish nursing through collaborative work between the Health Ministry Association and the American Nurses Association have defined and described the ideals of accountability through the *Scope and Standards of Parish Nursing Practice* (ANA, 1998). This document follows the nursing process and requires documentation in all phases of the nursing process. These documents must be developed by the community of professionals involved in the ministry of parish nursing practice and must be consistent and compatible with the parish nurse's actual practice to ensure their accuracy. Self-regulation and peer review are critical components to accountability. As professional registered nurses, parish nurses are called to be accountable to registered nurse professional ideals and any denominational or congregational ideal.

As the ministry of parish nursing practice holds the spiritual dimension as central to the practice, parish nurses recognize the existence of spirit as defined in their own beliefs and faith traditions. Judeo-Christian traditions recognize a transcendent power that calls humans toward the highest ideal. Parish nurses engage with those served in prayer, meditation, and healing services and may incorporate a variety of healing techniques. Embraced by parish nurses, spiritual care has a long history within nursing, dating back to Florence Nightingale (1994):

> Where shall I find God? In myself. That is the true Mystical Doctrine. But then I myself must be in a state for Him to come and dwell in me. This is the whole aim of the Mystical Life; and all Mystical Rules in all times and countries have been laid down for putting the soul into such a state ... (p. xiii).

> ... With regard to health or sickness, these are not 'sent' to try us, but are the results of keeping, or not keeping, the laws of God; and therefore, it would be 'comfortable to the will of God' to keep His laws, so that you would have health (p. xvi).

Parish Nurse Documentation

Parish nurses not only exemplify accountability through the ministry of parish nursing practice based on standards of practice but also are legally required to actualize accountability through documentation of their service to clients. State nurse practice acts, the ANA *Scope and Standards of Practice* (2004), and the *Scope and Standards of Parish Nursing Practice* (1998) all require parish nurses to document. As early as 1990, McDermott provided a rationale for documentation in the ministry of parish nursing practice. Over the years as parish nursing programs emerged, parish nurses have developed their own documentation systems with some guidance from the International Parish Nurse Resource Center. Institution-based programs also have looked to their sponsoring health system when developing a documentation system.

With the application of computer technology, documentation systems have been changing quickly. The familiar SOAP, PIE, DAR, and narrative charting techniques are disappearing in favor of computerized documentation systems. Hospital systems are moving to paperless computerized documentation systems that cross acute care, ambulatory care, and home health. These systems include click-off assessment forms and diagnosis, intervention, and outcome lists that incorporate terms from professionally recognized standardized taxonomies. Parish nurses have the opportunity to document in these systems if they are employees of the health system. These large, computerized documentation systems have the benefit of integrating care across the healthcare spectrum and aggregating data across health disciplines.

In the late 1990s, the Kellogg Foundation funded the development of a documentation system designed to reflect the ministry of parish nursing practice in a format that can be statistically aggregated using standardized nursing taxonomies. The documentation system manual, *Integration* (Burkhart, 2002), includes all the information to implement such a documentation system for parish nursing. *Integration* is available for purchase through International Parish Nurse Resource Center, Deaconess Foundation, or Eden Seminary Bookstore. Many different documentation systems can be used by parish nurses; however, for the purpose of illustration the *Integration* documentation system will be used in this chapter.

Because parish nurses must document, parish nurses can choose a documentation system that not only meets legal requirements but also can help facilitate the ministry of parish nursing practice and help communicate that ministry to both congregational leaders and healthcare system leaders. Documentation of parish nursing interventions can be an asset to the parish nurse in the following ways (Burkhart, 2002; Burkhart & Kellen, 1999):

- Assists parish nurses in tracking and organizing client health information, as well as providing quick access to historical and ongoing client information.
- Provides summary statistics—communicates what parish nurses do in a summary format to all audiences, such as church leadership, health systems, and funders.
- Supports the integration of parish nursing into a continuum of care.
- Addresses liability issues—documentation protects nurses, health systems, and churches from liability by providing evidence of care rendered.
- Fulfills a professional responsibility—documentation is a professional responsibility outlined in the *Scope and Standards of Parish Nursing Practice* (1998).
- Meets the requirement regarding recording client interactions for accreditation with the Joint Commission on Accreditation of Healthcare Organizations.
- Contributes to a further understanding of parish nursing.
- Can provide researchers in the future with a wealth of data on this new specialty practice.

Parish nurses who are not employees of a health system may need to use a stand alone documentation system. *Integration* is one example of a stand alone system. Figure 8-1 presents a sample brief encounter form used as part of the *Integration* documentation system that exemplifies a paper/pencil version of a check-off list (Burkhart, 2002). This change to the check-off forms offers parish nurses an opportunity to capture elements of the ministry of parish nursing practice in a form that can be statistically aggregated. The use of standardized nursing taxonomies facilitates a check-off format for documentation systems and uses language that is clear, meaningful, and professionally recognized by other nurses and providers.

Parish Nursing Services
Brief Client Interaction Form

Client Name: _____

DOB: _____   Age/Age Range: _____   Date: _____

Gender: M F   Marital Status: _____   Time: _____

Address: _____

_____

Phone: _____

Ethnic Heritage[1] (circle):   C   A   H   OA   NA   ME   FE   MC   U   O

Congregational Status (circle):   Parishioner   Non-Parishioner

Referral Source[2] (circle):   S   P   NP   PS   MD   HCP   M   O   PN   FAM

Location[3] (circle):   C   PNO   V   H   HV   NH   P   PA   M   Other

Progress Note: _____

_____

_____

_____

_____

_____

_____

_____

_____

_____

                                    Parish Nurse _____

                                    Congregation _____

☐ Has screening documentation

_____

[1]C=Caucasian; A=African American/Black; H=Hispanic; OA=Oriental/Asian; NA=Native American; ME=Middle Eastern; FE=Far Eastern; MC=Multi-Cultural; U=Unknown; O=Other
[2]S=Self; P=Parishioner; NP=Non-Parishioner; PS=Pastoral Staff; MD=Physician; HCP=Other Health Care Professional; M=Media; O=Other; PN=Parish Nurse; FAM=Family
[3]C=Church; PNO=Parish nurse office; V=Visit to HCP; H=Hospital; NH=Nursing Home; P=Phone; PA=Pantry; M=Mail, Other=Other
© This form cannot be modified or used without written permission from Lisa Burkhart. 1/02

Figure 8-1   Brief Client Interaction Form. (Copyright Lisa Burkhart.)

Continued

Client Name: _____

Nursing Diagnosis[1]

Life Principles

❏ Spiritual Distress

❏ Readiness for Enhanced
Spiritual Well-Being

❏ Decisional Conflict

Health Promotion

❏ Ineffective Health Maintenance

Activity/Rest

❏ Disturbed Sleep Pattern

Cognitive/Perceptual

❏ Disturbed Thought Process

Self-Perception

❏ Powerlessness

❏ Hopelessness

❏ Situational Low Self-Esteem

❏ Chronic Low Self-Esteem

Role/Relationship

❏ Interrupted Family Processes

❏ Impaired Social Interaction

Comfort

❏ Chronic Pain

❏ Acute Pain

❏ Social Isolation

Coping/Stress Tolerance

❏ Anxiety

❏ Fear

❏ Ineffective Coping

❏ Compromised Family Coping

❏ Disabled Family Coping

❏ Readiness for Enhanced Family
Coping

Safety/Protection

❏ Risk for Self-Mutilation

❏ Risk for Injury

Nursing Interventions[2]

Physiological Basic

❏ Pain Management

❏ Progressive Muscle Relaxation

❏ Sleep Enhancement

❏ Transport

Behavioral/Cognitive Therapy

❏ Bibliotherapy

❏ Music Therapy

❏ Mutual Goal Setting

❏ Patient Contracting

Communication Enhancement

❏ Active Listening

❏ Complex Relationship Building

❏ Conflict Mediation

❏ Meditation

❏ Socialization Enhancement

Coping/Spiritual/Religious

❏ Anticipatory Guidance

❏ Body Image Enhancement

❏ Coping Enhancement

❏ Counseling

❏ Crisis Intervention

❏ Decision-Making Support

❏ Dying Care

❏ Emotional Support

❏ Forgiveness Facilitation

❏ Grief Work Facilitation

❏ Hope Instillation

❏ Humor

❏ Mood Management

❏ Presence

❏ Recreational Therapy

❏ Religious Ritual Enhancement

Coping/Spiritual/Religious (cont.)

❏ Role Enhancement

❏ Security Enhancement

❏ Self-Awareness Enhancement

❏ Spiritual Growth Facilitation

❏ Spiritual Support

❏ Support System Enhancement

❏ Touch

❏ Values Clarification

Psychological Comfort Promotion

❏ Anxiety Reduction

❏ Calming Technique

❏ Simple Guided Imagery

❏ Simple Relaxation Therapy

[1]Diagnosis Labels reprinted with permission from NANDA.
[2]NIC labels reprinted with permission from Mosby.

Figure 8-1, cont'd   Brief Client Interaction Form. (Copyright Lisa Burkhart.)

In choosing a documentation system for the ministry of parish nursing practice, one must also choose a system that can capture the spiritual dimension of care. Three standardized nursing taxonomies have been tested in parish nursing practice and have been shown to capture the spiritual dimension of care: NANDA International nursing diagnoses (NANDA International, 2003), Nursing Interventions Classification (NIC) (Dochterman & Bulechek, 2004), and Nursing Outcomes Classification (NOC) (Moorhead, Johnson, & Maas, 2004). NANDA International is the oldest and most widely used system and is the only ANA-accepted standardized taxonomy that includes spiritual and religiosity nursing diagnoses. NIC has been shown to capture the spiritual dimension of parish nursing practice (Burkhart & Androwich, 2004). In an NINR-funded national study through the University of Iowa, the spiritual NOC outcomes demonstrated good reliability (Kappa >.8) and statistically significant validity in parish nursing (Moorhead, Johnson, & Maas, 2004).

Another consideration in choosing a documentation system for the ministry of parish nursing practice is that the system captures the uniqueness of parish nursing practice. A documentation system is an information system—that is, it represents how information moves through the ministry of parish nursing practice. To better understand how information flows in parish nursing, Advocate Health Care in Chicago, Illinois, sponsored research with parish nurses (Burkhart, 2002). Results from this research indicated the following five types of information flows in parish nursing (Burkhart, 2002):

- One-on-One Client Interactions and Follow-up. This is defined as the parish nurse working with individual clients or on behalf of individual clients. As a personal health counselor, the parish nurse discusses health issues and problems with individuals (e.g., assessing a client's spiritual well-being; visiting a client in the hospital or home; and providing care to a client over the telephone, in the parish nurse office, or in church. This also includes gathering information or coordinating activities for the client without the client being present.).
- Group Programs. This includes all activities associated with setting up a congregation-based

health program or meeting for a group of clients. A program is interpreted very broadly and includes all care or programs targeted to a group of clients. For example, as a health educator, the parish nurse coordinates educational programs promoting an atmosphere in which individuals of all ages explore the relationship between values, attitudes, lifestyle, faith, and health (e.g., wellness programs, seminars). Also, as a developer of support groups, the parish nurse facilitates the development of support groups for members of the faith community and people from the external community. In addition, parish nurses coordinate screenings, spiritual retreats, environmental/safety activities for the church (e.g., fire hazards, infection control, vermin precautions), and community outreach programs.

- Resource/Liaison/Networking. A parish nurse quickly becomes known to other community organizations as a source of information or as a community health leader. As a result, parish nurses can be seen as an information resource to other organizations or the parish nurse can participate as a liaison, performing networking or advocacy activities. For example, as a resource, parish nurses may provide information over the phone to other community groups, or the parish nurse can sit on community committees representing the faith community.
- Volunteer Facilitation. As a facilitator of volunteers, the parish nurse recruits, coordinates, and provides support to volunteers within the congregation who serve in various health ministries.
- Parish Staff Activities (including attending meetings, church functions, and performing office work). Many times parish nurses attend meetings or church functions to contribute to the health system, church, community, or parish nursing services. Parish nurses also spend time writing reports or grants for the church or health system while documenting and maintaining records and resource files.

One can spend a great deal of time documenting information. However, parish nurses choose this ministry of parish nursing practice to spend time with clients, not to document the care.

Therefore, it is important to discern what information must be documented. Legally, not all information must be documented. Prior to choosing a documentation system, parish nurses should identify what information must be documented and also choose what elements of client interactions are needed or desired for summary reports.

The elements required for documentation differ not only based on the law of each state but also may differ based on the nature of the service provided. Parish nurses are encouraged to discuss documentation requirements with those knowledgeable regarding documentation requirements for their state. Table 8-1 lists required documentation elements per type of service based on most nurse practice acts and the *Scope and Standards of Parish Nursing Practice* (ANA, 1998). The table also identifies suggested elements for statistical aggregation.

TABLE 8-1 Required Documentation and Suggested Statistical Variables Per Information Category		
Information Category	**Required Documentation**	**Information Useful for Statistical Reports**
One-on-One Interactions	Client name Date and time of interaction Assessment data Identification of a concern or issue being addressed Nursing interventions Outcome (what happened to the client given what the nurse performed)	In addition to required documentation: Age Race New/Follow-up client Parishioner/Nonparishioner Referred from Referred to
Screenings	Care only provided at screening Date and time of screening Client name Assessment data Identification of a concern or issue being addressed Nursing interventions Outcome (what happened to the client given what the nurse performed)	Number screened Number with abnormal findings Number of with abnormal findings not under physician care (potentially newly diagnosed)
Group Programs	None	Name of program, date, site of program Length of program and time in planning program Speakers, presentation outline, and objectives Number of people attended Target audience Evaluation Budget
Volunteer Coordination	None	Names of individual receiving service Name of individual providing service Services provided Date of service
Referral/Liaison/ Networking	None	Meetings attended Time
Office Work	None	Time and type of meeting Time and type of worship activity Time writing reports Time developing resources/maintain files Time documenting

This is an important time for those nurses who are serving congregations through the ministry of parish nursing practice. Each parish nurse has the opportunity to maintain the integrity of this specialty practice and document the journey of caring for others through the ministry of parish nursing practice. Parish nurses have an extremely vital role to play in reforming the healthcare system in the United States and abroad. This contribution is legitimized through creation and consistent use of a documentation system that incorporates standardized languages that can be understood by all healthcare providers

With the movement toward computerized documentation, not only will physician data be available but all healthcare data will become more available for study as the federal government calls for standardization of healthcare information. The federal government has endorsed one integrating database for healthcare documentation, the Systematized Nomenclature of Medicine, Clinical Terminology (SNOMED CT). SNOMED CT includes professionally accepted standardized taxonomies. Three of those nursing taxonomies—NANDA, NIC, and NOC—have been expanded to include language that allows for better documentation of spiritual and religious interventions (Burkhart, 2005). Parish nurses must be accountable for telling the story of whole person health through language that all will understand. Only through this work will whole person health become, in the words of Reverend Granger Westberg, "a workable method of operating within

healthcare and organized religion or become a passing fad of the 20th century."

Conclusion

Parish nurses are accountable to many different people, groups, and professional organizations as well as their own belief systems and sovereign God. This complex of accountabilities must be clarified and honored if the ministry of parish nursing practice is to mature and maintain a professional and ministerial integrity. The clients served by the ministry of parish nursing practice can be individuals, be they parishioners or other community members. Clients also can be groups, including families, support groups, people who attend an educational program, or those who read parish newsletters or bulletin articles. Clients can also be populations. Parish nurses play an important role in healthcare policy development, which affects large populations.

A primary accountability for all nurses, including parish nurses, is documentation. If one parish nurse chooses not to employ the use of a documentation system that facilitates reporting client services, both legal ramifications and potential hazards to the whole ministry of parish nursing practice arise. Think carefully of what it means to serve your congregation, your community, and your God as a parish nurse, for it has implications for the whole ministry of parish nursing practice.

REFERENCES

American Nurses Association. (2004). *Nursing: Scope & standards of practice*. Washington, DC: ANA.

American Nurses Association. (2003). *Nursing's social policy statement*, (ed 2). Washington, DC: ANA.

American Nurses Association. (2001). *Code of ethics for nurses with interpretive statements*. Washington, DC: ANA.

American Nurses Association. (1998). *Scope and standards of parish nursing practice*. Washington, DC: ANA.

Burkhart, L. & Kellen, P. (1999). Proposed diagnosis and interventions. In P.A. Solari-Twadell and M.A. McDermott. *Parish nursing: Promoting whole person health within faith communities* (pp. 257-267). Thousand Oaks, CA: Sage Publications.

Burkhart, L. (2002). *Integration: A documentation system reporting whole-person care*. Evanston, IL: Author.

Burkhart, L. (2005). A click away: Documenting spiritual care. *Journal of Christian Nursing*, 22(1): 6-12

Burkhart, L. & Androwich, I. (2004). Measuring the domain completeness of the NIC in parish nurse documentation. *CIN: Computers, Informatics, Nursing*, 22(2): 72-82.

Djupe, A.M. (1992). Accountability. *Proceedings of the Sixth Annual Westberg Symposium. Accountability: The foundation of parish nursing practice*. Northbrook, IL: National Parish Nurse Resource Center.

Dochterman, J. & Bulechek, G. (2004). *Iowa intervention project: Nursing interventions classification (NIC)* (4th ed.). St. Louis: Mosby.

Kirscher, G. (1992). Whole person accountability: Passing fad or promising future? *Proceedings of the Sixth Annual*

Westberg Symposium, Accountability: The foundation of parish nursing practice. Northbrook, IL: National Parish Nurse Resource Center.

Lundeen, S. (1992). An agenda for change: Issues of accountability. Proceedings of the Sixth Annual Westberg Symposium, Accountability: The foundation of parish nursing practice. Northbrook, IL: National Parish Nurse Resource Center.

McDermott, M.A. (1990). A rationale for documentation. In P.A. Solari-Twadell, A.M. Djupe & M.A. McDermott. Parish nursing: The developing practice. Park Ridge, IL: Advocate Health Care.

McDermott, M.A. (1999). Accountability and rationale. In P.A Solari-Twadell & M.A. McDermott. Parish nursing: Promoting whole person health within faith communities (pp. 227-232). Thousand Oaks, CA: Sage Publications.

Moorhead, S., Johnson, M., & Maas, M. (Eds.). (2004). Iowa outcomes project: Nursing outcomes classification (NOC) (3rd ed.). St. Louis: Mosby.

Nightingale, F. (1994). In J. Calabria, & M. Macrae. Suggestions for thought. Philadelphia: University of Pennsylvania Press.

NANDA International (2003). NANDA nursing diagnoses: Definitions & classification 2002-2003. Philadelphia: Author.

O'Brien, M.E. (2003). Parish nursing: Healthcare ministry within the church. Boston: Jones and Bartlett.

Plato (1993). Republic. (Trans. R. Waterfield). New York: Oxford University Press.

United States Department of Health & Human Services. (2003). Fact Sheet. www.os.dhhs.gov.Summer, 2004

Van Loon, A. & Carey, L.B. (2002). Faith community nursing and health care chaplaincy in Australia: A new collaboration. In L. Vandecreek & S. Mooney (Eds.). Parish nurses, health care chaplains and community clergy: Navigating the maze of professional relationships. New York. The Haworth Press.

Westberg, G. (1992). How accountable are we for whole person care? Proceedings of the Sixth Annual Westberg Symposium, Accountability: The foundation of parish nursing practice. Northbrook, IL: National Parish Nurse Resource Center.

Challenges to the Ministry of Parish Nursing Practice

9

Phyllis Ann Solari-Twadell
Mary Ann McDermott

Challenges to the ministry of parish nursing practice come from many directions. At times, given the nature of the known and unknown potential threats to the ministry of parish nursing practice, it is a wonder that it has grown and matured as it has over the last 20 years. The strength of the grassroots movement of the ministry of parish nursing practice substantiates that this is more the work of the Holy Spirit than of any human being. So mystical sacredness surrounds this ministry of parish nursing practice. We all are aware that anything of a sacred nature that is God orchestrated will be challenged. This chapter is directed to just a few of the challenges to this ministry.

Attendance at an all girls' Catholic high school leaves one with some interesting lessons. It was not uncommon for the Sisters to attend formal dances held at the school with boys. During the slow dances the Sisters would circulate. When finding a boy and girl dancing too closely together, the Sister would come up next to the couple and say "make room for the Holy Spirit," encouraging them to dance with more space between them. We all need that reminder, individually and collectively, as we work with and through these challenges to the ministry of parish nursing practice and as we foster Reverend Granger Westberg's dream, which in some respects has become our own, "of whole person care being a workable method of operating within healthcare and organized religion, empowering both healthcare providers and receivers" (Westberg, 1992).

Challenge: Unceasing Inspiration

Who are the Inspirational Vision Makers?

In 1999, at the 13th annual Westberg Symposium, *Parish Nursing: A Journey in Wisdom*, Margretta Madden Styles provided the keynote address. In her presentation, she identified that the parish nursing movement did not have a stated vision. She noted that although the movement seemed to be growing, the movement is likely to disappear without a clear sense of purpose (a mission) and a description of future intent (a vision). For many listeners this came as a revelation. We believe that the late Granger Westberg provided a vision for parish nursing. But Dr. Styles, in her wisdom, was right. The collective had developed no vision or mission for parish nursing. That work became the agenda for the 14th Annual Westberg Symposium. Dr. Judith Ryan provided the direction for the process in her keynote address.

Inspirational leadership in parish nursing thrives not just nationally but also internationally, regionally, and locally. This fact must not be forgotten. Parish nursing has been blessed with many visionary leaders. That is the gift of the Holy Spirit working amongst us, in us, and through us. So as the good Sisters said years ago, "make room for the Holy Spirit." We all need to tend to our development as spiritual leaders to foster growing self-awareness of our contribution to enhancing the integrity, availability, and understanding of the ministry of parish nursing practice.

Inspiration for the ministry of parish nursing practice is not a one-person responsibility. Each individual involved in the ministry of parish nursing practice should have as part of his or her "quiet time" an opportunity to journal personal "inspirational moments." We all have them; however, we may not in our busy schedules take the time to recognize them. If parish nursing is God's work, all need to be both seeking inspiration and providing inspiration to others to contribute to the divine plan for the ministry of parish nursing practice.

Challenge: Being Moldable, Yet Able to Maintain Shape

Change: The Ever-Present Constant

Change is always easier if, as a participant, I am open-minded and sense that the change is necessary and will contribute positively to the future. True change however, seems to just present itself and force new perspectives and corresponding actions. A humorous perspective on change: What makes God laugh? Our plans! A mindset of "being open" could be considered a prerequisite for parish nursing. In reviewing Chapter 2, it is amazing to reflect on how much has changed since the "**Daughters**" were working in parishes trying to foster whole-person health. This should be a lesson for us—an image of all that has gone before us and changed to bring us to this moment in time. "Change weaves experiences into the fabric of our lives. With change, we are invited to stretch ourselves beyond what was thought possible" (Solari-Twadell, 1994, p. 3). As we invite/ struggle/accept new ways of envisioning, describing and educating others on the ministry of parish nursing practice, there needs to be the recognition that the journey is the goal.

So how is it that we remain moldable yet not lose the integrity of who we are? How can we come to accept different ways of describing the ministry of parish nursing practice by using standardized languages rather than the historical seven functions? We challenge ourselves to be renewed. "Apathy and lowered motivation are the most widely noted characteristics of a civilization in decline. Those who believe in nothing change nothing for the better. They renew nothing and

heal no one, least of all themselves" (Gardner, 1981, p. xxi).

Challenge: Understanding There Will Never Be Enough

Resources for the Ministry of Parish Nursing Practice

We may experience episodes in our lives that we could describe as "a little slice of heaven." However, we know that we do not live in heaven but in a very imperfect world, a world of many needs. The congregation as a subset of a community has many needs, more than that to which a parish nurse can often respond through his or her ministry. Money, time, and people are never sufficiently available to match the need. Some parish nurses may think that if they were in more affluent parishes that the resources would be present to minister to all. It may appear that it would be easier for some parish nurses in larger parishes as there are more resources, but it seems that very few parish nurses ever feel that they have the resources they need to do their work well. Resources are important but are not the single solution. Clearly understanding what success means to you is important. One understanding of success is doing the best you can, with what you have, at the time.

Another perspective that may save a parish nurse from setting herself up for problems is to honestly determine the following: (1) What resources are needed? (2) What resources are available? (3) Which of the resources available are accessible to the parish nurse for the accomplishment of a specific effort or project? (4) Can the work of the project or program be accomplished with what is available and accessible? This kind of resource assessment can help a parish nurse come to a clear understanding of what is possible and to be aware in advance of consequences of projects undertaken without necessary resources.

On a larger scale, more and more parish nurses are choosing not to be paid or compensated in their ministry positions. Quite often this "choice" is made because of insufficient financial resources of the sponsor/s. A national survey of parish nurses who had completed basic parish nurse preparation revealed that 68% of the respondents were not paid in their parish nurse positions.

Of those not paid, 27% (n=315) indicated they would be grateful to be paid, whereas 39% (n=455) noted that they would not want to be paid (Solari-Twadell, 2002). The same survey also demonstrated that parish nurses who are paid are likely to work more hours and implement a greater number of nursing interventions than those in unpaid models of practice. There are some denominations that understand all ministries to be a service offered to the congregation, not as a position of paid employment. Nurses entering into this ministerial arrangement in providing parish nursing services need to develop personal clarity on what can be offered to the congregation, considering the additional responsibilities the nurse may have in paid employment, as well as family and other commitments. As the parish nurse becomes a resource to the congregation, all must understand parameters of the services he or she can realistically provide or this parish nurse could find himself or herself personally compromised. This does not mean that a parish nurse who is paid could not find oneself in a similar position.

Clarity of role, boundaries, and resources will always be challenges for the ministry of parish nursing practice. Needs will always outweigh resources—a challenge not unlike Jesus' own. Yet it is very clear. He did not heal everyone. He was a person of human limitations. So are we. As was He, we need to be clear about these limitations and work with them, not perceive them as problems that will be solved one day. This is a constant challenge, one faced by many in ministry. How do we move in our ministry of parish nursing practice while accepting this reality and yet not allowing that reality to compromise who we are and what we do? This challenge requires continual discernment, divine inspiration, and maybe at times divine intervention.

Challenge: Knowing What You Are Called to Do and What You Can Do

Role Clarity

Parish nursing is unique in the way services are offered and can look different from congregation to congregation depending on the needs of the people and the skills and talents of the nurse. However, everyone must understand role delineation.

The integrity of the specialty depends on it. The role of the parish nurse has never been more clearly described. The agreed-upon nature of the practice is found in the *Scope and Standards of Parish Nursing Practice* (1998). Research using the Nursing Interventions Classification system identifies the complexity of the role and sets the parameters for the basic preparation for the parish nurse (Solari-Twadell, 2002). Individual parish nurses practicing within congregations share a collective understanding that no one ministering in a congregation and using the title of parish nurse will take it upon themselves to violate the practice boundaries that have been determined by the whole. Violation puts the whole of parish nursing in jeopardy. It also can confuse the consumer. Parish nursing is about wholeness and calls each in the ministry of parish nursing practice to honor the integrity of other parish nurses by using nursing interventions consistent with the parameters of the specialty practice.

Challenge: Communicating Often and Clearly

Consistency in Presence and Message Reinforces Learning

Sometimes parish nurses are discouraged when a member of the congregation lacks understanding of the intent of the ministry of parish nursing practice. Education about the nature of the ministry of parish nursing practice must be communicated clearly and frequently. "New members join the faith community, lay leaders rotate in and out of positions and pastors come and go. This type of dynamic in congregational life calls for ongoing education" (Solari-Twadell, 1999, p. 8). The "dynamic nature" of the congregation demands that communication be clear and regular. Many stories could demonstrate where parish nurses got themselves into difficult situations because they assumed someone knew something or thought that someone else had communicated an important piece of information to another person on the staff or in the congregation. The parish nurse role is highly relational. The parish nurse is always talking to someone either at the church, on the phone, or perhaps through e-mail. This communication must be clear.

The parish nurse may also assist in the development of written communication regarding the ministry of parish nursing practice to be used by the institution or congregation. These written communications should be reviewed for clarity. This will help ensure that no one will misunderstand the purpose or services of the ministry of parish nursing practice.

Challenge: Learning How to Partner Without Assuming the Work of Others

Health Promotion Is Enhanced through Collaboration with Others

Reverend Granger Westberg (1987) from the beginning grounded parish nursing in the idea that health and well-being were easier to sustain in collaborative relationships than in isolation. Lloyd and Ludwig-Beymer (1999) identified two levels of collaboration: "(a) collaboration at the individual level and (b) collaboration at the group or collective level" (p. 109). They caution the following:

> True collaboration requires much more than merely saying that you believe in it or that you understand it as a concept. Furthermore, although it may seem to be a fairly simple concept to grasp, implementing and making collaboration an integral part of daily life may not be straight forward…Consistent and successful collaboration requires a strong sense of systems thinking, teamwork, nonlinear thinking and a willingness to be flexible (p. 109).

Again, communication must clarify collaborative arrangements and responsibilities. Without collaboration, the resources available to the community may not easily reach the people in the pews. Collaboration allows more people to access resources. Providing access to healthcare resources in earlier stages of illness is a benefit that a parish nurse can bring to congregants. Collaboration with other resources and agencies in the community may enhance the parish nurse's ability to provide this service.

Collaboration is only as strong as the relationship of the people involved. In Chapter 6, Blanchfield and McLaughlin provide the reader an excellent basis from which to understand the intricacies of collaboration. Inherent in their chapter is the importance of developing the skill to negotiate collaborative relationships with individuals and groups. However, as they noted, finding ways to maintain and enhance these relationships over time is equally important. It is through these relationships that new relationship possibilities are created. Do not underestimate the significance of the relationship that is developed with collaborators. It is the lifeblood of the mutual arrangements and can enhance service to others.

Challenge: Developing an Adequate Infrastructure to Sustain the Ministry of Parish Nursing Practice

Attending to the Basics

Establishing a solid infrastructure to support the functional integration and the longevity of a parish nurse program within a faith community is vital to the integrity and longevity of parish nursing ministry. Functional integration is the extent to which key support functions and activities are coordinated across an organization, adding greater overall value to the system (Shortell, Gillies, Anderson, Erickson, & Mitchell, 1996). The creation of an infrastructure for the ministry of parish nursing practice is a basic component in developing the ministry of parish nursing practice within a congregation. Unless the basics receive attention in the developmental phases of the ministry of parish nursing practice, a certain vulnerability will remain throughout its existence. At times of change, such as the placement or selection of a new pastor or the retirement or leave-taking of the parish nurse, the ministry could be in jeopardy of continuation. An infrastructure that integrates the parish nurse with the ministerial team and the congregation can help build bridges between the parish nurse and influential members of the congregation, the health cabinet, or grateful members of the congregation who will help ensure resources and continuity in times of change.

Self-care, spiritual formation, and accountability are some of the basics for parish nurses. Left unattended, these factors rob the nurse of some of the basic building blocks for the ministry from a personal perspective. Attending to these basics is tedious and time-consuming and requires patience.

Some people interested in parish nursing for their congregations want it *now*. Some nurses want the position to be created *now*. No one is served well when the foundation is lacking. The ministry of parish nursing is too important to the people it serves to fail to anchor it in the congregation. Sacredness is found in the intimacy between the parish nurse and his or her congregation. The infrastructure needs to protect this sacredness well before the parish nurse is selected. Yes, developing infrastructure may cause waves in "the way things have been done" in the congregation. But remember, the parish nurse ministry is not for the faint of heart. Parish nursing is intended to be a catalyst for change; given the proper foundation, the ministry of parish nursing practice will change the nature of how the congregation serves not only its own members but also the community at large.

Challenge: Continuing to Create the Body of Knowledge Particular to the Ministry of Parish Nursing Practice

The Need for Research, Publication, and Presentation Related to the Ministry of Parish Nursing Practice

Participants in the Westberg Symposium acknowledged early on that its continuing education presentations needed to be published in full. A proceedings book was one way of developing the body of knowledge particular to the ministry of parish nursing practice. The nurses' work was captured in a publishable format that could be made available to participants, as well as for purchase by those who could not attend the Westberg Symposium. Capturing and documenting what parish nurses and parish nurse coordinators have learned is invaluable to the growth and maturation of this movement. Publishing some of these presentations and stories about the practice of parish nursing in popular lay publications will enhance the visibility of this ministry.

A growing body of research related to parish nursing is being conducted today. Research uncovers new knowledge and understanding. The acquisition of new information is accompanied by the challenge to embrace the change in understanding. New research findings must be discussed, dissected, and digested so that it is integrated into the long-term understanding of the ministry of parish nursing practice. This digesting will mature and change the culture of parish nursing.

Publications by experts in parish nursing in peer reviewed, referenced nursing journals with broad readerships is equally important. It enhances the understanding of this specialty and offers other nurses greater understanding about providing spiritual care to their clients. This takes time, effort, resources, and some risk. However, without it, the ministry of parish nursing practice–and indeed the whole of nursing—may very well never realize its potential.

REFERENCES

American Nurses Association. (1998). *Scope and standards of parish nursing practice*. (9806st). Washington, DC: Author.

Gardener, J.W. (1981). *Self renewal: The individual and the innovative society*. New York: W.W. Norton and Company.

Lloyd, R. & Ludwig-Beymer, P. (1999). Listening to faith communities: Collaboration with those served. In P.A. Solari-Twadell & M.A. McDermott. *Parish nursing: Promoting whole person health within faith communities*. Thousand Oaks, CA: Sage.

Shortell, S.M., Gillies, R.R., Anderson, D.A., Erickson, K.M. & Mitchell, J.B. (1996). *Remaking health care in America: Building organized delivery systems*. San Francisco: Jossey-Bass.

Solari-Twadell, A. (1994). *Perspectives in parish nursing practice*. Park Ridge, IL: International Parish Nurse Resource Center.

Solari-Twadell, P.A. (1999). The emerging practice of parish nursing. In P.A. Solari-Twadell & M.A. McDermott. *Parish nursing: Promoting whole person health within faith communities*. Thousand Oaks, CA: Sage.

Solari-Twadell, P.A. (2002). The differentiation of the ministry of parish nursing practice within congregations. *Dissertation Abstracts International, 63(06)*: 569A. UMI No. 3056442.

Westberg, G. (1987). *The parish nurse*. Park Ridge, IL: National Parish Nurse Resource Center.

Westberg, G. (1992). How accountable are we for whole-person health? *Proceedings of the Sixth Annual Granger Westberg Symposium. Accountability: The foundation of parish nursing practice*. Northbrook, IL: National Parish Nurse Resource Center.

UNIT II

Educational
Preparation for
the Ministry of
Parish Nursing
Practice

You Teach Who You Are: A Lesson Plan for the Parish Nurse Educator

10

Mary Ann McDermott

You teach who you are! This is the premise of Palmer's *The Courage to Teach* (1998). Those readers who participated in the parish nurse educator preparation sessions I taught probably made acquaintance with Palmer's material at that time. The invitation to teach in those sessions some years ago provided me with a real challenge. What do you teach experienced college and university faculty? Certainly I would not be so bold as to lecture on how to teach. Although most had not been in a parish nurse role, all were to have completed the basic parish nurse course as a prerequisite. Consequently, plowing through the basic and coordinator curricula module by module also seemed ludicrous.

When the student is ready, the teacher will appear. That familiar maxim became truth for me just in time. At a large conference center that I was touring in New Orleans, I came upon a teacher convention book market. Palmer's book, a recent release, was featured in one of the booths. I was familiar with some of his other previous works (Palmer, 1981, 1983). I glanced through the table of contents; the teacher appeared; the sale was made. In the years since that purchase, my now well-worn copy has stimulated a great deal of personal reflection on the parish nurse educator's role, the role of every parish nurse as an educator, and my own role. Palmer's volume inspired the theme and generated many—but certainly not all—of the ideas for this chapter.

Have you ever considered that your involvement in the educator role, as Schwehn (1996) reminds us, is one of culture transmission and change across generations? "I touch the future; I teach" stated Christa McAuliffe (Exley, 1997, n.p.). You are a parish nursing culture transmitter! I believe that culture transmission, really good teaching, depends upon a great deal of self-knowledge. Parker (1998) put it this way: "good teachers share one trait: a strong sense of personal identity infuses their work" (p. 10). Williams (2002) points out that it is important to acknowledge that most of us desire to explore a range of concerns about ourselves.Williams (2002) argues, "We want to sort through our own desires and find out why we feel as we do" (p. 20). I have included several learning activities and reflections that I hope will enhance your self-knowledge, especially as it impacts your educator role.

Four Teachers in Your Life

Who do you think you are in the teacher role? All parish nurses, parish nurse coordinators, and parish nurse "educators" are teachers. We profess to be whole persons, and we speak to teaching and ministering to the health of the whole person. It follows that we are whole teachers. Menninger (Exley, 1997) said, "What the teacher is is more important than what he teaches" (n.p.). We are influenced by a great number of people in our

111

lives, consciously or unconsciously integrating qualities of some of them, making them our own. Although you can meet my first request by engaging in the activity by yourself, consider doing this exercise with another parish nurse, parish nurse coordinator, parish nurse educator, and/or a good friend.

This activity, attributed to the Sufi tradition, can be done as a spoken exchange. I guarantee, however, a much more meaningful experience with the following suggestions. To make this a meditative experience you might like to select and play some beautiful music on your CD player. The Native American flute music of R. Carlos Nakai (1998) is a favorite of mine for this activity. Gather some colored markers, some favorite old magazines, masking tape, a glue stick, and a scissors. Find a large piece of white "butcher" paper or brown wrapping paper about the length and width of your body. Lay down on the floor. Ask your partner to draw around you with a large colored marker to form an outline of your body. Take some time for this; switch, and complete the outlining of your partner. Rest quietly for a while and think about teachers in your life who have made a difference. These individuals do not have to have been employed as teachers. They can be living or dead; you might have had long- or short-term relationships with them; possibly they are people you have only read about, people you have never met.

Consider first someone who had a great influence on your intellect, the way you think. Did he or she model the life of the mind? What were the qualities about that person that made the difference in you? Your outlined head will be the symbol. Consider next a person who taught you a number of skills: household, a craft, a musical instrument, nursing skills. Was it the skill of the person or something else about him or her that influenced your skill development? Your hands will be the symbol. Thirdly, give thought to an individual who taught you to be a person of action, to move, literally, on your beliefs. Was this person a social or political activist in the sense of being a public figure? What behaviors did they demonstrate? Your feet will be the symbol. Lastly, in deep silence, listen to your heart, hear it beating, place your hand over your heart and feel it beating. Who in the world has most influenced

your way of being in this world? What attitudes, feelings, and/or values did they convey? Your heart will be the symbol.

Continue this activity in a quiet atmosphere. Attach your outlined contour to a bare floor or a wall with masking tape. Write or print your name somewhere on the drawing. Highlight with the colored markers the four parts on your body outline: head, hands, feet, and heart. Page through some of the magazines that you have gathered, find some images that relate to the four teachers and their respective gifts to you. Cut them out and glue them and/or design images or write a few words with your colored markers and place them onto the corresponding part of your body. Once you have finished, stand back from your image, and reflect on what you have created. Take turns speaking about your creations, your collective selves with your partner. Also talk about the process: How did it feel having someone draw around your body? Did you include anything, images or words, which surprised you?

Carl Jung states, "One looks back with appreciation to the brilliant teachers, but with gratitude to those who touched our human feelings" (Charlton, 1994, p. 94). Have you ever thanked in person or in a written note of gratitude the individuals you identified in the above activity? Consider doing so within the next few days; you can still write notes to those you are unable to locate or have died. The process of acknowledging and "getting in touch" with your sense of gratitude is the important feature of this gesture. Certainly, however, those who can be found and contacted will appreciate your thoughtfulness.

Role Models for Teaching from Life and from Scripture

Role-Modeling Theory

One tends to teach as one has been taught! This is an old maxim, but it consists of much truth. Much of teaching actually consists of modeling. I first came to learn about the concept of role modeling in graduate school when studying Bandura's Social Learning Theory. Bandura (1971) spoke of modeling or observational learning as the process through which individuals observe the behaviors of others, form an idea of the performance and results of the observed behaviors, and use that idea as coded information to guide behavior in the future. Bandura (1971) states, "Whatever their orientation, people model, expound, and reinforce what they value" (p. 211).

Favorite and Not-So-Favorite Teachers as Role Models

Alone or with a friend, tell about a favorite teacher, a great teacher in your life. Select one of the individuals you described earlier, or choose a different teacher, but one with whom you had a direct experience in a teacher-student relationship. Write a paragraph or two, compose a poem, and/or write some song lyrics about that teacher, about that experience, about the difference that person made in your life.

Modeling can be positive or negative. Consider for a few minutes a not-so-favorite teacher, a poor teacher in your life. Write a paragraph or two, compose a poem about that teacher, and/or write some song lyrics about that teacher, about that experience, about any difference that person made in your life. Someone should probably make a collection of these narratives and make them available to teacher education programs. Is there an entrepreneur among you?

Examine both writings. My experience over a number of years informs me that the narrative that describes the way in which the favorite teacher influenced you will name very specific characteristics. If you had been doing this exercise in a large group and we collated these characteristics, we would be able to identify some common characteristics. Those that are most commonly mentioned by my students: cared about, never gave up on me; enthusiasm, passion for their subject matter and the ability to pass that on; fully present in the moment; readily available and accessible in and out of the classroom. Schwehn (1996) states that during a similar activity teachers his students selected as good role models shared certain qualities of character: integrity, truthfulness, compassion, dedication, empathy, attentiveness, and love. Because teaching and learning are reciprocal activities, can you identify any qualities in your self that might have elicited great teaching? Speaking about the teacher and teaching in *The Prophet*, Gibran states,

"The teacher … gives not of his wisdom but rather of his faith and his lovingness. If he is indeed wise he does not bid you enter the house of his wisdom, but rather leads you to the threshold of your own mind" (p. 51).

The characteristics that my students used to describe poor teachers also had common themes. Many times these were directly opposite those used to describe their favorite teachers: did not seem to care about me; I was just a number or a name on an alphabetical class list. Perhaps worse yet were the following: would "ball me out" in front of other students, doctors, or even patients; lack of enthusiasm for subject matter; or even if the teacher was devoted to her subject matter privately, was unable to pass it on; seemed continuously preoccupied both in and out of the classroom or clinical area with other matters; lack of availability and accessibility; not in her office when she said she would be; never provided a way to get hold of her if we had a problem; would just disappear if there was a crisis on the unit. These teachers seemed to be conveying a message quite effectively: Knowledge is not virtue; do as I say, but not as I do! Since teaching and learning are reciprocal in nature, can you identify any qualities in your self that might have elicited such poor teaching? Discuss your write-ups with several others that have shared in carrying out this activity. Affirm your gifts and liabilities. Listen to and reassure one another. Do not retrospectively try to solve problems!

Christ as Role Model for Teaching

I spent one summer reading the gospels for lessons from Jesus as teacher, on teaching. I found many instances of Jesus modeling superior, large group lecturing talent. He knew all about small group discussion, right down to the size of the ideal small group as dictated in the education literature: twelve. His one-on-one tutoring skills displayed a deep understanding of "individualizing" instruction. In all instances, He used appropriate teaching techniques that exhibited His familiarity with a variety of learning styles. Quick to improvise and aware of audiovisual enhancements to learning, He used a stick in the sand to make His point. He knew about sharing a meal with the students to make the lesson go down a little easier.

Consider that one of His most important lessons has come down to us as the last supper, not the last class meeting. Don't you and your students often celebrate the last class with the sharing of food and beverage? Christ was a storyteller *par excellence*, using one parable after another. He believed in repetition. If the disciples did not seem to understand the material the first time, he found another way to teach the same lesson using a different story. I am sure most readers have heard me repeat an anonymous (I cannot remember where I first heard it), modified, and somewhat humorous contribution to some deep truths about Jesus as teacher and we as learners:

The Lesson Plan

Then Jesus took his disciples up into the mountains and gathering them together

He taught them saying: Blessed are the poor in spirit: for theirs is the kingdom of heaven. Blessed are they that mourn: for they shall be comforted. Blessed are the meek: for they shall inherit the Earth. Blessed are they who hunger and thirst after righteousness: for they shall be filled. Blessed are the merciful: for they shall obtain mercy. Blessed are the pure in heart: for they shall see God. Blessed are the peacemakers: for they shall be called the children of God. Blessed are they who are persecuted: for theirs is the kingdom of heaven.

And Peter said: "Are we supposed to be taking notes on this?"

And Andrew said: "How well will we have to know this stuff?"

And James said: "Will this be on the final?"

And Philip said: "How much will it count?"

And Bartholomew said: "Can we write a paper instead?"

And John said: "The other guys' disciples didn't have to learn this stuff."

And Matthew said: "Can we leave now?"

And Mark said: "I've got to go; is all this on your website?"

And Thaddaeus said: "Are there Cliffs Notes at the bookstore on this?"

And Luke said: "Could you go over that part about the meek again?"

And Thomas whispered: "I doubt if He knows what he's talking about."

And Judas muttered: "What does this have to do with the real world?"

Just then a tenured Pharisee walked up to the class and asked Jesus to show him his lesson plans and published scholarship; inquired about his terminal objectives in the cognitive domain, his research agenda and list of funded grants; and distributed some instructional accountability evaluation forms to the disciples. And Jesus wept.

Metaphor to Describe Teachers/Teaching

Metaphor (a figure of speech which makes implied comparisons between things that are not literally alike) and analogy (the resemblance in essentials between things) are powerful ways to think about things. For many years I had graduate students in a teaching course develop a personal metaphor for teaching. They had to write a short paper that extended the application of the metaphor. I had many students who wrote about teacher as farmer—working with the soil, seeding, watering, fertilizing, deadheading, and harvesting. I had students who wrote about teacher as artist, midwife, lapidary, travel agent, tour guide, and even as spelunker—a cave explorer! Some even wrote about teachers as fictional characters: Alice in Wonderland, Indiana Jones, etc. I always requested permission to save them and hope, maybe still, to publish them. Spoden (1999) preempted me! As part of an ongoing teacher appreciation project, he collected and published inspirational stories and poems by students to honor their teachers.

Spoden (1999) used eight metaphors to organize the narratives that were submitted for his collection:

1. The Healer, who offers comfort and assurance
2. The Thinker, who sparks a love of knowledge
3. The Sage, who assists students in discovering important truths about the world and themselves
4. The Maestro, who helps students express themselves in the arts
5. The Dancer, who makes learning an exciting, joyous experience
6. The Believer, who pushes students to find inner strength and determination
7. The Guide, who helps students find their life calling

8. The Torchbearer, who envisions teaching as passing something along from his or her own learning inheritance to the next generation.

Do you recognize yourself as role model/teacher in any of these descriptions? Have you already created or might you now create a metaphor for yourself as another expression of interest in self-knowledge as a teacher?

Teaching as Vocation

Schwehn (1996) asks us to remind ourselves often that teaching is a vocation; in fact, he argues, "teaching is a religious calling that involves the cultivation of certain moral and spiritual virtues" (p. 7). He points out that if we consider it otherwise we will risk making one of two fundamental errors: "We will either reduce it (*teaching*) to a set of methods or techniques … or we will mystify it by turning it into an occult practice that defies rational appraisal or description" (p. 6). My own very favorite image of vocation is Buechner's (1993) beautiful quotation of vocation as "the place where your deep gladness and the world's great hunger meet" (p. 119). I have often reflected on how fortunate we in the nursing profession—particularly those who have taken positions in parish nursing—are because of our easy access to that sensation of deep gladness. Personally, I have found my deep gladness in teaching nursing.

Palmer (2000) tells the story of his understanding, well into adulthood, that vocation or calling came from a voice external to himself. That idea created a lot of guilt about the distance between who he was and who he was supposed to be. He now acknowledges vocation as a gift, not a goal, and it comes from a voice inside "calling me to be the person I was born to be, to fulfill the original selfhood given me at birth by God" (p. 10). Gately (1981) has two lines in her wonderful poem "Called to Become" that reinforce Palmer's insight: "No one is called to become who you are called to be" (pp. 68-69).

Teaching holds a mirror to the soul; how does the quality of my spiritual life form or deform the way I relate to my students, my subject, my colleagues, my world? How do we go about listening to the Call, cultivating our own spirituality, our spiritual life? How do you attend to the teacher within? Palmer (1998) defines *spiritual* as "the

diverse ways we answer the heart's longing to be connected with the largeness of life—a longing that animates love and work, especially the work called teaching" (p. 5). As a response to that question, Palmer (1998) identifies the common spiritual practices of solitude, silence, meditative reading, walking in the woods, keeping a journal, and finding a friend who will listen (pp. 31-32). In Chapter 4, Taylor describes in-depth some of these practices. Are we also called, as educators, to spiritual leadership? Solari-Twadell offers us a model of spiritual leadership in Chapter 26, giving us a language for that concept and encouraging us to talk to each other about our inner lives.

When was the last time you talked with another parish nurse, parish nurse coordinator or parish nurse educator about teaching as vocation or even about teaching in any depth? How can a regional network of parish nurse educators or the IPNRC sustain and deepen our connection with one another around forming a community of parish nurse educators? Palmer (1998) talks about developing "communities of truth" that invite diversity, embrace ambiguity, welcome creative conflict, practice honesty, experience humility and become free by invoking the grace of great things (pp. 107-108). Let us take the invitation to invoke the grace of great things.

Born to Teach: An Experience of Deep Gladness

Another exercise! This activity, as well as the ones described earlier, makes for great journaling. Describe a teaching success or a time in the classroom or the clinical area when you could hardly hold the joy—a time when you knew, you just knew, you were born to teach! "I am not a teacher but an awakener," said Robert Frost (Exley, 1997, n.p.). When did you first/last experience that *aha* moment? Can you identify the factors for success, for experiencing deep gladness that were present? What made it all work?

I recall an instance in a health ministry class session several years ago when one of the students—I can still see her as if it were yesterday—responded to me from across the table and said, in an instant of transformation for her and for me, "I never thought about it that way before." She owned a new idea; she had new power.

I owned the moment, I had a new understanding in those few seconds of my vocation of teaching: to facilitate students to think about things differently. Deep gladness spread over me!

Born to Teach—Not!

Describe a teaching bomb, a less than optimal experience, a time in the classroom or the clinical area where you knew right then and there that you should have never taken this teaching position. You wanted to run away, out, anywhere! This could be a particular student interaction, class session, or clinical setting or occur over the course of an entire semester. Until you have a bomb—and there will be some and even some more—you have not lived; you have not taught long enough. Can you identify the factors for failure, deep anguish that were present? What was not working?

I recently experienced an entire semester that seemed to last into eternity. Undergraduate senior students in a leadership management course, I believe, may have hastened my decision to retire. To this day, I have not been able to identify all the factors that contributed to my anguish. Fortunately, the next semester, I had a new course and new students. Maybe that is the joy of teaching; you can always start again!

Evaluation: Expectations Influence Behavioral Outcomes

Parish nurse educators must subject themselves to regular evaluation of their teaching as a matter of justice and professional integrity. Perhaps *assessment* is a better word. *Assessment* comes from the Latin root *assidere*, meaning "to sit beside." That term seems less harsh. If we profess that evaluation seeks to provide direction, we will seek out evaluation as a means to improving our teaching. Creating evaluation tools that can provide the information we need to enhance the quality of our offerings is essential. Faculty are often expected or required to use the forms provided by their respective institutions that may or may not provide students the opportunity to provide us with the desired feedback. Although it is time-consuming, additional alternative evaluation formats can supplement the "required" form/s. In Chapter 16 Tippe urges parish nurses

to prepare a portfolio for evaluation purposes; it would behoove the parish nurse educator to do the same. Professional development as an educator can be documented in the portfolio. John Cotton Dana stated, "Who dares to teach must never cease to learn" (Charlton, 1994, p. 97).

Students enrolled in the parish nurse coursework need to be evaluated and provided with direction, as a matter of justice and professional integrity as well. Graded with a letter grade or pass-fail, students deserve to be validated in their classwork. Quite commonly this is not done objectively. Faculty, for the most part, have not required students write formal papers or take tests and exams. Subjective evaluation is not altogether inferior, for most parish nurse faculty are well-experienced teachers who are valued for their "educated" subjectivity; however, some combination of objective and subjective evaluation may be preferable.

Our observations of students in the classroom and around the coffeemaker are ordinarily linked to—are synonymous with—judgments. Palmer (1998) states that, not unlike in medicine, the way we diagnose our student's condition will determine the kind of remedy we offer. What kind of diagnoses have you been making lately? What do you do about "weeding out" the inappropriate potential parish nurse—in a kindly manner? Who and how do you need to notify, given guidelines about confidentiality, regarding your "subjective" assessment? Who among you has not had at least one "student from hell?" That wording is Palmer's designation (Palmer, 1998, p. 43)—certainly not mine! However, like the teaching experience/s that bomb, if you have not had one, you have not taught long enough. This is when the network, the community of parish nurse educators as resources to one another, can really help.

Best Parish Nurse Educator Practices

William Arthur Ward states, "The mediocre teacher tells. The good teacher explains. The superior teacher demonstrates. The great teacher inspires" (Exley, 1997, n.p.). How does one inspire students or, for that matter, family members and colleagues? Are there best practices in this area? At some risk, I have identified below several ideas as well as techniques and teaching strategies that might qualify for parish nurse educators to consider as best practices.

Creating the Space

How does one go about what I once called "stacking the deck" for learning? In recent years the literature has clarified the language for this idea. The teacher is requested to create the conditions, to create the space for learning. Palmer (1998) invites us to consider a set of paradoxes in his suggestions that the teaching and learning space should have the following characteristics: " (1) be bounded and open; (2) be hospitable and charged; (3) invite the voice of the individual and the voice of the group; (4) honor the little stories of the individual and the big stories of the disciplines and tradition; (5) support solitude and surround it with the resources of community; (6) welcome both silence and speech" (p. 74). He goes into some detail about the practicalities of implementing these ideas in creating this space.

I offer several other ideas for "stacking the deck." Most educators think a lot about how to best "spend" the time in the classroom. Assignments given in advance, even of the first class, to preread some materials makes the chances of fruitful discussion time much more feasible. Conducting an assessment of the group before—or certainly during—the first class meeting allows the parish nurse educator to "meet the learners where they are," a basic principle of teaching and learning. The teacher who starts class with introductions gets off to a much different start than one who starts with the course syllabus and detailed instructions of APA format for submitting written work.

Another consideration before a teacher ever enters the classroom is the parish nurse educator's reflection upon what the class participants really want to know. What do I believe they need to know that is not in the book, on the web, or in other formats that can be easily accessed? My question to myself has always been "what do they *gotta* know"? Can you reduce to a matchbook cover the "core" content of a class? Have you ever forgotten your notes and did just fine by reducing to the essentials, remembering to emphasize only what you recall as really important? I believe this

makes the way in which class time is "spent" much different.

Schwehn (1996) believes—and I agree—that teaching and learning are "acts of piety, arising from religious affections like awe, wonder, and gratitude in the presence of the gifted given-ness of creation" (p. 8). For this reason in thinking and planning for class, I always try to find appropriate ways to incorporate the arts: art, music, literature, and especially poetry into the content. Thinking ahead, I plan classroom time and assignments to elicit awe and wonder. As learning outcomes, these affections are even more evident when journaling—in or out of class—is assigned.

Teaching Strategies and Techniques

"Techniques are what teachers use until the real teacher arrives," states Palmer (1998, p. 5). That saying not only reinforces the entire theme of Palmer's book but also reminded me about the importance of process. I was introduced to Parker and Rubin's (1966) *Process as Content* shortly after arriving at Loyola while I was participating in a massive curriculum revision. Process, they say, is "the cluster of diverse procedures which surround the acquisition and utilization of knowledge ... is in fact the highest form of content" (p. 1). They point out, "Where the stress is upon process, the assimilation of knowledge is not derogated, but greater importance is attached to the methods of its acquisition and to its subsequent utilization" (p. 2). Although the content of the parish nurse curriculum is very important and the core has been selected based on evidence from current practice, it is *process* that is a major concern related to the delivery of the curricula. This issue has specifically been brought to bear in the discussions about its importance in the curricula's distance learning format.

Although I try to use a good deal of discussion when teaching the parish nurse curricula and have used a myriad of small group techniques, the best practice I want to share here is one related to lecturing. The ever-popular lecture always seems to be a fallback measure, a good way to be sure I "cover" the topic. I have to remember that, in truth, I am in the classroom to "uncover" the content. If I stay so close to the text or syllabus, the students might as well have stayed home.

Although primarily talking about music education, Ristad (1982) tells us, "As a teacher I sometimes delude myself into thinking I am speaking to a student's condition, when in reality I am only responding to an old compulsion to teach a certain thing at a certain time-to stuff certain truths into each student's bag.... I can also delude myself into thinking the student has learned what I thought I taught" (p. 128).

For a number of years I have used a formula developed by Weaver (1982) as a way to organize and deliver both speeches and lectures. He uses the acronym AIDA, a familiar word to some, unrecognizable by many. I have outlined his ideas with my modifications:

A, Capturing *Attention*: Provide some transition time, give a brief overview of the class. Begin with a story, a personal experience or a startling statistic. Howard's (2004) edited collection of essays on teaching includes his own essay, "Stories, Mon Amour," in the section entitled "Why We Teach" (pp. 12-31). Howard views his life as a professor at Notre Dame as being a creator and teller of really provocative stories. He reminds us that we live in and through stories. Share your stories and allow/encourage the students to tell their stories. Be autobiographical; be flawed. One caveat—be sure to relate them to the material at hand!

I, Holding *Interest*: Conduct an audience analysis; attempt to meet learners where they are. What do they *gotta* know, spoken of previously. Focus on a few points in depth. Try to provide a variety of kinds of information, in various formats, all while using some humor.

D, Creating *Desire*: Without your enthusiasm for the subject matter, nothing else matters. Demonstrate an active and emotional commitment to the topic.

A, *Action*: Weaver talks about teacher bodily action in the classroom. I have converted this to mean, "What do you want the students to do as a result of your teaching, as a result of this class session?" Audi (1994) said it eloquently: "One is

never *just* a teacher. One is always an advocate of a point of view, a critic of certain positions ... a person dealing with, and indeed responsible for, others in common tasks" (p. 35). Palmer (1999) says that "[a]n expressive act is one that I take not to achieve a goal outside myself but to express a conviction, a leading, a truth that is within me" (p. 24). By doing so, "I come closer to making the contribution that is mine to make in the scheme of things" (Palmer, 1999, p. 24).

Please note, I am not recommending lecture as the best way to "uncover" the parish nursing basic or coordinator content; but when and if you find yourself using this strategy, do think about AIDA. I would be remiss in not mentioning mentoring as a best practice, especially as we discuss the need to take action. The power of mentors is not necessarily in the models of good teaching they give us; rather, Palmer (1998) reminds us "their power is in their capacity to awaken a truth within us" (p. 21). Chapter 15, written by Rosemarie Matheus, mentor par excellence, covers this best practice in detail.

Conclusion

The exercises/activities described in this chapter hopefully have provided the reader with the opportunity to explore the landscape of the teacher within. Gaining an appreciation for the individuals who have influenced the way in which we are in the world of teaching also enhances our self-awareness. Acknowledging teaching as a calling immediately places our work, *our deep gladness meeting the world's great hunger*, in the spiritual domain. Viewing ourselves as role models (consciously or unconsciously) and as people of influence who exert spiritual leadership offers a new perspective on our roles within both academic and healthcare institutions as well as in parish nursing. I believe the need is clear to establish a supportive parish nurse educator community to invoke the grace of great things for the future!

REFERENCES

Audi, R. (1994). On the ethics of teaching and the ideals of learning. *Academe*, 85(5): 26-36.

Bandura, A. (1971). *Social learning theory.* New York: General Learning Press.

Buechner, F. (1993). *Wishful thinking.* San Francisco: Harper.

Charlton, J. (Ed.). (1994). *A little learning is a dangerous thing: A treasury of wise and witty observations for students, teachers, and other survivors of higher education.* New York: St. Martin's Press.

Exley, H. (Ed.). (1997). *Thank heavens for teachers.* New York: Exley Publications/Hallmark Books.

Gateley, E. (1981). *Psalms of a laywoman.* Chicago: Claretian Publications.

Gibran, K. (1936). *The prophet.* New York: Knopf.

Howard, G.S. (Ed.). (2004). *For the love of teaching.* Notre Dame, IN: Academic Publications.

Nakai, R.C. (1998). *Mythic dreamer.* Phoenix: Canyon Records Productions.

Palmer, P. (1981). *The company of strangers: Christians and the renewal of America's public life.* New York: Crossroad.

Palmer, P. (1983). *To know as we are known: A spirituality of education.* New York: Harper and Row.

Palmer, P. (1998). *The courage to teach: Exploring the inner landscape of a teacher's life.* San Francisco: Jossey-Bass.

Palmer, P. (1999). *The active life: A spirituality of work, creativity and caring.* San Francisco: Jossey-Bass.

Palmer, P. (2000). *Let your life speak: Listening for the voice of vocation.* San Francisco: Jossey-Bass.

Parker, J.C. & Rubin, L.J. (1966). *Process as content: Curriculum design and the application of knowledge.* Chicago: Rand McNally.

Ristad, E. (1982). *A soprano on her head: Right-side-up reflections on life and other performances.* Moab, UT: Real People Press.

Schwehn, M. (1996). The spirit of teaching. *Conversations on Jesuit Education*, 10: 5-18.

Spoden, J. (Ed.). (1999). *To honor a teacher: Students pay tribute to their most influential mentors.* Kansas City: Andrews McMeel.

Weaver, R.L. (1982). Effective lecturing techniques: Alternatives to classroom boredom. *New Directions in Teaching*, 81(7): 31-39.

Williams, C. (2002). *The life of the mind: A Christian perspective.* Grand rapids, MI: Baker Academic.

Parish Nurse Curricula

Mary Ann McDermott
Phyllis Ann Solari-Twadell

The rapid development of the concept, role differentiation, the increasing breadth of the role, and international geographic expansion of parish nursing since 1984 led to the need for appropriate preparation for individuals desirous of using their gifts in the ministry of parish nursing practice. In this chapter the historical development of curricula for parish nursing will be reviewed. Readers will be asked to appreciate the difficulty of identifying accurate descriptive language not only as it applies to the practice, especially the ministerial perspective, but also to the development of standards and curricula as well. The current status of curricula updates, management and offerings will be discussed. A case for continuing to develop evidence-based curricula to adequately reflect current and anticipated future parish nursing practice will be made. An organizing framework for that process, based on research, concludes the chapter.

Historical Overview of Curricula Development

Early Origins at Lutheran General Hospital

More than two decades have passed since 1984 when Granger Westberg (1990) approached the administration at Lutheran General Hospital (LGH) about the idea for a pilot project for his concept of parish nursing. Once implemented, Granger went about the country, popularizing the idea. It was not long before hospital, clergy, and nursing leaders wanted more information about this innovative role. With no published material available, these individuals were curious and chose to come visit and spend some time with the six original parish nurses. The parish nurses were enthusiastic about sharing their experience but were still in the very early stages of role definition. Time out from the practice to speak with interested outsiders had to be curtailed.

Out of Vice President Reverend J. Wylie's Office of Mission and Church Relations at Lutheran General Health System, the Parish Nurse Resource Center was initiated in 1986 and Ann Solari-Twadell appointed director. Subsequently the center became the national, and still later to reflect the growth of the practice, the International Parish Nurse Resource Center. The center's purpose was development of quality parish nurse programs and study of organizational models, functions, educational preparation, and denominational affiliations of the nurses (Lloyd & Solari-Twadell, 1994).

The resource center began to offer the first formal continuing education program on parish nursing, and in 1987 these programs evolved into the annual Westberg Symposium on parish nursing. The resource center initiated a two and a half-day "Orientation to Parish Nursing" continuing education programs in 1989. Interested nurses received basic information on the concept, a plan to get a program started in their congregation/area, and a chance to discuss with experts the legal as well as the ministerial facets of this new role. The orientation included a half-day on-site with a practicing LGH-sponsored parish nurse. These sessions were discontinued by the resource center in 1996 when a lengthier evidence-based curriculum for basic preparation became available.

Parish Nurse Resource Center as Consultant and Convener of Curricula Development

During the late 1980s and early 1990s, the director of the resource center served as a consultant to both Georgetown University and Marquette University in developing credit-bearing and continuing education offerings. Small (1990) provides a strong rationale for curriculum development but acknowledges that at the time, "educational preparation is being defined more by participation and the sharing of experiences than by a curriculum based on a theoretical framework" (p. 237). Small (1990) describes the program that she developed at Georgetown as "an example of a curriculum designed to prepare the parish nurse at the advanced nursing practice level and reflects a philosophy of specialized nursing practice and graduate education" (p. 246). Small (1990) was clear that in "designating the master's level of preparation for the parish nurse does not imply that only those nurses prepared at this level should practice as parish nurses" (p. 247). The Marquette Parish Nurse Institute, under the able direction of Rosemarie Matheus, was initiated in 1989. Coursework, both credit-bearing and as continuing education, were offered on-site in Milwaukee. Maybe more importantly, Matheus traveled the country, taking herself and her parish nursing preparation to every nook and cranny of our land.

The director of the resource center served as a catalyst in 1991 by convening a "spiritual think tank," according to Dahm (2003, p. 10). This was a meeting for representatives from several seminaries and four schools of nursing in the Chicago area (Loyola University Chicago, North Park University, Xavier University, and Rush University). The discussion centered on the possibility of a collaborative effort in the development of curricula aimed at developing joint competency for those in healthcare, particularly nurses, who saw their work as a ministry and who sought to gain additional preparation in this area. An informal consortium was formed to offer three courses in health ministries and consequently to develop a prototype of a combined MDiv./MSN degrees program. This consortium has continuously offered course work and three other programs (Lewis University, Elmhurst University, and the University of Illinois) have joined the group. Interestingly, the cohort of faculty have become a community of colearners, along with the students interested in enhancing their own knowledge of spiritual care and health ministries (Dahm, 2003).

Early Diversity of Educational Programming

In addition to the diversity of offerings described earlier, by the early 1990s the Resource Center documented 52 educational offerings in the United States (McDermott, Solari-Twadell, & Matheus, 1998). Thirty-two of these were sponsored by healthcare institutions; 12 were university-based; one was housed in a seminary; and the remainder were provided through parish nurse networks or congregational sponsors (McDermott et al, 1998). Programs included daylong and weeklong orientations, continuing education workshops and seminars, the first distance learning programs, and credit-bearing courses over an entire semester. Some diversification in educational offerings was anticipated and even encouraged early in the development of parish nursing. The variety of offerings seemed to best reflect the differences of geographic regions and the distinctive attributes of denominational sponsorship. Differences were apparent in selection and prioritization of content, faculty background, and the number of classroom and/or practicum hours. A concern that a wide variation in application of the parish nurse role might cause confusion among program sponsors within the national and local healthcare community and, most importantly, among the congregation and those they serve in the community was expressed (McDermott et al, 1998).

Initiation of a Self-Regulatory Process

By the nature of its status in society, every profession, especially those related to health, needs to protect itself and the consumer from unqualified practitioners. The profession of nursing is ethically responsible for the quality of care delivered to the public in the name of parish nursing. One of the ways this has been historically carried out is by developing and monitoring the education of its members. In response to the growing concern related to parish nurse preparation and at the recommendation of nurse leaders and educators, the resource center initiated a self-regulatory process in June 1994. The aim of the project was to ensure the educational foundation for the future of parish nursing practice. Invitations were extended for a two and a half-day colloquium to develop beginning guidelines for parish nurse education. Twenty-six parish nurses, parish nurse educators, and clergy from across the country worked diligently to draft a philosophy of parish nursing. The guidelines differentiated between programming that provided overall orientation to the concept of parish nursing and the site-based orientation for a role in a specific congregation. Guidelines were also developed for continuing professional development of parish nurses and for coursework in degree-granting institutions (Solari-Twadell, McDermott, Ryan, & Djupe, 1994).

Partners for Curriculum Development

As a natural aftereffect of the colloquium, the center carried out an educational programming needs assessment. Begun in 1996, a convenience sample of 50 parish nurse coordinators known to the center were queried regarding the content of their own educational offerings to prepare their parish nurses. They were also asked to identify additional educational experiences in which they had engaged to prepare themselves for the coordinator role and/or what content they would identify as being most helpful or ideal to implementing their role. Comments on the specifics of that preparation: site, length, and cost were requested. The findings from the needs assessment process served as the basis for a collaborative curriculum development and implementation venture between Marquette University, Loyola University Chicago, and the International Parish Nurse Resource Center.

Collaboration during the first year focused on taking the needs assessment data to identify core content and a curriculum format for both basic preparation and coordinator education programming. Three thousand readers of *Perspective in Parish Nursing Practice*, a publication of the center,

were asked to submit the names of content experts who could develop curriculum modules of the content topics that had been identified previously by the 50 coordinators. Detailed modular syllabi were subsequently created and peer-reviewed by the content experts who functioned as partners in the first evidence-based parish nurse curricula process. The modules were written at the baccalaureate level of professional nursing education. It was acknowledged that options should exist for both continuing education units and undergraduate credit.

A second invitational education colloquium was sponsored by the center in April, 1997. The purpose of the colloquium was to critically review all pre-peer–reviewed and submitted curriculum materials. Attending were the developers of the syllabi as well as a panel of external, nationally recognized nurse and ministerial leaders and educators. Representatives were present from the American Nurses Association and the National League for Nursing as well as reviewers from Canada and Australia. All those attending endorsed the curricula.

A great deal of dialogue occurred at the colloquium, not so much on the issue of content, but on the "process as content" of the parish nurse and parish nurse coordinator's educational experience. Process was/is seen as differentiating the curricula from other educational programming. A nurturing setting, the use of humor, and opportunities for play, both structured and nonstructured, were highlighted. The beginning and end of each day/class period and meal times should be used for shared devotional time. The coursework should have opportunities for the participants to plan and implement worship experiences, including a healing worship service when possible. A final celebratory ritual that could include family, friends, and clergy was thought essential for providing closure. This ceremony is an opportunity to emphasize the value of this ministry to the nurse as well as to those who have supported her in the past and will support her in the future. All of these elements of process make the coursework distinctive.

Pilot programming and further refinement of the curricula for both the basic parish nurse preparation and for the coordinator role was conducted in 1997 and 1998. To educationally mainstream parish nurse education, the decision was made to distribute the curricula through partnerships with colleges and universities.

Parish Nurse Educator Preparation and Partnering

Parish nursing coordinators and faculty who were known to have or could arrange an affiliation with a college and/or university were invited to participate in a pilot of a parish nurse educator program during the summer of 1998. A prerequisite was the sponsorship of their participation in the program by the affiliated institution. The potential faculty members were responsible to identify in advance individuals in their respective schools who could/would be the local content experts to teach specific core modules of the basic and coordinator curricula. The institution could use the curricula in either CEU or for-credit programming. The fees charged would help to cover the costs of the curriculum development process, as well as a copy of the entire curriculum. Subsequently, a small annual fee was also charged to cover listing in marketing materials/website related to available parish nurse educational programming.

Approximately 200 faculty, including several from other countries, have participated in the educator preparation. The faculty vary in their familiarity with parish nursing; some have practiced in the role, whereas others only recently enrolled in a basic parish nurse preparation course themselves. The program has been modified over the years both in content, process, and length. Time together is not spent teaching the educator to teach nor covering every module in the curricula; rather, much of the time has been used to reflect on teaching this distinctive content and to build an educator community.

Finding Meaningful Language for the Curricula

The invitational colloquium in 1994 brought to the attention of all those participating the difficulty of coming to agreement of what one means—what is conveyed—by the use of certain words and terms. Everyone thought the definition of orientation to parish nursing was clear: It should consist of "whatever I had been doing that I called *orientation*." As a result, "orientation" was divided into what became 1) orientation to the concept of parish nursing generally; and 2) orientation that

was congregation specific. What does "basic" mean to you? Probably not the same as it means to someone else. Basic parish nurse preparation, agreed upon at the second colloquium, was core knowledge needed by every nurse to function minimally in the role when holding the title: parish nurse. It was agreed that faculty/schools/programs could add additional modules to the basic curriculum; however, they were not to subtract or drastically modify the content or the agreed upon time allotment of modules from the basic curriculum. A number of programs have added modules on content that may be locally or denominationally relevant.

A very problematic word has been the choice of "endorsed" for the curricula. What does *endorsed* mean? Endorsed by whom? Must I attend an endorsed curriculum? Does this endorsement allow or inhibit other groups from developing their own curriculum? Sponsors of some educational programs preparing parish nurses not using the center's endorsed curricula experienced a decrease in revenue. The term *endorsed* grew out of the second colloquium. A celebratory ritual was held to provide closure to the process, in keeping with the beliefs of the group about the importance of and valuing of process. The ceremony invited participants to come forward and sign a beautiful calligraphed scroll, endorsing their work: the curriculum. Within a brief period and forever after, the term became problematic. Our colleagues from the ANA and the NLN had signed—what did that mean?

What does *standardized* mean to you? The development of the curriculum had been an effort to bring some standardization to the education of parish nurses. "Cookie cutter" said some. Endorsed or standardized, the curriculum development process was and continues to be an effort to assure the public that when the title *parish nurse* is used, the nurse has received the necessary preparation to function in this specialized role.

Other words that remain ambiguous, confusing, and at times controversial include receiving a "certificate of completion" (meaning that one has completed a course or a program) and being "certified" (an external professional group through peer review and testing has deemed the individual certified). Having the appropriate "credential/s" (educational and experiential qualifications) to be a parish nurse is different from being "credentialed" (at this point in time the national professional organization has not determined the prerequisites for parish nurses to be credentialed by their body). The term *joint competency* (nursing and ministry) is a desirable characteristic of the parish nurse. It can be achieved in a number of ways. Cross describes her journey through joint graduate degrees programs in Chapter 12. Is that an expectation for all parish nurses? Certainly not!

Scope and Standards of Parish Nursing Practice

Writing about curriculum development for parish nursing, Small (1990) pointed out "the need to begin discussions on standards of practice" (p. 235). She made the case early on that the standards needed to be broad in scope so as to be inclusive of diversity, but specific enough to define accountability to the consumer. Small was a leader in the Health Ministries Association (HMA) in the development of the ANA's *Scope and Standards of Parish Nursing Practice* (1998). The standards were reviewed and revised by a committee of the HMA and submitted to the ANA for publication in 2005. The document will have new language for what has been known as parish nursing. Faith Community Nursing, first used by Van Loon (1999) in Australia, is thought by some to be more inclusive. The new document, discussed in several other chapters of this book, will facilitate role development, define accountabilities, inform the discussion of competencies, and provide direction for future parish nursing curriculum development.

Curricula Update and Revisions

The International Parish Nursing Resource Center sponsored a third invitational colloquium in April, 2000. Thirty curriculum writers were invited to attend. Once again external reviewers were asked to participate in the process. The previous year, individuals from across the country who had completed the endorsed curricula—basic and/or coordinator—were asked what was most and least helpful about the curricula. These findings were circulated to the invitees. Before attending, participants were requested to review those findings and all modules, examining them for accuracy,

currency, and relevancy and to submit their comments to the center. These evaluations were summarized and distributed at the colloquium for discussion and action. As a consequence, a number of modules were modified, especially through updating of references. Several modules were deleted and/or combined. Two new modules were added. Time allotted to each module was also reviewed and modified.

A great deal of discussion centered on the development and use of "competencies" for describing and evaluating the parish nurse in the basic coursework as well as in practice. Competency language was introduced into the rewrite of modules of the basic curriculum. Both the current status and the future potential for distance learning as a delivery system for parish nursing education were discussed. The concern regarding inclusion of process elements was acknowledged and addressed. Gustafson, an experienced distance learning parish nurse educator, prepared a paper on that topic for that colloquium. Gustafson discusses current issues that surround this topic in Chapter 17. An external reviewer, Dean Sheila Haas, Loyola University Chicago, Niehoff School of Nursing, made the case for considering the language of "role dimensions" rather than parish nurse functions; however, participants determined they were not ready to accept that language. The external review representative of the ANA made a presentation to the group on the potential for future development of a credentialing process for parish nursing.

International Parish Nurse Resource Center

Transfer of Ownership

After almost a decade of on and off discussion, a full-asset merger of Lutheran General Hospital (LGH) and Health System with the Evangelical Health System (EHS) occurred in 1995 to become Advocate Health Care (Advocate). The organizations had congruent missions and values. The ministry of parish nursing practice at its LGH birthplace was already in place at EHS. Parish nurses from both organizations came together under a director of parish nursing services for the new system. The International Parish Nurse Resource Center became a cost center of the newly formed organization. The director of the center was responsible to the new office of mission and spiritual care. All previous initiatives of the center proceeded on schedule for several years. As the economics of healthcare, specifically reimbursement, changed and faltered, the leadership of Advocate took on a number of cost-cutting measures. Programs were downsized or cut completely. In the case of the resource center, partnerships—both local and national—were sought to share the cost of operation. After almost a year of exploration, an administrative decision was made in October, 2001 to transfer the assets of the center to the Deaconess Foundation in St. Louis, Missouri. It is important to publicly acknowledge that this was a transfer of assets, not a sale of the center, as has been published elsewhere in Smith (2003) (p. 56). The "assets," however, did not entail transferring the staff. Deaconess Foundation, which had sponsored parish nursing in the St. Louis area for some time, had both the access to philanthropy and a knowledgeable staff willing and able to take on this challenge, thus ensuring the ongoing vitality of the center.

Current Program Management and Offerings

The center, now located in St. Louis, has continued to provide uninterrupted services to the parish nurse educator community. *Parish Nurse Perspectives*, a newsletter for parish nursing, is published quarterly. Educational programs from throughout the country and the world that offer the basic parish nurse and the parish nurse coordinator courses are listed on their website (www.parishnurses.org). The staff provides consultation and is active in promoting parish nursing through speaking and publication. A chat room has been set up for parish nurse educators. A curriculum update was sponsored by the center in 2003 and 2004. Educators were contacted and invited to participate in the process. Curricula were reviewed and revised as appropriate. Annual preparation of parish nurse educators, both old and new, has been continued and remains the primary means of distributing the curriculum. Educators are facilitated in their networking by the center at the annual Westberg Symposium.

Future Development of Evidence-Based Curricula

The findings from the research *The Differentiation of the Ministry of Parish Nursing Practice in Congregations* (Solari-Twadell, 2002) are described in part in Chapter 3. The Nursing Intervention Classification System (NIC) was instrumental in this research. The use of NIC was central to the identification of those nursing interventions that were most commonly used by parish nurses on a daily/several times a day, weekly, and monthly basis and those nursing interventions that the parish nurses believed core to the ministry of parish nursing practice.

Advantages to using NIC for this research particular to education and curricular development, as noted in Chapter 3, that NIC "standardizes and defines the knowledge base for curricula and practice" and "assists educators to develop curricula that better articulate with clinical practice" (McCloskey & Bulechek, 2000, p. x).

As noted in Chapter 3, the taxonomy of nursing interventions is "structured into three levels: domains, classes, and interventions (McCloskey & Bulechek, 2000, p. xix). Each intervention "in the classification is listed with a label name, a definition, a set of activities to carry out the intervention and background readings" (McCloskey & Bulechek, 2000, p. 3). For example, the nursing intervention *spiritual support* is found in the *behavioral domain* and the *coping assistance class*. The nursing intervention of *spiritual support* is defined as "assisting the patient to feel balance and connection with a greater power." The activities listed to "carry out" the intervention are the following (McCloskey & Bulechek, 2000, p. 607):

- Be open to patient's expressions of loneliness and powerlessness.
- Encourage chapel service attendance, if desired.
- Encourage use of spiritual resources, if desired.
- Provide desired spiritual articles, according to patient preferences.
- Refer to spiritual advisor of patient's choice.
- Use values clarification techniques to help patient clarify beliefs and values as appropriate.

- Be available to listen to patient's feelings.
- Express empathy with patient's feelings.
- Facilitate use of meditation, prayer, and other religious traditions and rituals.
- Listen carefully to patient's communication and develop a sense of timing for prayer or spiritual rituals.
- Assure patient that nurse will be available to support patient in times of suffering.
- Be open to patient's feelings about illness and death.
- Assist patient to properly express anger in appropriate ways.

The background reading for these interventions follows the information detailing the activities for the intervention. The detail offered in this taxonomy provides a structure for a parish nurse curriculum. The activities identify the content that needs to be taught for each of the interventions.

Once the frequently used and core interventions were identified by the researcher, it was important for Solari-Twadell to determine how this information could be organized to educate parish nurses. In analyzing the current parish nurse curricula four major themes that current parish nurse curriculum models followed were identified: role/function, contextual, organizational/administrative, and process. The role/function theme offers learning that pertains to the integration of the functions of the parish nurse role. The contextual theme focuses on the context for the ministry of parish nursing practice including the role of the congregation in health, theology, ethics, the ministerial team, and legal considerations. The organizational/administrative theme addresses initiating programs, grant writing, documentation, and assessment. The process theme emphasizes worship, self-care, spiritual leadership, humor, and resource sharing.

The second outcome emerging from Solari-Twadell's curricula analysis was the realization that the parish nurse can absorb only so much new learning at one time. The basic "endorsed" preparation for the parish nurse already totals a minimum of 43 continuing education units. Therefore by creating a phase II for parish nurse preparation, the parish nurse will have an opportunity to return to the congregation and implement some of the learning from the basic preparation. The development of a phase II set of content topics supports the continuous learning of the parish nurse by offering education on other subjects related to the commonly used and core interventions for parish nursing. Once phase II is completed, a series of advanced seminars, identified by the researcher/respondents as requiring extended periods of time to focus in depth on just one topic, could be offered. The suggested structure and content for this projected parish nurse education plan is included in Appendix 11A.

Dissemination of Findings

The results of the research *The Differentiation of the Ministry of Parish Nursing Practice in Congregations* (Solari-Twadell, 2002) were presented at the August 2002 parish nurse educators event sponsored by the International Parish Nurse Resource Center. It was called *Hearing the Call, Nurturing the Spirit* and was held at the Pallottine Renewal Center in Florissant, Missouri. Over 60 parish nurse educators attended this presentation. After the presentation and discussion, a survey was distributed to the participants. The intention of the survey was to determine the support for the use of this framework for the next revision of the parish nurse curriculum. The results of the survey indicated strong support for the revision of the basic parish nurse curriculum using the Nursing Interventions Classification system along with the proposed curricula structure, format, and content.

Conclusion

The intention of the basic preparation course for the parish nurse is to prepare the nurse for the future. Use of the Nursing Interventions Classification system as the foundation for a future curriculum revision for the ministry of parish nursing practice will expand the current parameters of the content. The justification for the expansion of content is based on national research of parish nurses that have been prepared in the current basic parish nurse preparation and actively practicing in the ministry of parish nursing. The results of this nursing research provide an evidence-based rational for revision of the current basic preparation for parish nurses and presents a strong case for attention to this framework for such "re-visioning."

Major curriculum revision is costly and time-consuming; to be done properly, it must be well planned and executed. A major revision of the parish nurse curricula done inclusively, as past curricular revisions were, requires planning and an enthusiastic embrace by those who manage the process. The question before parish nurse educators is one that will be significant to the growth and maturation of the ministry of parish nursing practice. Will parish nurses of the future be prepared to use content consistent with the language that will be used by all health professionals or by the past descriptors of the hypothesized seven functions of the parish nurse? This is a critical choice point, one that will carve out the direction and integration of the ministry of parish nursing practice into the continuum of care far into the future.

REFERENCES

American Nurses Association. (1998). *Scope and standards of parish nursing practice*. Washington, D.C.: Author.

Dahm, J. (2003). The nurse as health minister. *Chart: Journal of Illinois Nursing*, 100(6): 10-11.

Lloyd, R., & Solari-Twadell, P.A. (1994). Organizational framework, functions, and educational preparation for parish nurses: National survey 1991 & 1994. *Proceedings of the 8th Annual Westberg Symposium*. Park Ridge, IL: National Parish Nurse Resource Center.

McCloskey, J.C., & Bulechek, G.M. (2000). *Nursing interventions classification (NIC): Iowa intervention project*. St. Louis: Mosby.

McDermott, M.A., Solari-Twadell, P.A., & Matheus, R. (1998). Promoting quality education for the parish nurse and parish nurse coordinator. *Nursing and Health Care Perspectives*, 19(1): 4-6.

Solari-Twadell, P.A. (2002). *The differentiation of the ministry of parish nursing practice within congregations*. Dissertation Abstracts International 63(06), 569A. UMI No. 3056442.

Solari-Twadell, P.A., McDermott, M.A., Ryan, J., & Djupe, A.M. (1994). *Assuring viability for the future: Guideline development for parish nurse education programs*. Park Ridge, IL: Lutheran General Health System.

Solari-Twadell, P.A., & McDermott, M.A. (1999). *Parish nursing: Promoting whole-person health within faith communities*. Thousand Oaks, CA: Sage.

Small, N. (1990). Curriculum development for parish nursing: An educator's perspective. In P.A. Solari-Twadell, A.M. Djupe, & M.A. McDermott (Eds.). *Parish nursing: The developing practice*. Oak Brook IL: Advocate Health Care.

Smith, S.D. (2003). *Parish nursing: A handbook for the new millennium*. Binghamton, NY: Haworth Press.

Van Loon, A.M. (1999). The Australian Concept of Faith Community. In P.A. Solari-Twadell, & M.A. McDermott (Eds.). *Parish nursing: Promoting whole-person health within faith communities*. Thousand Oaks, CA: Sage.

APPENDIX 11A

Proposed Format for Curriculum Revision of the Basic Parish
Nurse Preparation Course

Topics Based on Paradigm of the Functions of the Parish Nurse Role	Content of the Modules Based on the Use of NIC	Contact Hours
PHASE I: BASIC PREPARATION		
1. Integrator of Faith and Health	Presence	2
	Active Listening	
	Coping Enhancement	
	Spiritual Support	3
	Spiritual Growth Facilitation	
	Touch	1.5
2. Health Educator	Health Education	1
	Exercise Promotion	
	Energy Management	
	Teaching: Disease Process	1
3. Referral Agent	Referral	1.5
	Decision-Making Support	
	Health System Guidance	
	Health Care Information Exchange	
4. Personal Health Counselor	Emotional Support	3
	Anticipatory Guidance	
	Counseling	
	Self-Awareness Enhancement	
	Grief Work Facilitation	2
5. Coordination of Volunteers	Working with Volunteers	1.5
6. Developer of Support Groups	Support Groups	1.5
7. Health Advocate	Support System Enhancement	2
	Hope Instillation	
Subtotal CEUs		20

Continued

Proposed Format for Curriculum Revision of the Basic Parish Nurse Preparation Course—cont'd

Topics Based on Paradigm of the Functions of the Parish Nurse Role Topic	Content of the Modules Based on the Use of NIC	Contact Hours CEUs
II. CONTEXTUAL		
The Role of the Congregation in Health, Healing, and Wholeness		3
Theology of Health, Healing, and Wholeness		2
Ethics in Parish Nursing		1.5
Functioning within a Ministerial Team		1.5
Legal Considerations for Parish Nurses		1.5
Subtotal CEUs		9.5
III. ORGANIZATIONAL/ADMINISTRATIVE		
Assessment: Individual, Family, Congregation		1.5
Getting Started		2
Grant Writing		1.5
Documentation		1.5
Subtotal CEUs		6.5
IV. PROCESS		
Self-Care		1
Worship		1
Humor		1
Spiritual Leadership		2
Resource Sharing		2
Subtotal CEUs		7
Total CEUs for the Basic Preparation Course for Parish Nurses		43 CEUs

Proposed Format for Curriculum Revision of the Basic Parish Nurse Preparation Course—cont'd

Topics Based on Paradigm of the Functions of the Parish Nurse Role NICs	Content of the Modules Based on the Use of NIC	Contact Hours CEUs
PHASE II		
Dying Care		2
Self-Esteem Enhancement		2
Health Screening		2
Vital Signs Monitoring		
Caregiver Support		2
Family Support		2
Consultation		3
Telephone Consultation		
Telephone Follow-up		
Program Development		2
Religious Ritual Enhancement		2
Health Care: Information Exchange		1.5
Total CEUs		18.5
ADVANCED WORKSHOPS		
Teaching:		8
Individual		
Procedure /Treatment		
Prescribed Medication		
Prescribed Diet		
Learning Facilitation		
Learning Readiness Enhancement		
Nutritional Counseling		4
Weight Reduction Assistance		
Forgiveness Facilitation		4
Environmental Management: Safety		4
Fall Prevention		
Religious Ritual Enhancement		8
Documentation		
Family Involvement Promotion		8
Family Integrity Promotion		8
Family Support		
Caregiver Support		
Values Clarification		8
Truth Telling		
Dying Care		8
Total CEUs		60

Developing Dual Competencies: A Personal Perspective

Reverend Sheryl S. Cross

Just months into my first year as a new parish nurse, it was obvious to me that more than 20 years of experience as a registered nurse was not adequate preparation for the challenges of the ministry of parish nursing practice in the unique setting of a faith community nursing. For competent practice as a parish nurse, I needed more professional pastoral skills, confidence, and credibility that come with a broad foundation of in-depth theological education. Spiritual care is central to parish nursing. All that a parish nurse does in "seeing, hearing, and being" integrates skills of spiritual care.

Certainly a public health or community health nurse could be quite helpful in the setting of a faith community by promoting wellness; early detection of illness and intervention through physical assessments, health screenings, and health education; and referrals to other resources in the community, etc. Such a nurse may be very caring, but if he or she does not consciously relate to faith or spiritual concerns as well, he or she is not fully embodying the intention of parish nursing. Parish nursing, like all specialty or advanced practice areas of nursing, requires an advanced, special body of knowledge and skills. Many skills needed for this setting are not a part of basic nursing education or practice experience; these needed skills come from disciplines other than nursing, particularly theology and pastoral ministry.

Before serving as a parish nurse, I had many years of experience as an active member and lay leader in the church. This contributed to development of a mature faith and appreciation for the dynamics of the church setting and organization, yet the understanding and skills acquired for ministry and spiritual care were limited. Nowhere in my undergraduate nursing education were there opportunities to acquire skills for spiritual care to be offered in traditional nursing settings, much less in the less familiar setting of a faith community. This does not deny that we were repeatedly told that nursing care should address concern for the whole person, including body, mind, *and spirit*. Yet even in a church-affiliated, traditional faith-based nursing program, the nursing curriculum was already full with other essential areas to cover. There seemed to be no time to learn how to be intentional about spiritual care beyond contacting the chaplain or the patient's priest, rabbi, pastor, or other spiritual mentor. It was assumed that all students would consider the spiritual needs of patients intuitively, yet the means of delivering that care was ambiguous.

Before development of any comprehensive or standardized curricula for parish nursing, in the early 1990s, "orientation" to parish nursing courses were helpful in introducing "spiritually mature," experienced professional registered nurses to the developing concepts of whole person care within the context of faith communities (e.g., churches, congregations). Many of these courses successfully communicated the uniqueness of parish nursing by emphasizing the aspects of being a specialized area of *ministry,* as well as nursing practice. The early courses and those developed since that time recognize that the practice of a nurse "placed" to work in a church is quite different from that of a nurse prepared to serve in the ministry of a faith community. Reverend Granger Westberg (1990) described the nurse as the professional that can effectively stand with a foot in two places as a bridge between professions: one in the world of science and healthcare and the other within humanities and the faith community amidst its religious traditions and belief systems. Because of the collaborative demands of this setting, this parish nurse hungered for the ability to function competently with confidence at the level of a recognized church professional, as well as a health professional. Most particularly there was the need to know more about "doing ministry."

In Pursuit of Excellence

One aspect of professionalism is the ongoing search for knowledge and development of skills to maintain and increase one's level of expertise and competence in practice. With professional commitment, my quest for dual competencies in nursing and ministry led first to Clinical Pastoral Education (CPE), which provided a reflective and process-centered opportunity different from any previous nursing course encountered. CPE provided the supervision and mentoring to sharpen interpersonal communication skills and psychosocial and spiritual assessment skills, along with the heightening of self-awareness and a greater spiritual sense of self, God, and others. An appetite was whetted for broader theological grounding and practical ministry skills having found the learnings of CPE immediately applicable and very helpful in the practice of parish nurse ministry. When I was discerning the first steps of this journey as preparation for ministry as a parish nurse, the desired level of professional competence pointed to the need for graduate education. Through the following eight years, the quest continued toward eventual completion of separate master's degrees in both nursing and in divinity.

At the time (in the mid 1990s) there were no programs available close to home in the St. Louis area that offered a curriculum appropriate or specific to a degree in parish nursing. My conversations with Eden Theological Seminary and the nursing department of Webster University (both located in Webster Groves, Missouri, a St. Louis suburb) led to an informal agreement that allowed simultaneous course work with registration at both institutions. The institutions and I both understood that this was for the purpose of attaining dual competencies in both nursing and ministry as preparation for the multidisciplinary, advanced practice of parish nursing. After carefully pondering and comparing the curricula content, choosing one degree over the other was not appropriate because of major components from each curriculum that I considered important for parish nursing.

This chapter is written from the personal experience and Christian perspective of a seasoned parish nurse having completed both an MSN (Master of Science in Nursing) and M.Div. (Master of Divinity). Moving to completion of these degree programs in nursing and ministry seemed to be the next step toward serving as an advanced level parish nurse. My intention was to broaden the parish nursing role, never to transition away from it. The primary aim of this journey was preparation for the broader responsibilities of a position that might combine the roles of parish nurse along with the ministry of Word and Sacrament as an associate pastor. Other future employment possibilities considered were roles in institutional or academic settings. Now, several years after graduation, I serve as a health ministries consultant and parish nurse educator within the United Church of Christ and other ecumenical health ministry organizations. I am also an ordained clergyperson serving as the solo pastor of a rural church close to the metropolitan area of St. Louis—a wonderful situation, albeit different from those imagined when deciding to pursue the dual degrees. One never knows what incredible things will happen when open to the possibilities and work of God's Spirit. From this perspective this chapter speaks to the following:

- Rationale of dual competencies for the ministry of parish nursing practice
- Educational opportunities beyond basic preparation for parish nursing
- Key elements to development of dual competencies
- Advantages and disadvantages of developing dual competencies

- Conclusions concerning dual competencies (drawn from personal reflections and conversations with others involved in parish nursing and health ministry education.)

Rationale for Dual Competencies

Assumptions and Philosophy of Education in Preparation for Parish Nursing

Just shortly before his death while speaking at one of the symposiums that bears his name, Reverend Dr. Granger Westberg said he believed the future of parish nursing lay in maintaining its spiritual focus. This statement has grounded, informed, and formed this writer's practice and ministry as well as the assumptions and philosophy of education of parish nurses as preparation for ministry as a nursing professional. I have come to understand parish nursing as the following:

It is a specialized area of ministry which blends, calls forth, and uses the gifts of experience, faith, education, and skills of a professional registered nurse in the context of pastoral care and ministry of a local faith community or congregation. It is inspired by the faithful work of deaconesses of the early Christian church and others throughout the history of the church, such as nuns, monks, Deaconess sisters, and others who have consecrated their lives and service to promoting health and wellness as well as caring for the sick, poor, and vulnerable.

Spiritual care with integration of faith and health is central to parish nursing, as "Christian religious education" in its broadest sense. This is based on my understanding of Christian religious education as, at its best, the broad, whole person, and dynamic sharing (teaching, instructing, and socializing) of the redeeming "good news" of the Gospel, to facilitate spiritual formation, "bringing to faith" individuals and the community, in ways relevant to everyday life, implicitly and explicitly integrating the meaning of faith (as trusting relationship and awareness of God's presence) into all aspects of life as a disciple and diaconal community of Jesus Christ.

With a whole person approach and faith-based perspective, parish nursing focuses on health promotion within a faith community and those it serves through education, counseling, advocacy, resource and referral consultation,

and facilitation of small groups and ministry volunteers—that by one's presence, particular care, and embodied faith, others may come to know the compassionate love and grace of Jesus Christ.

As a specialized area of ministry and an advanced practice of professional nursing, parish nursing requires a unique body of knowledge and skills beyond basic nursing education and practice experience. As preparation for this blended vocation, parish nursing education must be multidisciplinary, including concepts of person, health, nursing, and environment along with theological concepts of ministry, pastoral care, healing, and wholeness.

Development of dual competencies (particularly in nursing and theology/ministry) permeates all levels of parish nursing preparation. Based on adult learning theory and models, parish nursing education occurs at levels including baccalaureate, continuing education, master's, and post-master's to support and nurture lifelong learning, professional development, and personal spiritual formation. In my experience, students participating in parish nursing education are adult learners, typically aged 40 to 65, who are highly motivated and vocationally oriented; from diverse life situations and faith traditions; with a variety of nursing experiences, most having worked five or more years. Their levels of nursing education include those from diploma, associate, baccalaureate, master's, and post-master's programs. Commonality among learners is that all are registered nurses with a particular interest in the integration of health, faith, and spiritual care. Many verbalize a sense of "being called" to parish nursing, whereas others are only beginning to explore the ideas inherent in the role.

One goal I have as a parish nursing educator seeking to promote dual competencies is to facilitate individuals' understanding of parish nursing along with discernment of their call to ministry. The parish nurse educator is needed to do the following:

- Provide critical feedback.
- Guide, affirm, and encourage.
- Provide essential information.
- Promote development of basic ministry skills needed to begin to practice effectively within parish nurse roles.
- Nurture students' spiritual growth.
- Role-model creative teaching.
- Support the development of a parish nurse community.

Although learner-focused teaching is ideal, curriculum planning and implementation must address the parish nurse role expectations as defined by the *Scope and Standards of Faith Community Nursing* (2005), with a particular focus on aspects of spiritual care.

The term *faith community nursing,* which has been used in Australia for many years, is being used increasingly in the United States and Canada to include more faith groups for which the term "parish" may be confusing or seem inappropriate. Faith community nursing includes those who may use the title *parish nurse, congregational nurse,* or *health ministry nurse.* For purposes of this chapter, the traditional term parish nurse in its generic sense is used because of its current familiarity.

All courses for parish nurses need not be multidisciplinary but should provide educational opportunities for parish nurses in a collegial learning environment, which is essential to the development of dual competencies. Cross-cultural dialogue among different professionals—particularly students of theology, ethics, pastoral studies and counseling—increases respect for the gathered wisdom and the unique body of knowledge of each discipline. Whether for continuing education or for academic credit, the small group dynamics of four to 16 participants provides for the most effective teacher-learner interaction and group discussions, both of which are essential components for the content and transformative process of parish nursing education. A variety of formats and methods honor learner needs, interests, and learning styles and incorporate opportunities for group sharing, personal reflection, integration, and transformative (literally life-changing) content and process. Specific teaching strategies to promote dual competency may include: reading assignments (with written reflection required) that reflect the body of literature from the disciplines of theology, pastoral studies, and ethics as well as nursing. Lectures; small and large group discussions; role play; case studies; journaling; student presentations as individuals or groups; videos; overheads; handouts; guest lecturers from a variety of health ministry-related disciplines; opportunities to meet practicing parish nurses, health ministers, and clergy; individual mentoring; meditation; worship and prayer, including opportunities to plan and lead, can also

be used. Opportunities to learn "in community" need to be balanced by opportunities for personal introspection and reflection.

According to Ramshaw (1988), using music, art, poetry, and other multisensory modalities, including rituals that incorporate the fine arts (e.g., drama and dance) as a mode of expression, is an attempt to momentarily concretize the abstract, which is particularly helpful concerning spiritual issues. Use of the fine arts promotes cultural sensitivity while also providing variety in the learning activities that are auditory, visual, and kinesthetic and recognize a variety of individual learning styles. For those who will lead worship in the future as an intervention to promote healing, the experience of using the fine arts and multisensory modalities provides helpful models of how to relate to the varied learning styles of worshipers.

One would be remiss in ending a statement on the philosophy and assumptions of parish nursing education without mentioning the importance of evaluation in developing dual competencies. Perhaps one might say it is *dually* important. For nursing and/or ministry education, ongoing evaluation of the educational process (via verbal feedback from teaching colleagues and learners before, during, and in the process as well as formal ending evaluation forms) provides feedback for continuous quality improvement. Because a multidisciplinary experience is more complex, ongoing evaluation is critical. Evaluation generally is extremely valuable and recognizes that teaching and learning are lifelong experiences. Because the focus of parish nursing is whole person, intentional care of both flesh and soul, education for parish nursing must be preparation for a nursing specialty as well as preparation for professional ministry, demanding dual competencies in basic and entry levels as well as advanced levels of the practice.

Personal Professional Competency as Both Nurse and Minister

Some have asked "Why a Master of Science in Nursing degree and a Master of Divinity degree?" As mentioned previously, each curriculum offered components this parish nurse considered important for advanced practice in parish nursing. The 36-hour (plus clinical hours) nursing degree consisted of all required nursing courses with the exception of two or three electives. The Webster University graduate curriculum focus is on Family Nursing (a perfect fit with parish nursing) with secondary focus options in nursing education or clinical practice. The choice to work on a master's degree in nursing was in part because an MSN is considered a minimal requirement to teach in any academic institution's school of nursing; appropriately, the electives in educational strategies, teaching methodologies, and curriculum development were taken. Besides the capability for more complex assessment, critical analysis, and practice at an advanced general nursing level, the nursing graduate studies also helped develop skills needed for writing, assisting with research, consultation, and mentoring of new parish nurses.

Completion of my graduate nursing degree did not include courses in pastoral care, scriptural studies, or studies in ministry, liturgy, theology, homiletics, or ethics. To gain competence in ministry on a professional level, seminary course work (81 credit hours plus 7 units of Field Education) was pursued. For many Christian denominations as well as in Judaism and other faiths, it is a tradition to value well-educated spiritual leaders, including clergy and other persons in ministry, such as pastoral counselors, ministers of music, youth ministers, and congregation administrators. In some denominations, parish nurses are now also expected to have some theological and ministry studies as part of their preparation for ministry. Completion of a degree may not be required, but minimally introductory studies in scripture and pastoral care are highly recommended.

Ecclesiastical Recognition and Authorization of Ministry

A number of faith groups and/or denominations have developed criteria and processes for preparation and entry into ministry as a parish nurse. In some cases, the expectations are minimal, but they do provide for a public celebration and acknowledgement of the parish nurse's service and gifts as recognized by the faith community. In other cases, requirements for authorizing parish nurse ministry are only slightly less than are expected for ordained clergy.

Just as a kaleidoscope of traditions in liturgy, worship rituals, polity, and creeds among ecumenical and interfaith groups exist, a similar variety is reflected in the ecclesiastical recognition and authorization of parish nursing/faith community nursing. This is reflected within just a few models in St. Louis, including the United Church of Christ, Missouri Synod Lutheran Church, and the Episcopal Church. Within the United Church of Christ, parish nurses serve in both paid and unpaid positions. Some work as few as several hours each week, whereas others work full time. Those who work in at least half-time positions and who are paid generally are those interested in seeking standing as "professionals" in ministry. Although doing so is optional, the individual may decide—with the congregation's support—to seek standing as a minister in the United Church of Christ.

Within the UCC, three types of recognized and authorized ministry—commissioned, licensed, and ordained—exist. Ordained ministry is the lifelong standing conferred on clergy who have the broadest responsibility for church leadership, including administering the sacraments, preaching, teaching, and pastoral care. The position requires seminary education with completion of a Master's of Divinity, with only a very few exceptions. Licensed ministers, although they have not completed a seminary education, are granted limited authorization to perform the ordained functions of Word and Sacraments, for a particular location and time period. Commissioned ministers are recognized and authorized for a particular specialized area of ministry (such as parish nursing) that requires special education—but not the broadest preparation as for ordained ministry. Although each local association determines its specific criteria (some expect extensive course work; others a minimal amount), all comply with the minimal denominational guidelines. As parish nurses become aware of the option of commissioning, they may choose to become a commissioned minister for the personal growth as well as the recognition and credibility it brings to the ministry of parish nursing. As commissioned ministers, some parish nurses may be eligible to participate in the benefit plans or seek a new position through the denomination search and call system.

The Missouri Synod Lutheran Church has an approved certificate program in parish nursing, offered through Concordia University in Mequon, Wisconsin, which prepares parish nurses, whether paid or unpaid, for what is recognized as diaconal ministry. The Episcopal church also has had an elaborate educational process that parish nurses may pursue to seek standing as ordained deacons, a consecrated position. This recognizes and authorizes one for service or diaconal ministry, which includes ministry of the Word, the preaching and proclaiming of the Gospel, but it does not authorize ministry of the Sacraments. Other denominations and faith groups have similar ecclesiastical processes, whereas others have no expectations or established plan for recognizing the ministry of parish nurses.

Ecumenical, Interfaith, and Multidiscipline Settings

The importance of dual competencies extends into *ecumenical, interfaith, and multidiscipline settings* common to many parish nurse ministerial settings. A background in theology, church history, and world religions is helpful for interpretation and collaboration in a culturally sensitive and congruent manner, as the parish nurse may need to be the facilitator of bridge-building dialogue. Other times the parish nurse may be called to a prophetic or advocate role, as one who speaks to the community, calling it to live into the vision and mission of their faith. As a multidiscipline professional, the parish nurse uses his or her healthcare expertise to facilitate access through the healthcare system while also "translating" as necessary for church members who trust the parish nurse as one of their spiritual caregivers.

Personal Sense of Call

Among the reasons to develop dual competencies, over and above one's philosophy of parish nursing education and quest for personal professional competence, is the personal sense of call or desire to live out a vocation of healing in the broadest sense of whole person care. The desire to incorporate healing modalities of the sacraments and rituals of worship and preaching as spiritual care may compel one to seek dual competencies in nursing as well as ministry.

From more than a decade in ministry, I have learned that renewal of one's own spirit, energy, and focus comes only by again and again grounding and centering one's self through meditation and study of scripture and prayer. Although the wider responsibility and demands of being a clergyperson can be very stressful and wearisome, an advantage of being a pastor is that in preparing to preach and lead worship at least weekly one is "forced" to spend time studying and meditating on scripture and in prayer as preparation. As a parish nurse, personal devotions, scripture study, and prayer often got squeezed out while I attempted to make another visit or plan another program. Without the constant intentional re-grounding, renewal, and nurture of faith as well as acquiring adequate skills to sustain oneself in ministry, one's sense of call may become confused and even deteriorate to a sense of burnout and compassion fatigue.

Credibility of Parish Nursing

Development of dual competencies for parish nursing is important to promoting the credibility of parish nursing within the profession of nursing as well as within the faith group/church denomination. Because many denominations value and expect persons in ministry to be well educated, theologically grounded, mature in faith, and effective communicators, it is important for parish nurses to be well prepared as church professionals to be taken seriously. Besides the ability to communicate well with church and community members, it is advantageous if the parish nurse is theologically articulate—able to think and speak the language of theologians and clergy.

Nearly all parish nurses and coordinators of parish nurse programs will agree that good working relationships with the clergy are essential for effective health ministries. When the parish nurse is capable of using and understanding technical language and concepts of theology, the depth and quality of pastoral care is enriched.

Professional and Personal Faith Development

Coursework in ministry studies or theology is very helpful to develop one's personal systematic theology. To be prepared to respond to the church member that asks, "If God loves me, why I am suffering?" requires having worked through many of those same questions for oneself. Being a theology student provides the opportunity to struggle with the "God questions" and issues of life with an organized and intentional approach to explore and ponder questions concerning the Divine. Such opportunities are not part of one's nursing education.

Beyond the critical thinking and assessment skills of graduate nursing courses, ministry requires an understanding of church and world history for perspective, particularly in ecumenical and interfaith encounters. Also learning a variety of hermeneutical tools allows for identification of the interpretative lens of the client and self as caregiver asking, "What do I bring to this situation, and in what ways do my biases influence my care and ministry with this person?" It is a professional goal to be able to evaluate a client's needs while being aware of how one's own foreknowledge, limitations, and boundaries may influence assessment, evaluation, and subsequent care.

Studies in ministry and theology for the parish nurse develop one's own spiritual disciplines for a lifetime of spiritual formation and grounding. Seminary level courses provide the advanced level for those who are spiritually mature, yearning for more in-depth knowledge as one's faith seeks understanding and ongoing renewal and strengthening.

When taking seminary level course work to develop dual competencies, the parish nurse can develop advanced skills to integrate faith and healthcare. Rarely are spiritual care skills *per se* taught (if they are at all) as part of undergraduate or graduate nursing curriculum. In some cases, a limited number of electives may be used to include pastoral care studies or other practical or applied theology courses. Such opportunities develop skills for spiritual care and allow the student to recognize spiritual and theological issues at stake, such as the meaning of life or death, one's relationship with the Divine, issues of good and evil, and existence of suffering and pain. These studies also make it possible to be scripturally grounded in one's care and ministry, prepared by having intentionally thought through one's own faith understandings and beliefs, have a sense of self with integrity, to have something of substance to offer in the "care of souls."

Educational Opportunities for Parish Nursing Beyond Basic Level

Pursuing a seminary degree is one option in light of the limited availability of advanced educational programs specific to parish nursing. Most advanced offerings are for continuing education rather than academic credit. Advanced degree-bearing programs relevant or specific to parish nursing have been slow in development for several reasons. Budgets to grow and maintain both schools of theology and schools of nursing remain tight, without additional resources for new program start-up, particularly if there are insufficient numbers of enrollees to cover program costs. With parish nursing being a fairly young nursing specialty less than two decades old, a limited number of qualified, multidisciplinary faculty experienced in parish nursing exists. As the shortage of nursing educators grows in general because of retirements and fewer younger nurses entering nursing education, how this trend will affect the future of parish nursing as well as nursing as a whole is of great concern. Despite these challenges, many possibilities exist for developing innovative, academic programs that will prepare parish nurses as leaders within faith communities. The key seems to be collaboration and partnerships between faith groups, schools of nursing, schools of theology, and funding bodies that value the integration of faith and health for the well-being of individuals and communities.

Embodiment of Integration: Four Keys to Success

Four keys to the successful journey of developing advanced level dual competencies through completion of academic degrees (such as the combination of MSN and M.Div. degrees or other graduate or post-graduate degrees such as in Christian Ministry, Pastoral Studies, or a Master of Arts in Health Care Mission) are process learning/reflective thinking, institutional/denominational support, financial support, and a personal support system.

Process Learning and Reflective Thinking

Including a strong process-learning component with both reflective thinking and group interaction is important for the ministry of parish nursing practice, but they appear to have limited or be lacking in MSN programs. For theology students the experience of "ministry seminar" provides the opportunity to reflect on one's own practice of ministry and how theology is applied. Written guidelines are the starting point for reflection, self-evaluation, peer critique, and group discussion.

When participants in CPE and Ministry seminars come from more than one discipline (e.g., chaplain, parish nurse, medical social worker, parish pastor, counselor), the multidiscipline exposure and interaction can be tranformative and integral to this learning process. An interdisciplinary approach (or dialogue *between* disciplines) that may occur in the presence of one or more disciplines (*multi*disciplinary) is reliant on overlapping skills and knowledge of more than one discipline, thus resulting in synergistic effects in which outcomes are enhanced and more comprehensive than possible from input of a single discipline.

A good example of the value of interdisciplinary discourse comes from the ancient wisdom story of the blind men who attempt to describe an elephant, each contributing from his own limited perspective various attributes of the elephant. No individual on his or her own holds the entire truth but together can come very close to an accurate description, and so it is that interdisciplinary dialogue enhances the learning process in preparation for the practice of parish nursing and ministry.

Institutional and Denominational Support

Without a doubt, the encouragement and openness of the academic institutions and the denomination with which the student is affiliated are key to successful development of dual competencies at advanced levels. The capability to be creative and innovative begins with the willingness to "think outside the box," to consider ways other than how things have traditionally been done. This requires that both academic and ecclesiastical administrators are confident and clear in their understanding of the vision and goals of the student who is seeking advanced competencies in nursing and ministry. These administrators also must have a high level of trust and comfort with the particular student's character, professionalism, and reasons for initiating such a collaborative endeavor.

Financial Support

Graduate and postgraduate programs are costly. Given the reality that the majority of active parish nurses practice in unpaid situations or in very low "below market" levels of income (considering what nurses in other settings are paid with equivalent education and experience), individuals that consider graduate study generally find it necessary to seek funding and/or financial sponsors. For support to be adequate, monies may need to come from a combination of sources, which may include healthcare institutions' employee tuition benefit plans, professional nursing organizations, not-for-profit philanthropic individuals or organizations particularly interested in promoting health and wellness and/or faith and health connections, seminary scholarship funds, denominational grants, and local congregations.

Other creative financing strategies may include entering into a "work study covenant." This arrangement involves a mutual agreement in which the student works a certain number of hours for the academic institution in turn for a waiver of a specified number of credit hours of course work. It was such a covenant with Eden Theological Seminary (Webster Groves, Missouri) that covered a major portion of the 81 credit hours plus field education costs toward completion of my Master of Divinity degree. Over a 6-year period both the seminary and I benefited by this agreement because the hours served were in the role of the seminary parish nurse. This was a new position that brought insights to the seminary community of students, faculty, staff, and their families (many of whom lived on campus). All had access to the parish nurse, and I fulfilled all usual parish nurse roles via regular office hours and less formal presence on campus as a classmate and part-time professional staff person. Not only did this work-study covenant make a seminary education financially feasible for me, but the seminary community also grew in its awareness of congregational health ministry possibilities as well as some increased awareness of personal health consciousness with little or no negative impact on the seminary's operating budget.

Although the data collected during those years has not been processed in any methodical way to date, the overall response to the parish nurse presence was very positive and affirming. One example is the feedback from a variety of faculty members, including Reverend Dr. Hale Schroer, then Eden's Dean of Students, who noted the incidence of flu and serious respiratory infections had been significantly less than previous years. He attributed this to the parish nurse arranging for flu shots on campus and follow-up teaching. In addition to one-on-one consultation, the flu campaign included campus newsletter articles, flyers posted in restrooms and other public gathering places, and lunchtime mini-workshops on lifestyle tips, including the importance of good hand-washing, adequate sleep, regular exercise, and intake of fluids (particularly those high in vitamin C). Unfortunately after I completed coursework in 2002 and no longer needed a tuition waiver, the seminary budget could not accommodate continuing the parish nurse position.

Personal Support System

The support of family and close friends is critical in the quest for dual competencies as an academic journey. Commitment to pursue dual master's degrees or postgraduate studies, simultaneously or separately, involves many sacrifices. Besides the enormous amount of time for class and study taken away from family activities and household responsibilities, the financial impact may be significant. Even in cases in which a major portion of the educational expenses are covered by grants, scholarships, or other sources, the student's income, if any, is usually very small and therefore limits the amount contributed to the family income. This economic reality and its stress on the family must be considered, particularly because it is highly probable that the parish nurse simultaneously may have children of college age who are looking to family for financial support for education.

Beyond the time and money, the emotional and psychological support is even more significant to the parish nurse's success academically as well as generally in this unique multidiscipline practice and ministry. A personal support system is foundational, and all else is built upon it. Besides friends and family members, the faith community

that the parish nurse student claims as "home" has an important role in offering affirmation, encouragement, and prayer that facilitate the embodiment of the vision and push the dream to fruition.

Curriculum Integration

When evaluating curricula for advanced competency development in parish nursing, one needs to find opportunities to explore the many intersections between community and public health concerns and those named as social justice and theological issues. Having the freedom to discover and name these connections that extend from one discipline into others is essential. In such an environment that pushes toward making these connections, the student develops complex, critical thinking behaviors that translate readily toward integration.

One example from personal experience is the use of family systems theories as the basis for the *seminary* course Pastoral Care and Family Dynamics. Several graduate nursing courses and practicum experiences that also used these theories to hone interviewing techniques as interventions followed. Each of these courses had immediate application to my current parish nursing practice and ministry.

In recent years, several institutions have developed integrative models with parish nursing and health ministry in mind. Eden Seminary developed its Master of Pastoral Studies (MAPS) degree that provides a broad foundation for types of ministry that do not require ordination. It is well suited for those interested in areas such as Christian education and parish nursing. Unless the student comes with a master's in nursing or is concurrently enrolled in a nursing program, no advanced nursing course work is included in the program. However, a student can seek out complementary graduate nursing courses as electives from a nursing school such as the neighboring Webster University, with whom Eden has a long-time history of various collaborations. Although relationships between these institutions are cordial, programming can hardly be described as "seamless" and requires meticulous planning and communication by the student. Schools of nursing and schools of theology in other locations certainly have a similar familiarity and history of accepting course work from one another.

Other institutions have programs for nursing and divinity degrees that are within its own system and therefore can accommodate dual competency programs more seamlessly. These include Loyola University (Chicago, Illinois), North Park Covenant Seminary (Chicago, Illinois), Boston College, and Duke University (Durham, North Carolina). Some students have completed dual degrees in nursing and theology or ministry through these programs since their inception. Students have completed graduate-level certificate programs such as that offered at Andover-Newton School of Theology (Newton Centre, Massachusetts), which offers an inter-disciplinary curriculum designed as preparation for congregational health ministry. Many of its students are registered nurses, but the program also includes social workers, psychologists, and chaplains as well as those working toward their Master of Divinity or Pastoral Studies degree. Other health ministry-related programs are being developed similar to that at Aquinas School of Theology (St. Louis, Missouri), which offers a Master of Arts in Health Care Mission designed specifically for health-care professionals.

Reflections

It seems appropriate to conclude such a chapter as this by reflecting upon the challenges, advantages, and disadvantages of developing dual competencies. As mentioned earlier, the financial considerations are significant and are the primary deterrent to pursuing dual competencies.

Some may choose to forego advanced degrees because any significant financial investment into parish nursing education has little or no potential for financial payback. Grant and scholarship resources are limited and not as obvious as for other areas of graduate or doctoral studies. The parish nurse student must be innovative and assertive to attract funding.

Finances are one hurdle; the time and personal effort are also more than many are willing to commit. Working on dual degrees simultaneously lengthens the time to complete either degree when done separately. My degrees were completed in 7 years. The first 3 years were dedicated to seminary studies alone, whereas the last four years involved course work for both the M.Div. and MSN. Although the simultaneous work allowed for extraordinary opportunities for ongoing multidisciplinary integration, the sequence and availability of courses at times was "out of sync" when spread out over more time than that required for the full-time student of theology or nursing. A student pursuing either of these programs part time would complete it in 3 to 4 years at the most.

Access to a theological seminary as well as access to a graduate nursing program in some locations is a challenge. Fortunately, some graduate-level health ministry programs are being offered online, such as those offered through North Park Covenant Seminary and Loyola University Chicago. More basic level parish nurse preparation courses are also going online. Some are credit-bearing but are primarily offered for continuing education units.

Lack of familiarity with or openness to parish nursing and health ministry on the part of administration, faculty, student peers, and colleagues can at times feel very lonely, frustrating, and wearisome in the repeated interpreting of the vision and goal of the "pioneering" effort of multidisciplinary education. Answering the question of "why someone would do that" also includes explaining reasons for choosing to complete two master's rather than an equivalent (or somewhat less) amount of work to complete a doctoral degree. Asking programs directly about how the student can integrate education in the two realms is important. If the program cannot answer the question, the student may choose to continue the search for a program. Academic institutions may consider it financially risky to invest in development of a curriculum to accommodate dual degrees in nursing and divinity/theology because the current demand for such dual programs is limited. However, interest appears to be growing with the maturing of parish nursing as a specialty practice.

A very practical and desirable aspect of simultaneous and/or collaborative dual degree work is keeping in touch with the newest concepts and best practices of the nursing profession. By far the greatest advantage of developing dual competencies is the enhanced quality and professionalism of practice. The very presence of the parish nurse student in a dual program brings a multidisciplinary perspective to student colleagues, administration, and faculty, who otherwise may be unfamiliar with the ministry of parish nursing practice. The dual degree nursing and divinity student has the opportunity to introduce and increase awareness of health ministries concepts through papers and presentations and written reflections upon integrating both nursing and theological texts and course work. One example is the paper I presented at The Thirteenth Annual Westberg Parish Nursing Symposium, "Worship and Ritual as Wise Parish Nurse Interventions." Adapted from a paper written for a liturgy and worship seminary course, this paper explored and developed the rationale for incorporating concepts of worship and liturgy into the ministry of parish nurse practice reflecting on the family systems theory.

Along with the freedom to explore, process, and continually integrate new insights and knowledge, the manner in which scheduling is handled is critical. Both personal and institutional flexibility is an absolute requirement and in many cases is the only practical way for some in ongoing practice and ministry to pursue any graduate work, much less the more complicated endeavor of dual degrees. Part of the necessary flexibility is the openness to "trade" or accept some electives between schools. This optimizes the use of valuable time, energy, and financial resources.

Conclusion

All parish nurses should have some theological course content within their orientation and parish nurse basic preparation courses, with the purpose of preparing specifically for the unique setting of faith communities and ministry. Realistically, more advanced seminary-level or graduate nursing course work may not be practical or necessary. It depends on the particular setting and level of practice as well as personal resources and life situation. All parish nurses, however, are expected to practice at a minimal level of competency in both nursing and ministry as defined by the ANA *Scope and Standards for Practice for Faith Community Nursing* (2005).

Those who feel called and who desire preparation for congregational ministry at a level as defined by the traditions and expectations of their denomination may choose to pursue dual degrees. Others may see dual degrees in nursing and ministry to be highly valued and sought after for positions of management and administration of parish nursing programs and other health and human service church-sponsored institutions. Healthcare professionals with theological, pastoral care, and/or health ministries degrees are prepared appropriately to uphold traditions of the sponsoring faith group and maintain its vision and mission of compassionate care. Others may feel compelled to pursue dual competencies in response to the challenge within the ANA *Scope and Standards of Faith Community Nursing Practice* (2005) as a personal contribution to promote the ongoing professional development of parish nursing as a relatively new nursing specialty. Yet others cite among their reasons preparation for future parish nursing certification through the ANA. This credentialing process may be many years away, if it ever arrives. The number of parish nurses requesting this credential will need to grow substantially as the financing to begin the development and maintenance of a certification process is quite expensive. Ultimately, the primary reasons for developing dual competencies are for the preparation of ministry and fulfilling Westberg's vision for the future of parish nursing by maintaining its spiritual focus.

REFERENCES

American Nurses Association. (2005). *Scope and standards of faith community nursing practice*. Washington D.C.: Author.

Cross, S.S. (1999). Worship and ritual as wise parish nurse interventions. In *Proceedings: Thirteenth Annual Westberg Parish Nursing Symposium: A journey in wisdom*. Itasca, IL: (pp. 241-250). International Parish Nurse Resource Center. Advocate Health Care.

Ramshaw, E. (1988). *Ritual and pastoral care*. Philadelphia: Fortress Press.

Westberg, G. (1990). *The parish nurse*. Minneapolis: Augsburg.

Competencies in Parish Nursing Practice

Jayne Britt

13

Whether ministry within a congregation or a professional nursing practice, people are more concerned today about the competency of the person providing the service. Consumers are more knowledgeable and informed. Many different religious denominations have formation programs, certificates in ministry, or other mechanisms for ensuring that those that are providing service on behalf of the denomination/congregation have a level of competence to do so.

Historically, the profession of nursing and individual nurses within the profession have accepted an inherent responsibility to demonstrate effectiveness and expertise in the duties performed. Professional nurses strive to "do no harm": to provide safe, competent care. A concerted effort helps to protect patients from injury and promote their optimal health and well-being by understanding the implications of the care provided and the potential consequences of substandard care. The professional nurse, since Florence Nightingale, has been accountable for continually upgrading skills and knowledge, being aware of standards of care, and recognizing the responsibility for assessing and maintaining a safe level of practice. This accountability has been demonstrated through measurements such as registration, credentialing, licensure, certification, and accreditation as well as tools such as orientation checklists or skill inventories. Recognition of the need to demonstrate and measure competency has reached a pragmatic level in today's society. The global market includes frequent movement of professionals between locations, including institutions, regions, and even countries, thus increasing current interest in validating nursing competencies.

Nursing practice has become more complex. Nurses in all roles must have knowledge in multiple dimensions—including financial, political, technical, sociocultural, and ethical—as well as leadership and communication skills (Krejci, Wessel, & Malin, 1997). Recognition of the need to accurately demonstrate competency has drawn focus from accrediting organizations, such as the Joint Commission on Accreditation of Healthcare Organizations (JCAHO, 2003), which now includes review of competency policies and validation in their survey standards. Permeating all of this is a current, general increase in the public's interest and awareness of the need for accountability in all areas of the marketplace. And this search for accountability is perhaps especially strong in relation to the delivery of health services, no matter what the setting.

Parish nurses find themselves in a unique, independent practice and ministry situation. They practice in a multitude of program model situations: paid, unpaid, institution-based, and so on. But in all situations and practice models, the parish nurse maintains a responsibility to self, professional practice standards, the *Scope and Standards of Parish Nursing*, the faith community served, patients, and God, to develop and maintain competency in the ministry of parish nursing practice. Because the parish nurse maintains a certain level of independence in all practice models, determination of learning and competency needs will more consistently be self-directed. Institution-based models of parish nursing will, at times, require that new information or skills be learned by all employees, or by certain parts of the organization, very often to maintain compliance with regulatory requirements. Examples of this are patient confidentiality training related to Federal HIPAA regulations, CPR certification, Safety, and Infection Control training. Other than this institution-based example, parish nurses will most often be responsible for assessing and defining their own educational, core, ongoing, and specific practice needs and will also be responsible for formulating methods of compliance to demonstrate identified competencies.

Defining Competency

But how is competency defined? Definitions of competency are numerous. Although each group or organization should develop its own definition, some examples are the following:

- The specification of knowledge and skill and the application of that knowledge and skill to the standard of performance required in the workplace (AQTFS, 1999)
- The effective application of knowledge and skill in the work setting (delBueno, Barker, & Christmyer, 1980)
- The attributes of knowledge, abilities, skills, and attitudes that underlie competent performance (Gonczi, Hager, & Oliver, 1990)

Key terms in these or any definition of competency are *performance and application* of knowledge and skills. Competency is not only the understanding of a process, procedure, or technique; but it is also the demonstration of the ability to *effectively* apply knowledge or skill in situations such as a work setting. In this respect, effectiveness and competency are not synonymous. Effectiveness denotes the ability to produce a satisfactory result, based on a predetermined action. Competence is an integral component of effectiveness, as one must have competence to produce effective results. In nursing, "competence underlies the ability to be professionally effective" (Deane & Campbell, 1985, p. 7).

If one looks at the components of competence as building blocks, personal characteristics and abilities, along with acquired skills, knowledge, and information, meld to form a base or foundation that presents itself in behavior and performance. Formalizing and giving structure to the assessment of the end behavior and performance then translates into competency assessment (Figure 13-1).

Dimensions of Competency

Because of the complexity of overall nursing practice, numerous dimensions are included in nursing competence. One framework for nursing competencies that uses a broad-based professional competency model includes the dimensions of conceptual, technical, contextual, interpersonal communication, integrative, and adaptive areas of

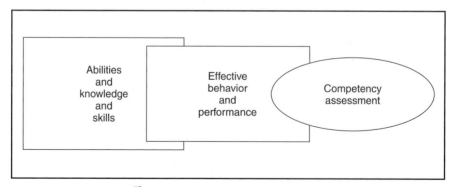

Figure 13-1 Competency Assessment.

Clinical/Technical	Critical Thinking	Interpersonal
Cognitive skills	Problem solving	Communication
Knowledge	Time management	Customer service
Psychomotor skills	Priority setting	Conflict management
Technical understanding	Planning	Delegating
(ability to follow	Creativity	Facilitating
directions, carry out	Ethics	Collaborating
procedures, etc.)	Resource allocating	Directing
	Fiscal responsibility	Articulating
	Clinical reasoning	Understanding diversity
	Reflective practice	Team skills
	Learning	
	Change management	

Figure 13-2   Basic categories in each of the three competency domains. (From Wright, D. [1998]. *The ultimate guide to competency assessment in healthcare.* Eau Claire, WI: Creative Healthcare Management, p. 18.)

competency (Illinois Articulation Initiative, 2004). These areas may be more easily grouped into the three dimensions or domains of cognitive/critical thinking, psychomotor/technical, and attitudinal/interpersonal (Wright, 1998). Figure 13-2 illustrates some basic categories in each of the three domains.

Types of Competency

Competency assessment for healthcare professionals is an ongoing process, ultimately designed toward a commitment to meet patients' needs.

Educational Competencies

The competency process begins with educational competencies embedded in the educational system. Each healthcare-related profession defines its own educational competencies, based on the knowledge and skill development required to perform within the discipline. In a broader view, the 2003 Institute of Medicine (Tanner, 2003) provided direction for clinical education by identifying five competencies in which all clinicians, regardless of their discipline, should be proficient. They are the following:

- Providing patient-centered care
- Working in interdisciplinary teams

- Using evidence-based practice
- Applying quality improvement
- Using informatics

This kind of movement toward interdisciplinary educational competency for all healthcare providers may be seen as a favorable attempt to affect the overall system in its provision of safe, consistent, and effective patient care.

Hiring Competencies

Hiring competencies are determined by the organization, department, or individual responsible for employee hiring. Hiring also may be influenced by compliance with regulatory requirements from local, state, or federal levels. Hiring competencies may include review of such items as education, previous experience, licensure, registration, and/or other interview criteria.

Core Competencies

The application of the basic skills, knowledge, abilities, and understanding required to perform and fulfill a specific job description are considered core competencies and are reviewed and considered—but not fully assessed—in the initial hiring process. These core competencies may be exceeded by an individual but are considered minimally accepted demonstration of the ability to perform effectively after being placed in the role within a specific time frame (e.g., 6 months or 1 year). Core competencies are developed for a position and are job description-specific.

Annual or Ongoing Competencies

Annual or ongoing competencies are designed to meet specific needs that have been identified on an annual or ongoing basis. These often reflect an identified problem, high-risk situation, learning deficiency, or desire to acquire new skills or knowledge by a group or individual. However, they may also be a response to such things as training needs for a new policy, procedure, or equipment. Annual/ongoing competencies that are organizational or organization-wide should have content tailored to apply to specific roles and job descriptions, thus making the competency job- or practice-specific.

Age-Specific Competencies and Cultural Competencies

Age-specific competencies and cultural competencies identify characteristics, needs, and traits that are unique within specific age and cultural groups and assess the ability of the healthcare worker to understand these diversities and apply this knowledge to their practice, in both tasks and situations. Age-specific and cultural competencies may be assessed by themselves, as stand-alone competencies, or may be incorporated into core or annual/ongoing competencies in practice-specific procedures or situations.

Competencies of all kinds must be viewed as components of an ongoing process, which fold into and compliment each other. Beginning with the definition of knowledge and skill training required by the educational system, continuing with assessment of basic (core) skills and abilities, and progressing to ongoing measurement of application or performance of skills/knowledge as well as assessment of new skills and knowledge, competency assessment is now viewed as part of the professional lifecycle and an integral part of an ongoing healthcare quality process.

Competency Development

Development of a competency begins with a *measurement of current practice* and the *identification of learning needs* or previously acquired skills and knowledge, which need to be demonstrated. This identifies the purpose or intent of the competency being written. Ask what area of practice or what learning need has been identified and will be measured. As an example, are basic/core competencies to be assessed? These are developed from the core elements of the scope of practice and job description, which will serve as guides in their development. Or will it be an annual/ongoing competency, based on the identification of a specific learning need? In this case, the need identified will be the basis for development of the competency.

Once intent and purpose of the competency have been defined, the *practice skill/knowledge or practice change/improvement to be demonstrated* should be defined. What specific learning is needed? What skill must be acquired? And *what must be accomplished* to fulfill the need and meet the competency? The domain should also be identified. Does the competency fall in the dimension of critical thinking, interpersonal, or technical? Or does it overlap two or more of the dimensions?

Last, how will the *competency be demonstrated and verified*? What method of verification will show effective application of the skill/knowledge, either previously acquired or new? Various verification methods may be selected for any given competency. Many different verification methods need to be selected—including post-tests, case studies, exemplars, peer review, observation of work, and return demonstration. Selecting a verification method appropriate for the competency and keeping in mind that "no one verification method can assess all three skill domains" is important (Wright, 1998, p. 51) (Figure 13-3).

Some questions to summarize and guide the process for development of a competency are the following:

- What is the need, intent, or purpose for the competency?
- How was the need determined?
- What type of competency is it?
- What skill and/or knowledge must be learned and demonstrated?
- What is the dimension(s) of the competency?

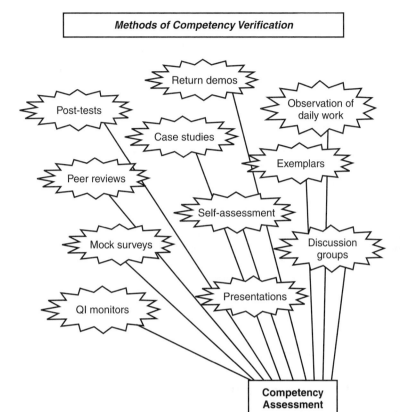

Figure 13-3 Competency Verification Methods. (From Wright, D. [1998]. *The ultimate guide to competency assessment in healthcare.* Eau Claire, WI: Creative Healthcare Management, p. 51.)

- What must be done to prove or acquire the skill, ability or knowledge?
- How will it be verified?

These questions are depicted as a process in Figure 13-4.

From these steps, a simple template can be readily designed for individuals or organizations, which would assist with and standardize the process of competency development. A sample template might look like that in Figure 13-5.

Using a system for competency development and going through predetermined steps such as those described assists in clarifying the learning need and defining what needs to be done and what the desired outcome will be, thus simplifying and demystifying the process.

In addition to being self-directed, the parish nurse includes multiple dimensions of patient care in the scope of the ministry of parish nursing practice. For a registered nurse in a healthcare

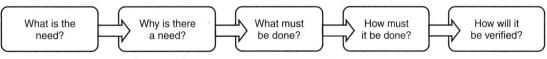

Figure 13-4 Competency Development.

Parish Nurse Competency

Name: _____

Church: _____

Type of competency: _____

Identified learning need: _____

_____

_____

Anticipated skill/knowledge improvement: _____

_____

_____

Competency domain (circle):   *Critical thinking*   *Interpersonal*
                                          Clinical/Technical

Skill/Knowledge will be accomplished by: _____

_____

_____

Competency will be verified by: (method) _____

Figure 13-5 Sample Parish Nurse Competency Template.

setting, items such as changes in the healthcare system that affect practice situations, advances in medicine, technology or equipment improvements, disease management, and others offer a continuing pool of learning needs and opportunities for competency development. Continuing education offerings are available in numerous methods and formats: from lectures and seminars, to periodicals and books, to the Internet and e-courses that meet such competency fulfillment. However, the scope of the ministry of the parish nurse includes more than tangible, physical needs. Parish nurses address whole-person needs; therefore, the parish nurse must consider body-mind-spirit in self-assessment, self-development, and competency development. Body, mind, and spirit needs must be considered and treated as integral components of the individual ministry of parish nursing practice, the faith community served, and the personal and individual needs of the parish nurse. Following are examples of components that could be considered in *body-mind-spirit competency assessment*.

Body

- Physiologic, disease-specific knowledge and information
- Infant care and information for new parents in the church
- Pathophysiology of substance abuse and addiction
- Age or culture concerns within the faith community
- Infection control measures in the church's nursery or preschool
- Publication of revised B/P guidelines
- Several new diabetic patients in the congregation

Ask:

- What situation has made me feel unprepared?
- Am I able to _____?

Mind

- Emotional/behavioral aspects of self or the practice
- Dynamics of interpersonal relationships
- Communication skills
- Current information regarding depression, ADD/ADHD, anxiety, stress, bipolar disorders, etc.
- Age/culture issues relating to behavioral health
- Working with clergy
- Working with congregations
- Developing a health ministry team

Ask:

- What situation has made me feel unprepared?
- Am I able to _____?

Spirit

- Theological reflection and personal spiritual development
- Spiritual formation exercises
- Spiritual direction opportunities
- Age/culture issues relating to religious diversity
- Recognized need for self—time, reflection, meditation, prayer
- Recognized need to feed and renew your spirit
- Spiritual retreats

Ask:

- What situation has made me feel unprepared?
- Am I able to _____?

Because parish nurse competency development is self-directed, it is easily structured with use of resources.

1. Developing competencies for the ministry of parish nursing practice begins with identification of the need for basic educational preparation specific to the practice (such as the International Parish Nurse Resource Center Basic Preparation). Completion of a basic preparation course in parish nursing and familiarity with the *Scope and Standards of Parish Nursing* (ANA, 1998) will provide a new parish nurse the educational and core competencies needed to initiate a ministry of parish nursing practice.
2. From this starting point, using the body-mind-spirit approach, with honest self-reflection, analysis, and prayer, the nurse can identify learning needs. These identified learning needs become annual or ongoing competencies.
3. A competency development format or template can then be used for structure and focus.
4. Using available resources, including peers in the ministry of parish nursing practice, will make completing and validating the competency an uncomplicated process.

An example of some competencies that have been implemented by some parish nursing programs are cultural competency, HIPAA, state child abuse reporting requirements, age-specific competencies, infection control, advanced directives, parish nurse documentation, change management, interpersonal relationships, setting boundaries and recognition of personal gifts. Figure 13-6

Parish Nurse Competency

Name: _Sally Nurse_

Church: _Faith Church_

Type of competency: _Annual_

Identified learning need: _1. Ongoing need to understand and incorporate cultural_ _and religious considerations in interpersonal relations. 2. New church members of an_ _ethnic minority group._

Anticipated skill/knowledge improvement: _Awareness and sensitivity to_ _ethnic diversity._

Competency domain (circle): *Critical thinking* *(Interpersonal)* *Clinical/Technical*

Skill/Knowledge will be accomplished by: _View video: "Communicating Across_ _Boundaries"_

Competency will be verified by: _Discussion at church staff meeting._

Figure 13-6 Completed Sample Parish Nurse Competency Template.

demonstrates the use of the parish nurse competency template.

Competency Measurement

Just as no single best definition of *competency* itself exists, no single best method adequately measures competency. This is due mainly to a general lack of consensus on what available method most accurately measures competency.

In addition, no single measurement method can accurately measure *all* competencies.

The measurement method chosen may be as simple as a selection choice of aware/knowledgeable/proficient or as complex as devising an instrument for evaluation of qualitative or quantitative measures and data. Quantitative measurement, such as objective test questions, has been criticized as too task-oriented; whereas qualitative measurement, such as subjective situational observation, may be said to lack definition (Bartlett & Simonite, 2000).

The goal in selecting a measurement method for any given system of competency assessment is that the method chosen be clearly defined, meaningful, and workable for the specific competency. For parish nurses, this translates to matching the competency measurement method to the specific parish nursing situation. Peer review, for example, might have the greatest validity and meaning in measurement of a parish nurse's competency in documentation. On the other hand, a post-test and exemplar might be most effective in measuring a competency related to the federal regulation on patient confidentiality (HIPAA) and how it affects the church setting.

Reviewing the competency dimensions in the process of selecting the measurement tool/instrument is helpful. Is the dimension in the area of critical thinking, interpersonal skills, or technical? The qualitative or quantitative nature of the dimension may then assist in determining what type of instrument might be most valid, meaningful, and workable for the competency being completed. See Figure 13-3 for a selection of measurement and verification methods.

Conclusion

As professional nurses invested in the growth, development, and maturation of the ministry of parish nursing practice, a continued accountability is needed for all that is done to provide safe, competent care to clients while maintaining high standards of practice. The American Nurses Association in collaboration with the Health Ministries Association offers the *Scope and Standards of Parish Nursing Practice* (ANA, 1998), and the International Parish Nurse Resource Center (IPNRC) offers support and resources such as the *Core Curriculum for Parish Nursing Practice* and the *Philosophy, Root Assumptions, and Strategic Vision of Parish Nursing* and many other items, all providing a solid foundation and framework for the ministry of parish nursing practice. Although

they work in a very self-directed capacity, parish nurses maintain an obligation to the profession and a personal responsibility to God and to those served to ensure the highest possible level of competence in care delivered.

It has been proposed that six competencies are required for self-directed learning: "self-assessment of learning gaps; evaluation of self and others; reflection; information management; critical thinking; and critical appraisal" (Patterson & Crooke, 2002, p. 25). How accurately these apply to and how freely they should be embraced by parish nurses in developing competencies for their own ministry of parish nursing practice! Although the competency movement has incurred debate, in the end, it is nurses who will define nursing, and parish nurses who will define the ministry of parish nursing practice. Many parish nurses will have no impetus or requirement to develop competencies in their personal ministry of parish nursing practice. However, the following factors must be taken into account when deciding whether pursuing personal competency development is valuable:

- Learning is a lifelong activity. One must continue to learn and grow as individuals and human beings to remain positive and functional.
- The process of developing self-competencies facilitates learning, personal growth, and motivation.
- As professionals, the nurse must be personally committed and responsible to himself or herself, the profession of nursing, and the ministry of parish nursing practice.
- Called to serve, parish nurses have an obligation to maintain high standards and to further advance the ministry of parish nursing practice in His name.

Competency assessment, development, and implementation is an effective means to demonstrate confidence and ensure full use of all the methods and tools God has given us to perform effectively in caring for all God's people through the ministry of parish nursing practice.

REFERENCES

American Nurses Association. (1998). *Scope and standards of parish nursing practice.* (9806st). Washington, DC: Author.

Australian Qualifications Training Framework Standards. (1999). *Training package for assessment and workplace training.* Assessment Validation Strategies: Australian National Training Authority, Brisbane, QLD4001, Australia.

Bartlett, H. & Simonite, V. (2000). A comparison of the nursing competence of graduates and diplomats from the nursing programmes. *Journal of Clinical Nursing,* 9(3): 369-379.

Deane, D. & Campbell, J. (1985). *Developing professional effectiveness in nursing.* Reston, VA: Prentice-Hall.

delBueno, D.J., Barker, F., & Christmyer, C. (1981 Feb). Implementing a competency-based orientation program. *Journal of Nursing Administration,* vol II (2): 24-29.

Gonczi, A., Hager, P., & Oliver, L. (1990). Establishing competency-based standards in the professions. *NOOSR Research Paper no. 1.* Canberra: AGPS.

Illinois Articulation Initiative. (2004). Illinois baccalaureate majors curricula. *Nursing Competencies.* www.itransfer.org/IAI/Majors/Nur/

International Council of Nurses. (2003). ICN offers guidance on global nurse competencies. *ICN Framework of Competencies for the Generalist Nurse.* February, Geneva Council of Nurses.

Joint Commission on Accreditation of Healthcare Organizations. (2003). *Standards and Performance Measures.* Oakbrook, IL: Author.

Krejci, J. Wessel & Malin, S. (1997). Impact of leadership development on competencies. *Nursing Economics,* 15(5): 235-241.

Patterson, C. & Crooks, D. (2002). A new perspective on competencies for self-directed learning. *Journal of Nursing Education,* 41(1): 25-31.

Redman, R. (1999). Competency assessment: Methods for development and implementation in nursing education. *Online Journal of Issues in Nursing,* September 30.

Tanner, C.A. (2003). Building the bridge to quality. *Journal of Nursing Education,* 42(10): 431.

Wright, D. (1998). *The ultimate guide to competency assessment in healthcare.* Eau Claire, WI: Creative Healthcare Management.

Learning to Pray

Annette Langdon

Lord Jesus Christ, come and abide in my heart more and more. Fill me with your Holy Spirit and teach me to pray. Help me receive your great compassion that I may know your grace and confidently share your healing love with those you place in my path.

—Annette Langdon

Introduction

Parish nursing is a melding of nursing and ministry. As the nurse incorporates practices of ministry into the practice of nursing, he or she discovers the incredible importance of prayer and ritual. The parish nurse soon recognizes the need to grow in this area. Knowledge and conversation around the physical aspects of health are familiar. Scripture, prayer, and issues of faith may not be.

As a new parish nurse, I knew my pastor expected me to pray with the people I visited at the hospital. I understood the importance of prayer and intended to pray, but I was too shy to let any of the healthcare staff hear my awkward prayers. I would visit with a parishioner until I thought no one else would be nearby; then I would try to quickly move into prayer. This worked for a while until the day I visited a man who was hard of hearing. He repeated my brief prayer in a very loud voice! God was nudging me to be more concerned with my prayer conversation than with who might be listening.

Student nurses learn to provide privacy when needed: to pull the curtain around the patient or close the door. As parish nurses, we learn to pull the mental curtain around an interaction to create a holy space in which to pray. It takes practice to focus and share a verbal prayer with others, but the value of prayer spurs us to learn.

"Clara," a faithful 80-some year-old member of the congregation, asked me to come and take her blood pressure. "Clara" is one of those people that has sunshine beaming from her face and a big heart full of concern and care for others. Her faith is deep, and her prayer life is active.

I stopped in at "Clara's" apartment, and we chatted for a few minutes before I took her blood pressure, which was within normal range. Our conversation briefly centered on the care of our physical bodies and then moved on to other topics such as family and her activities. After a cup of coffee and more enjoyable conversation, I asked if I could pray with her before I left. She agreed, but when I asked what she would like to pray about, she said, "You just pray." So I prayed. I do not remember what I prayed about, but I do remember that during the prayer, tears came into her eyes. She didn't want to talk about those tears. Brushing them away, she sent me on my way. As I left, I pondered this event. What was it that brought those tears? They didn't come with the close physical contact of a hug or during conversation, even with wonderful open-ended questions. They only came during prayer.

Prayer is a valuable tool offering therapeutic benefits for those the parish nurse encounters and for the parish nurse. Prayer is easily adapted to any given situation or setting and is useful with individuals, small groups, and large gatherings. The action of prayer visibly communicates the integration of faith and health, which is one of the distinctive activities of the parish nurse.

Parish nurses are at various stages of comfort with prayer. Some employ it with ease, whereas others struggle to use it at all. Regardless of where the reader is in her or his prayer life, there is always more to learn about prayer. This chapter encourages the reader to continue growing in her or his use of prayer, personally and professionally.

Exploration of Prayer

Prayer, very simply, is conversation with God. It involves talking and listening. Our expression to God can take many different forms. We may speak, think, sing, write, or dance our thoughts and feelings to God. We may also find expression through painting or playing a musical instrument. The means are endless. Henri Nouwen (1995), a Catholic priest, professor, and author, shares in his book on prayer entitled *With Open Hands* the notion that prayer is a process of opening ourselves to God. Indeed, our life is a prayer.

Our choice of prayer style will vary throughout our lives and with what our hearts are compelled to share with God. At times we will sing praises to God for many blessings or we may speak a need or desire. Sometimes we will shout a word of thanksgiving, whereas other times we will scream with rage at the pain we suffer. In prayer, we can share with God whatever we are experiencing, in whatever manner is comfortable.

Why We Pray

Scripture instructs us to pray. "Pray continually" (1 Thess. 5:17, NIV, 1995, p. 1827). "Ask, and it will be given to you; seek, and you will find; knock, and the door will be opened to you" (Matthew 7:7, NIV, 1995, p. 1448). "Pray for each other so that you may be healed" (James 5:16, NIV, 1995, p. 1884). God wants to be in conversation with us, to hear our praise, our questions, our doubts, our confessions, and our words of thanksgiving. God invites us into a relationship that includes dialogue. How incredible that Jesus tells us to "Ask and you will receive, and your joy will be complete" (John 16:24, NIV, 1995, p. 1625).

If you ask a group of people to reflect for a moment and then share some words that would describe an experience of prayer, the responses are words like peace, comfort, healing, love, affirming, cleansing, nurturing, powerful, calmness, acceptance, gratitude and hope. These are therapeutic thoughts that come through the simple use of prayer.

In the last several decades, there has been a resurgence in the interest in prayer secularly and medically. Polls of the general public disclose that 90% of Americans pray, and scientific research studies reveal the therapeutic value and the use of prayer in healthcare (Gallup, 1999).

One of the first studies on therapeutic use of prayer, "Positive Therapeutic Effects of Intercessory Prayer in a Coronary Care Unit Population," was conducted by Dr. Randolph Byrd (1988) and reported in *the Southern Medical Journal*. It demonstrated that the patients who were randomly selected to be prayed for experienced fewer complications than the control group. This work has been replicated with similar results.

In the early 1990s Larry Dossey, a physician of internal medicine, set out to disprove the mounting research on prayer. He reviewed 130 scientific studies and became convinced of the power of prayer. His book, *Healing Words: the Power of Prayer and the Practice of Medicine* (1993), is interesting to read, as he shares his review of research and his thoughts about the application of prayer in the practice of medicine. In recent years many other publications have confirmed Dossey's beliefs.

As a parish nurse, I find the research on prayer to be fascinating. It is, however, not the motivating factor for my use of prayer. My prayer life flows out of a relationship with Jesus Christ, not out of the most recent research. We may learn many things from scientific research, but our faith needs to be centered in God. See Appendix 14C for questions for further reflection and/or discussion on exploration of prayer.

Embarking on the Journey

For Starters

The best way to learn how to pray and to grow more confident is to do it. Like learning to ride a bike, you can read all you want about how to ride, but at some point, you just need to get on the bike and try it. With prayer, you may want to begin by setting aside 5 to 10 minutes a day to be quiet and pray. In this time, talk out loud or journal your thoughts to God. The physical act of talking or writing will help you focus your thoughts. Then be still for a minute or two and listen. By that, I mean "be open to hear what God would want to tell you."

One commonly used formula for prayer is ACTS, which stands for Adoration, Confession, Thanksgiving, and Supplication (Galli, 1999). These terms are defined in the following ways:

- *Adoration*: praising God for who God is and what He has done.
- *Confession*: asking God for forgiveness.
- *Thanksgiving*: thanking God for blessings and answered prayer.
- *Supplication*: praying for specific needs for self or others.

Another method, TRIP, developed by the Mount Carmel Ministries (2004), is to pray in response to a verse in scripture. It comprises the following components:

- *Thanks*: What in this verse makes me thankful?
- *Regret*: What in this verse causes me regret and moves me to confession?
- *Intercession*: What does this text lead me to pray for?
- *Plan of Action*: What action does this text encourage me to take today?

In whatever manner you pray, make your listening active. Yearn to hear God's voice and what God has to say to you. Psalm 95:7-8 exhorts us, *O that today you would listen to his voice! Do not harden your hearts* (NRSV, 1989, p. 550). Be open to hear what God wants you to pray. We can pray about many things, but to pray in synchronicity with God's will and desire requires listening.

Resistance

There is always resistance to praying. Thoughts such as: *Doesn't God already know everything I'm going to tell him? I don't have time! Why would God want to talk to me? I want to stay in control and I trust myself more than God.* These responses are age-old experiences of pride, self-righteousness, fear, and doubt. They represent obstacles that taunt us even after years of experience.

Then comes all the extraneous thoughts! As soon as you begin to be quiet, they come screaming for attention: *Gotta remember to pay the bills. Don't forget to call .... I wonder how so and so is doing. Remember to pick up....* It takes some discipline and determination to clear one's mind of all the clutter. Closing your eyes, being in a quiet space, and taking some deep breaths can be helpful. Learn to set aside these noisy thoughts by letting them go and gently return your focus to the conversation with God.

Forming Prayer Habits

Like forming any new habit or lifestyle, a daily routine is helpful. Set aside a specific part of the day for prayer, ideally a quiet time when you are least distracted. You may also want to choose a special chair or place where you will pray. A mother of small children used a doily and a candle to help her change her focus from the house to prayer. Setting out the doily and lighting the candle became her preparation for prayer. Once you become used to a routine, you will find yourself moving into prayer automatically, as you come to this designated time and space.

If you have the opportunity to be in a prayer group where you can listen to others pray, it will encourage your prayer life and language. When I first started out as a parish nurse, a small group of women met at the church once a week to pray for those in need. As I listened to their prayers, I learned about faith and God, as well as ways to connect and communicate. I also remember having some prayer time with a retired pastor and his wife. I prayed for their expressed needs, but when they began to pray I felt as though the heavens were opened and we were ushered into God's loving presence.

As you choose a time and place for prayer, you also need to consider a style of prayer that fits you personally. Some people are more suited to a reflective type of prayer, whereas others need some kind of activity to accompany their prayers. A visual person may find art, religious icons, and guided imagery to be what moves them to pray. Someone who is auditory will enjoy listening to scripture and prayers that are read. Another person will appreciate experiential types of praying, such as prayer walking.

Much has been written about the types of prayer that relate best to specific personalities. The Myers-Briggs Personality Indicator (Keating, 1999) is useful, and the findings are intriguing.

Even with the wisdom of such indicators, the journey to self-awareness is sometimes slow. What's important to remember is that there is no single way to pray. What moves one person may or may not be inspirational for another. Be patient with yourself and keep the goal of connecting with God primary. God is faithful. Trust God's faithfulness and God's love for you.

Prayer is hard work and difficult to sustain alone. Regular worship, daily reading of scripture or devotionals, and the support of others will encourage the growth of your prayer life.

Prayer is a lifelong conversation reflecting your relationship with God. Like any relationship, there will be ups and downs, times of closeness and times of distance. What's important is to keep talking, keep praying. Find ways to keep your conversation fresh and interesting (see Appendix 14A for 21 ways to refresh your prayer life).

Lectio Divina

Lectio divina is a type of prayer that is appropriate for all personality types (Michael & Norrisey, 1991, pp. 31-37). It means "divine reading" and can be done in one sitting or spread out over several days. The four steps are the following: reading (lectio), meditation (meditatio), prayer (oratio), and contemplation (contemplatio) (Box 14-1). For ease in remembering the steps, you can think of reading, reflecting, responding, and resting.

First, read aloud a portion of scripture slowly. Savor each word and phrase. Pause or repeat parts that seem to speak to you. Second, meditate on this passage by repeating it over and over. You may want to put emphasis on different parts, to draw out new meaning. Let the scripture touch your heart and speak to your personal needs. Have a notebook ready to jot down insights or reflections. Third, respond to God by sharing whatever you are sensing—gratitude, confession, joy, sorrow,

praise, or petition. You may want to use the ACTS formula to do this. Listen and respond to God as long as you like. Fourth, rest in God's Word for you by simply waiting for whatever God will send your way. This means being still and silent as you wait for the Lord to bring further understanding to your heart or mind. *"Be still and know that I am God"* (Psalm 46:10, NIV, 1995, p. 826).

The steps in *lectio divina* are not so much sequential steps as a dance of dialogue. God leads, and we respond. We pray, and God replies. Follow the leading of the Holy Spirit back to reread the passage, then to prayer, back to the passage, or quiet waiting and listening. There are no rehearsals, no script, only an invitation to enjoy the dance. For further reflection and/or discussion, see Appendix 14C.

Use of Prayer

Learning to Pray with Others

Prayer is very intimate. It takes us to the heart of people's concerns. It is powerful, and tears are not uncommon. It is important to provide privacy and give respect to the tender ground of the heart.

Praying for others is called *intercession*. It is when one stands in the place of another, when one goes before God on behalf of others. It is what we do when we care about others, especially when they are suffering or experiencing difficulties.

When a parish nurse comes to understand the value of prayer and wants to make use of it with others, she often encounters mental obstacles. *What if they don't want to pray? What if I pray the wrong thing? How will I know when to pray and what to say?* With the polls showing that 90% of Americans pray (Gallup, 1999), the parish nurse will err less often by offering prayer than by avoiding it. With practice these questions subside and prayer becomes easier.

To begin, the parish nurse may want to practice at home with a family member or a friend. With parishioners, she or he may want to start by simply holding their hand and praying the Lord's Prayer or by using a prayer from a hymnal or prayer book. Be assured that God will use whatever is offered.

Process of Praying with Individuals

Listening is crucial for knowing what to pray. While visiting with a parishioner, keeping prayer

---

BOX 14-1   Lectio Divina
(Divine Reading)

Reading *(Lectio)*
Meditation *(Meditatio)*
Prayer *(Oratio)*
Contemplation *(Contemplatio)*

concerns in mind will give some insights. Asking parishioners what they want to pray for will give more specific direction. Keeping an ear open to God during the visit or beginning the prayer time with a bit of silence to listen for what God would want you to pray for will give you yet more to put into prayer language.

Introduce the use of prayer with something like, "Prayer is helpful to many people. Would it be alright if I share a word of prayer?" Make it clear that you will speak the prayer and that you do not expect them to pray aloud. Depending on the person's comfort level, she or he may join you in verbally praying, but at the beginning, you can lessen anxiety by offering the prayer.

Identify the concerns to be mentioned in prayer by asking what they would like to pray for. As you have listened, you may have a running list of concerns, but often unexpected requests emerge when you ask specifically. They may want to focus on the needs of their spouses or families or the nurses and doctors who care for them. Give them a few minutes to think about what they would like to include in prayer.

When Jesus met blind Bartimaeus in Mark 10:51, he asked him, *What do you want me to do for you?"* (NIV, 1995, p. 1513). This is a wonderful open-ended question that we can transfer to those we encounter in our parish nurse practice. Here is the Son of God asking for our input. He wants to hear from us, to know what's on our minds. How incredible and encouraging to hear this question from Jesus!

When learning to pray with others, many parish nurses worry about praying the wrong thing. Generally the recipient of prayer will not remember the specifics, but they will remember the experience. Just be yourself. Talk as you would to a dear friend, knowing that prayer is an ongoing conversation. What you pray for today may change by tomorrow. If you are unsure of what to pray, then pray about your uncertainty. If there are no particular concerns, you can always pray a blessing or a prayer of thanksgiving. The general purpose is to be honest before God and to place the one you are praying for into the light of Jesus, to invite God's loving care.

There are many books with prayers that can be a resource for the parish nurse. Hymnals, devotional writings, and denominational prayer books contain some beautiful prayers that can be very meaningful. Being familiar with these resources and the prayers will help the parish nurse select an appropriate prayer.

It is comforting to know that all is not dependent on our meager efforts. Romans 8:26 reminds us that "the Spirit helps us in our weakness. We do not know what we ought to pray for, but the Spirit himself intercedes for us with groans that words cannot express," (NIV, 1995, p. 1720). Pray with assurance that God hears and will make good use of whatever you offer in prayer. Box 14-2 presents the five steps of the process of praying with individuals.

Consider the use of touch with the experience of prayer. The parish nurse may simply clasp the hand of the client or put a hand on the client's shoulder or head. The physical touch will communicate God's love in a gentle, yet powerful, manner. Jesus often reached out and touched those who were suffering and those who were considered unclean, untouchable. A caring touch seems to break through barriers that are unspoken. It communicates in a physical manner, while words speak to the mind. Out of respect for the individual and for the intimacy of prayer, it is essential to obtain permission before proceeding to touch anyone.

Posture may vary in prayer as the position of our body also communicates meaning. There may be times that kneeling is the most appropriate posture, expressing great need or submission. A parish nurse may ask clients to sit with hands upward on their laps, which expresses openness.

BOX 14-2   Process of Praying with Individuals

1. Listen to individual and to God
2. Introduce the use of prayer—"Prayer is often helpful. Would it be okay if I pray for you?"
3. Identify content—"What would you like to pray for?"
4. Consider posture and the use of touch
5. Focus your thoughts—draw a mental "curtain" to create a holy space

At times of gratitude, standing with hands raised is a physical sign of praise. The posture of the body is like an unspoken prayer.

Dealing with Obstacles

Obstacles come in various forms. Sometimes they relate to our faith. Sometimes they come from others or the environment. What's important is to keep your focus on God.

When you are about to suggest praying with someone, doubts may arise. *Who am I to think that I can pray? They aren't going to want to pray. I'll wait until next visit.* These thoughts and many others may come to deter you from moving into prayer. Some discernment is necessary, as there are times when it is inappropriate to suggest prayer. If these thoughts are inner chatter, brush them away and return your thoughts to God.

The environment may also pose a barrier to prayer. The TV or radio may be on. Other people may be in the room or coming in and going out. Do what you can to minimize the distractions. Ask if you may shut the door or turn off the TV or radio. Inform others of your desire for a few minutes without interruption. Just as when you do patient teaching, you want a conducive environment with minimal disturbances.

Regardless of where the parish nurse encounters people in need, there can be a time of prayer. In a noisy narthex, busy hospital hallway, or a quiet corner, the parish nurse can mentally draw a curtain and focus on one individual and his or her concerns. It will become a holy place where God is met. The specific words and surrounding environment are less important than the prayer from the heart.

Praying Scripture

Praying scripture can be very meaningful. After reading a portion of scripture, fold all of it or phrases of it into a prayer that specifically addresses the client's needs. Several resources or books offer this for specific situations or needs (Copeland, 1997). They take a Psalm or Bible passage and turn it into a prayer. (See Appendix 14B for a list of topics and scripture.) Box 14-3 presents one example of praying scripture.

Isaiah 43:1-4 can be personalized by inserting a name in place of Jacob and Israel: *"But now thus says the Lord, he who created you, O_____, he who*

BOX 14-3   Praying Scripture

Psalm 41:3:   The Lord sustains those on their sickbed; in their illness you, Lord, heal all their infirmities.

Prayer: Lord, sustain (person) in these days and hours before surgery. Heal (his/her) sickness and other weaknesses and make (him/her) strong.

Source: Person, G. (2001). *Psalms for healing: praying with those in need.* Minneapolis: Augsburg.

---

formed you, O _____: Do not fear, for I have redeemed you; I have called you my name, you are mine. When you pass through the waters, I will be with you; and through the rivers, they shall not overwhelm you; when you walk through fire you shall not be burned, and the flame shall not consume you. For I am the Lord your God, the Holy One of Israel, your Savior. …You are precious in my sight, and honored, and I love you" (NRSV, 1989, p. 672).

Another example is using Philippians 4:6-7: *"Do not be anxious about anything, but in everything, by prayer and petition, with thanksgiving, present your requests to God. And the peace of God, which transcends all understanding, will guard your hearts and your minds in Christ Jesus"* (NIV, 1995, p. 1810-1811). From this passage, one can pray, *"O Lord God, we admit that we are anxious and worried. Forgive us. We now pray for (name), and specifically ask for (requests). We trust this into your care and await your peace. In Jesus' name. Amen."*

One of the ways to discover biblical passages meaningful to the client is to ask them. When I visited an elderly man who had been in the hospital and extended care setting for several months, I asked him if there was any particular scripture that spoke to him during this difficult time. He responded quickly, "Psalm 13!" I turned to the psalm, not knowing it, and read *"How long, O Lord? Will you forget me forever? How long will you hide your face from me?"* (Psalm 13:1, NIV, 1995, p. 790). This psalm spoke poignantly of the man's pain and affirmed for him that God indeed understood what he was going through.

Praying with Families

When family members are present, the parish nurse may want to involve them in praying for the client. Consent to do so is advised if one is unsure of the status of the relationships. Inviting the family members to hold hands or place hands on their loved one gives them permission to come close and to express their care through touch. It may also acknowledge their own pain in watching their loved one experience difficulties.

When I visited a woman dying of cancer, her father sat in a chair by the door and watched her sleep. When the woman was alert and ready to pray, we invited the father to come closer. He brought his chair to the bedside and then folded his hands. I then invited him to hold his daughter's hand as we prayed. He gently did this and tears came to all our eyes. This was one of the last times he touched his daughter before she died.

Praying from a Distance

An older woman confided that her only child, a daughter, had been diagnosed with a terminal disease. Their relationship was rocky, and the daughter was not welcoming of her mother's care or presence. The inability to care for her daughter when she was in such need greatly distressed the mother. After conversation, we talked about how she could still care for her daughter through prayer. She could envision her daughter and see Jesus sending his love and light to the daughter. If any specific needs came to mind, she could ask Jesus to take care of these for her. This gave the mother much comfort and allowed her to express her love for her daughter.

Prayer and Ritual

A ritual is a solemn ceremony or act that offers meaning to life experience. The simple act of lighting a candle or playing sacred music can move one into a time of worship. Prayer may or may not be part of a ritual. Parish nurses can make use of rituals from their particular denomination, or they may create a ritual that is meaningful and healing.

Billy was a developmentally disabled child. He was the youngest in the family and brought much joy to everyone who knew him. After his death, one of his siblings had difficulty coming to the church building and had missed many weeks of confirmation classes because of it. After several months, the confirmation coordinator, one of our pastors and I discussed the situation. We decided to invite the family to come to the church for a time of prayer. We hoped this would give them a new memory of the church and help them through a tough part of their grief.

We invited the family and also one of the prayer groups of the congregation. After introductions, we talked about Billy and the difficulty of coming into the church where they last saw him. We talked about grief, the love of God, and some of our own experiences of grief work. We then invited the family to envision Jesus holding Billy and to entrust him into God's loving care. We asked them to kneel together, and we literally surrounded them and prayed. There were tears and then hugs. Since that time, the family has been coming to church regularly, and the daughter is back attending confirmation classes.

Another ritual can be used when moving out of a beloved home. When my mother was ready to sell the house that I knew as a child, I began to grieve the loss of this wonderful place that held so many memories. When our family was gathered at the house, we lit a candle and read Psalm 90:1, *"Lord you have been our dwelling place throughout all generations,"* (NIV, 1995, p. 875). We moved from room to room, sharing memories, tears, laughter and prayer. We prayed, thanking God for all the blessings and asking—for the family who would move into this dwelling—that they, too, would be blessed. It was in the prayer time that I felt most comforted and began to feel excitement for the family that would soon own my childhood home.

Rituals can be simple and are easily adapted for personal or specific needs. Some denominational resource books have prayers and rituals for ordinary events that occur in the family. These can be adapted for various needs of individuals or families.

Prayer in Small Groups

The parish nurse can use prayer with small groups, such as a health ministry committee, support group, or a study group. Having devotions and praying for God's guidance as the group meeting begins brings everyone's focus to the same place and invites openness to God. The parish nurse may also initiate a time for shared prayer, where the whole group can lift up personal concerns or those regarding the work at hand. A popcorn style of prayer works well: one person starts the prayer, and others can "pop" with their prayer thoughts at any time. Another method is to hold hands and go around the circle, squeezing the hand of the next person when finished praying or wanting to pass. Both these methods provide the invitation to pray without demanding it.

There are many ways to pray in a small group. We are limited only by our creativity. One small group began their meeting with silent prayer, which was surprisingly powerful. Another group ended their meeting time with sentence prayers of thanksgiving. Praying together as a group invites God's presence and builds the relationships of those praying. See Appendix 14C for questions to further reflect and/or discuss the content in use of prayer.

Involving the Faith Community

The parish nurse can encourage the involvement of the faith community in prayer in many ways. A few of these that are most applicable to the role of the parish nurse include prayer chains, prayer shawls, prayer walking, and prayers for healing.

Prayer Chains

Many churches have prayer chains that pass on a prayer request to a group of individuals by telephone or by e-mail. The parish nurse is often in a position to ask people if they would like the support of the prayer chain. With permission, the parish nurse can be the one who communicates the request to the prayer chain and can also share updates as time passes. Knowing that others are praying brings great comfort to people in a time of crisis, and sharing updated information keeps the prayers encouraged and motivated. Guidelines that will ensure confidentiality and a swift movement into prayer are important.

Over the course of 2 years, the e-mail prayer chain at my church received periodic requests from a woman who was dealing with infertility. She had been able to conceive but had experienced several miscarriages. We prayed for her to become pregnant, and when she did, we prayed for a full-term healthy baby. She kept us informed during crucial times and this kept us praying. It was a joy to be able to praise God with thanksgiving when a healthy baby was born.

Prayer Shawls

Prayer shawls are knit or crocheted by someone who intentionally prays for the recipient of the shawl, known or unknown. When completed, the shawl is delivered to someone in need of comfort or care. A woman, dying of cancer, received a prayer shawl and always wanted it to be covering her. Another woman, whose son was killed in a car accident, found comfort in the prayer shawl, which caught many of her tears. It was especially helpful when she was alone. It was a tangible reminder of God's presence.

The prayer shawl ministry blesses those who receive it, as well as those who create it. The knitters talk of feeling God's peace flowing through them as they knit or crochet, and they are moved to pray. Further information on prayer shawls can be found on the Internet at www.shawlministry.com.

Prayer Walking

Prayer walking can be a wonderful way that the parish nurse encourages both physical and spiritual exercise. It may be done alone, with a walking partner, or in a group. The physical activity offers a different way to listen and talk to God. If you are walking alone, don't think about anything, but let God direct your attention to what God wants to reveal to you. If you are walking with a partner or a group, begin with prayer, or pray as you walk.

Prayer walking can be useful for various purposes. Sometimes a congregation will have members walk around the neighborhood of their church and pray as they prepare for a time of outreach into the community. Another church may offer a prayer walk to engage people in exercise and to help them find prayer walking partners. On a retreat, people may be encouraged to take a prayer walk alone to reflect on the topics that have been discussed.

There is something about walking that opens the mind. I asked my son one day if he wanted to walk along with me to a nearby nature center. I had envisioned a quiet walk, knowing that he isn't much of a talker. I was totally surprised when we got passed the driveway and he began to talk, chatting the whole way! As with my son, prayer walking may do the same for us in our relationship with God.

Prayers for Healing

More churches are offering a specific time of prayers for healing. This may be during or at the end of a worship service or a service with the sole focus of hope and healing. Some churches offer this once a month or quarterly, whereas others have people available for prayer support every Sunday. It is a time of seeking God, the One who heals us, as expressed in Exodus 15:26, where God says, *"I am the Lord, who heals you"* (NIV, 1995, p. 109).

A service of prayers for healing can be created for one person or for many. It may be general or focused on a particular experience such as grief, miscarriage, divorce, or cancer. The format may include singing, a sermon or homily, anointing with oil, and the laying on of hands. The format depends largely on the specific church and denomination. In some denominations, the anointing with oil is a sacrament exercised by the clergy. In other denominations, lay or clergy are involved in anointing with oil and speaking the prayers. Generally, those involved have been trained in prayers for healing.

The prayer time for individuals can be done in a variety of ways. Some churches have people come forward and each individual receives anointing with oil and the laying on of hands with the same general prayer spoken over each one. Other churches offer the laying on of hands, with or without the anointing with oil, and a spontaneous prayer that responds to the individual's spoken concerns. The recipient may kneel, sit, or stand. However it is done, permission for touch and anointing is advised, to avoid any discomfort in the one asking for prayer.

Most prayers for healing are done with a team of at least two people. This arrangement allows for sharing the challenge of prayer and also gives the opportunity for one person to specifically listen for God's direction while the other may be speaking the prayer.

The laying on of hands is an ancient tradition of the church associated with prayers for healing. It is so natural to reach out and touch those who are hurting. After receiving permission, lay your hand gently on their head or shoulder. You may want to begin by saying something like "We lay our hands on you in the name of Jesus Christ," and then proceed with the prayer.

The use of oil comes from directions given in James 5:14: "Are any among you sick? They should call for the elders of the church and have them pray over them, anointing them with oil in the name of the Lord" (NRSV, 1989, p. 231). In the history of the church, the use of oil is associated with baptism and prayers for healing. Olive oil is used with frankincense and myrrh or some other fragrance. It is generally placed on the person's forehead with such words as "I anoint you in the name of the Father, Son, and Holy Spirit." The oil and fragrance offer a sensory communication of God's presence.

The parish nurse may be involved in prayers for healing, either in a leadership or supportive role. The parish nurse's involvement will lend credibility to the experience, especially in a church that has not had prayers for healing. It is good to remind those coming for prayer that healing comes in a variety of ways. Sometimes it comes through ordinary means like a good night's sleep or a long conversation with a dear friend. Sometimes it comes in ways that we understand, like through surgery or medication or counseling. And sometimes it comes in ways that we do not understand, but it is all God's work of healing.

The parish nurse can encourage people in need of healing to attend a service or ask for prayers for healing. Such people would be those who are dealing with a broken or strained relationship, a physical illness, upcoming surgery, depression, unemployment, grief, or other difficulty. People may also come for the peaceful time of prayer, to ask for a blessing or to pray for a loved one in need.

The hardest part about prayers for healing is that we have no control. As nurses, we know what kind of response to expect when we give a specific medication or treatment, but we do not know for sure the outcome of our prayers. As Christians, we are called to pray, to lift up the needs of others, but the outcomes are up to God. And God is a mystery that we do not always understand.

Sometimes I hear people pray, "Lord, *if* it be Your will, please heal so and so…." This way of praying calls into question God's willingness to heal. It may be a statement intended to express relinquishment of control, as in "Your will, not mine, O Lord," but it reveals the doubt that God is who God says He is: "the One who heals us."

In Matthew 8:1-4, a man with leprosy kneels before Jesus, saying, *"Lord, if you are willing, you can make me clean."* Jesus responds with a touch of his hand and the words, *"I am willing. Be clean"* (NIV, 1995, p. 1449). And the man was cured. In this passage, Jesus revealed his willingness to heal. In other passages, Jesus underscores this willingness by being the one who initiates the work of healing.

After studying the healing work of Jesus and recalling that God says "I am the One who heals you," I am convinced of God's willingness to heal. Relinquishment is still important, so I find it helpful to instead pray, "Jesus, heal (person), *according* to your will." This second way of praying leaves intact, our trust in God as Healer. See Appendix 14 C for questions to ponder or discuss on involving the faith community.

Prayer Practices for Self-Care

Many prayer practices can provide support and sustenance for the parish nurse. Staying connected to God is like keeping hold of a lifeline in turbulent waters. Personal prayer time prepares the parish nurse for ministry, and prayer with others lightens the burden of ministry.

Lifting Burdens

When the parish nurse prays with those she visits, the burdens shared are placed in the hands of God, who can handle them. They no longer weigh down the parish nurse, leaving her free to care for others. By the end of any given day, the parish nurse has met with many people who are suffering or struggling. Praying is one way of coping with the amount of pain encountered.

Make use of others who pray. If you visited someone and prayed with them and later still feel heaviness in your heart, ask someone to pray with you for the person and situation. This could be the clergy you work with or the church secretary. It needs to be someone who is bound by confidentiality; otherwise, you can pray without names. Pray until you sigh and know that it is in God's hands. You will feel the burden lifted. If the heaviness of heart comes again, know that you are

to return to prayer for the person or the situation. This is the Holy Spirit's nudge to pray.

Praying with a Labyrinth

Sometimes changing our way of praying can refresh our conversation with God. It helps us hear in a new way. An old tradition of praying with a labyrinth may be one such prayer experience. A labyrinth is like a maze that may be in or out of doors. You follow the path, walking until it leads you to the center and then back out. The focus on the path and the pausing in the center may allow you to listen in a different manner. For many, this way of praying is found to be relaxing and refreshing.

Prayer Support

It is wise to establish a system of prayer support for the parish nurse and the ministry. This can be either one person or several who covenant to pray daily for the parish nurse, his or her family, and the ministry. Keeping this person or people informed of specific prayer requests will help them stay in touch and motivated. These people can pray for your faith struggles and personal struggles as well as ministry issues. They are ministry confidants, going before you in prayer, covering you with protection and helping you grow and mature in your faith (Maxwell, 1996).

Having this kind of prayer support makes a huge difference to me. I know that I am not alone, that there are others who care and are lifting me up. Many days I know it is their prayers that give me the strength and guidance needed.

Praying for Protection

When you are involved in ministry, it is wise to pray for protection everyday. Put on the armor of God from Ephesians 6. Regularly receive the sacrament of Holy Communion. Make the sign of the cross and ask for the protection of the Holy Spirit. This is like putting on your seatbelt. You don't know what the day will bring, or what pain or conflict you will encounter. The ride may be easy or rough. You need God's protection and strength. There is no need to be a Lone Ranger. God has asked you to be a partner in ministry. Rely on your Partner!

Spiritual Darkness

Sometimes there is spiritual darkness—times when it is hard to pray and nothing seems to make a difference. God may seem absent, and your prayers feel like they go nowhere. You may feel despair, discouraged, or even hopeless. This desolate time may be from weariness, depression, sin, hardship, or the "dark night of the soul."

Taking care of yourself physically, mentally, and spiritually may alleviate this dark time. After a few years of being a parish nurse, I came to a time of darkness and despair. I no longer had energy or excitement for life. This did not leave me until I took a week off to rest and refill my own soul.

Resting, treating depression, or confessing hidden sins may lighten the darkness. A time of hardship or "dark night of the soul" may simply have to be endured. Whatever the cause, this is a time to trust God as more than the emotion we feel. Keep praying. Wait for God's presence with expectation. Trust that God is still at work, deepening your relationship.

Personal Prayer Retreat

At times, the only way to hear God is to withdraw from the world. Find a retreat center or place where you can be undisturbed. The time away can be as little as 2 hours or as much as a week. Rest, sing, pray, read. Do whatever you find helpful. *"Draw near to God and he will draw near to you"* (James 4:8, NRSV, 1989, p. 231). Jesus did this often when he withdrew to a lonely place to pray. This time away is crucial for staying connected to God and on track with where God has called you to serve.

After 7 years of serving a large metropolitan church, I felt empty. I thought it was perhaps time to think about doing something else. Then I went to a convent for 24 hours. My plan was to establish some goals for my work as a parish nurse and for myself personally. I did neither. I simply reconnected with God. I sang, napped, walked, and prayed. I rested in the presence of the Lord! It was like a marriage encounter with God! I returned refreshed and renewed for service.

Some people appreciate structure for a retreat. You may join a retreat that is offered at a church or retreat center or find some guidance in a book. Several books offer topics and examples for short or longer retreats. You may also consult with a spiritual director, who can help guide you through a personal retreat or as part of ongoing spiritual formation (see Chapter 4). See Appendix 14C for questions to further reflect and/or discussion on prayer practices for self-care.

Conclusion

Prayer is a vital instrument for the parish nurse personally and professionally. It is a means of care for those the parish nurse encounters. It keeps the parish nurse connected to God in work or rest or play. Through prayer, God offers the parish nurse strength and guidance, peace and healing, and all that is needed. Regardless of one's level of experience, prayer offers such a depth of opportunity that there is always more to learn. May God inspire us to continue to learn and grow!

Holy God, we are grateful for prayer that you allow us to speak to you. Help us to stay connected. Protect us from drifting away and from all that would harm us. Teach us how to be your instrument of love and healing to those you call us to serve. Open our hearts and our minds to your Holy Spirit, that we might serve you faithfully. In Jesus' name. Amen.

REFERENCES

Byrd, R. (1988). Positive therapeutic effects of intercessory prayer in a coronary care unit population. *Southern Medical Journal,* 81(7), 826-9.

Copeland, G. (1997). *Prayers that avail much: a handbook of scriptural prayers* (Vol. 2). Tulsa: Harrison House.

Daily texts. (2004). Alexandria, Minnesota: Mount Carmel Ministries.

Dossey, L. (1993). *Healing words: The power of prayer and the practice of medicine.* New York: HarperCollins.

Galli, M. & Bell, J. Jr. (1999). *The complete idiot's guide to prayer.* Indianapolis: Macmillan.

Gallup, G. Jr., (1999). *As nation observes national day of prayer, 9 in 10 pray, 3 in 4 daily.* Retrieved June 30, 2004 from http://www.gallup.com

Holy Bible, New Revised Standard Version (NRSV). (1989). Nashville: Thomas Nelson.

Keating, C. (1999). *Who we are is how we pray: matching personality and spirituality.* Mystic, CT: Twenty-Third Publications.

Lee, B. (2004). *21 ways to refresh your prayer life.* Prayer Ventures Inc. Retrieved April 2004 from www.prayerventures.org

Maxwell, J. (1996). *Partners in prayer: support and strengthen your pastor and church leaders.* Nashville: Thomas Nelson.

Michael, C. & Norrisey, M. (1991). *Prayer and temperament: different prayer forms for different personality types.* Charlottesville, VA: Open Door.

NIV study bible. Barker, K. (Ed.) (1995). Grand Rapids, Michigan: Zondervan.

Nouwen, H. (1995). *With open hands.* Notre Dame: Ave Maria.

Person, G. (2001). *Psalms for healing: praying with those in need.* Minneapolis: Augsburg.

APPENDIX 14A

21 Ways to Refresh Your Prayer Life by Betsy Lee

1. Sing a Psalm. Many of the psalms were originally composed on David's lute. Make up your own melody and sing or hum the words.
2. Take a prayer walk—around a lake, in a park, or through the neighborhood. Imagine Jesus walking beside you like a friend. Feel free to share your heart. He will listen.
3. Use a picture calendar for a devotional focal point. You might enjoy ocean scenes or gardens or mountainscapes. Imagine yourself in the scene; commune with God there.
4. Kneel as you pray. It will increase your humility and attitude of reverence and worship.
5. Dance to the Lord as David did (2 Samuel 6:14). Make up your own steps while listening to praise music. Clap your hands or lift them up as you sway to the music. Release your *whole body* to be an instrument of worship!
6. Pray while lying down outstretched on the floor.
7. Be completely silent. Silence is restful, and it allows us to rest in God's love. Empty your mind of pre-occupations and let God fill you up with Himself.
8. Rest your hands on your lap, palms up, ready to receive what God has to give in prayer.
9. Light a candle. Focus on the flame. Let its quiet beauty still your mind. Draw close to God, and He will draw close to you.
10. Personalize scripture. For example, hear God speak these words personally to you: "I will exult over *you,* (insert your name), with joy, I will be quiet in my love, I will rejoice over *you* with shouts of joy" (Zephaniah 3:17). Drink the words in deeply. Or you could pray this for a friend: "Lord, exult over *Jane* with joy; be quiet in your love, rejoice over her with shouts of joy!" Imagine your friend drinking these words in deeply.
11. Type out a verse of scripture and tape it to the steering wheel of your car. When your eyes glance down at it while waiting at a red light, ponder it and let God speak to you through those words. Let God's Word nourish your spirit.
12. Pray while engaging in a relaxing activity: pushing your preschooler in the backyard on a swing or jogging or gardening. This will slow your praying down to a more leisurely pace.
13. Use the outdoors to inspire your prayers. For example, as you drive down the highway, gaze at the sky and recall this verse, "For great is your love, higher than the heavens; your faithfulness reaches to the skies" (Psalm 108:4). Thank God for His vast, immeasurable faithfulness to you.
14. Journal as you pray. If a particular scripture verse seems to strike a chord in your heart and it seems that God is speaking those words directly to you, He probably is. Jot the verse down, reflect on it, let it unfold in your thinking over weeks, even months. Little by little, the full intent of what God is saying will be revealed.

21 Ways to Refresh Your Prayer Life by Betsy Lee—cont'd

15. Use concrete objects to focus your prayers. For example, if you need to give God a burden or heartache, hold a small wooden cross in your hand and let the pain literally be transferred from you to Jesus. Jesus invites us to do this: "Cast your cares upon me," He says, "because I care for you" (1 Peter 5:7). If you need to let someone go in your life, hold a miniature basket in your hand and imagine putting that person in the basket as Moses' mother put her son in a basket and let him go, trusting him to God.

16. Use life-size objects, too. For example, if God is calling you to take a step of faith, think of your ottoman in the living room as an altar; place your shoes on the ottoman to signify your willingness to be fully yielded to where He is asking you to go.

17. Organize your prayer life by focusing on different subjects every day of the week. You could pray for family members on Monday, your church on Tuesday, missionaries on Thursday, etc. Be sure to reserve Wednesday just for praise, no petitions. Nothing overcomes a mid-week slump like a surge of worship and praise!

18. Pray thematically. Use the theme from a single verse to guide your prayers: "I am the light of the world" (John 8:12). Pray that Jesus would infuse the lives of those you love with His light; ask for His light to illumine a confusing situation you are wrestling with; imagine the light of His presence bathing a dark place in the world.

19. Step into a scene of scripture. Experience through your senses the actual sights, sounds, and smells of the setting of a Gospel story. Imagine yourself in the story face to face with Jesus. Let Him touch the leper in you, heal your blindness, call you back to life like Lazarus.

20. Draw pictures in the margins of your Bible or in a notebook as you pray. If you are a visual person, this is a powerful way to process prayer and let it do its deep work.

21. Listen. Listen. Listen. God speaks in many ways: through pictures, dreams, impressions, words of scripture, circumstances, other people.

APPENDIX 14B

Bible Verses that Address Specific Situations

When you are:	Find help in:
Discouraged	Psalms 43, 130
Anxious	Philippians 4: 6-9
Stressed	Psalm 46
Facing a crisis	Joshua 1:5-9, Psalm 3
Grieving	1 Corinthians 15, Revelation 21-22
Unsure of the future	Romans 8:31-39, Psalm 121
Needing forgiveness	Psalm 51, Romans 7:19-25
Fearful	Isaiah 41: 10, 13
Seeking God's will	1 John 4:7-21, Matthew 7:7-12
Lonely	Isaiah 43:1-4, Isaiah 58:9
Worried	Philippians 4:19, Psalm 32:7
Hearing bad news	Psalm 112:7
Tempted	James 1:2-6, Psalm 139
Afraid of death	John 11, 17, 20
	2 Corinthians 5, Revelation 14:13
Guilty	Psalm 103:12, 1 John 1:9
Needing peace	John 14:27, Psalm 85:8
Needing hope	Lamentations 3:21-23, Psalm 71:5,1 Peter 1:3

RESOURCES FOR TOPICS IN THE BIBLE

The Bible Promise Book, Barbour Publishing
American Bible Society, 1865 Broadway, New York, NY 10023, www.forministry.com

APPENDIX 14C

Questions for Reflection or Discussion

INTRODUCTION

1. Think about some experiences you've had with prayer—what have they taught you about yourself?
2. What would it mean for you to think about prayer as God-centered and not self-centered?
3. Pretend you are visiting someone. What are some "core" concerns to pray for?

EXPLORATION OF PRAYER

1. When has prayer captured your heart and brought healing and hope?
2. How does the research shared help those who may be skeptical of prayer?
3. Practice using different types of prayer. With which do you feel most comfortable?

EMBARKING ON THE JOURNEY

1. As you read through this section, what was helpful for your own prayer journey?
2. What is intimidating about praying for yourself or others?
3. Who would be a good prayer mentor for you and how could you learn from them?

USE OF PRAYER

1. How does it make you feel to know the Holy Spirit is the most active participant in your prayers?
2. When do you feel most weak in prayer?
3. Which rituals and traditions involving prayer have been meaningful for you or others?
4. Who do you know who could use a special prayer right now?

INVOLVING THE FAITH COMMUNITY

1. How does your worshiping community gather for prayer?
2. In what way do you or could you support the prayer ministry of your faith community?

PRAYER PRACTICES FOR SELF-CARE

1. What are some prayer practices that you do regularly? How do they help you?
2. Reflect and share or journal on the idea of a prayer retreat for self-care.

Mentoring the Parish Nurse

Rosemarie Matheus

15

The Oxford English Dictionary first cited the word *mentor* in 1750. Its origin is credited to Homer's *Odyssey* when Odysseus left his son in the care of his friend, Mentor. From this relationship the word mentor came to mean friend, teacher, trusted advisor, wise person (Shea, 1997). Earlier accounts of mentor relationships are recorded in China, Egypt, and Ireland. *Abbas* and *Ammas* were titles given to early Egyptians, Syrians, and Palestinians known for their holiness, wisdom, and knowledge. They filled roles similar to the Greek mentor. Chinese kings developed a mentor role called *shan jang* as early as 2333 BC (Huang & Lynch, 1995). The medieval guild masters provided mentoring for apprentices in social, religious, and personal matters. The process of mentoring was first mentioned in the nursing literature in 1977 (Vance & Olson, 1998). Mentoring as a strategy in business and management became popular in the 1970s and 1980s (Morton-Cooper & Palmer, 1993).

Current definitions of mentoring only agree that it is a relationship between two people. Huang & Lynch (1995) describes mentoring as a dance in which the mentor and the mentee each give and receive. A mentoring relationship is reflected in how a person's spirit is cherished but goes beyond religious God-talk (Vance & Olson, 1998; Sellner, 1990). Shea (1997) quotes developmental psychologist Levinson, who writes: "mentoring in its most fundamental sense is about transformation… helping someone else encounter his or her deeper self, which Jung calls the larger and greater personality maturing within" (p. 15). More pragmatic definitions describe mentoring in terms of desired outcomes and tasks. Murray (2001) defines mentoring as "a deliberate pairing of a more skilled or more experienced person with a less skilled, less experienced one, with the mutually agreed goal of having the less skilled person grow and develop specific competencies" (p. xiii). When a mentoring program for parish nurses is developed, the elements of these definitions should be reflected in the relationship of the mentor and the parish nurse as mentee. This may require institutions and parish nurses to rethink and clarify their previous concepts of mentoring.

Characteristics of the Mentor

Appropriate characteristics describing a mentor include advocate, advisor, teacher, listener, counselor, guide, compassionate, nurturer. Words not characteristic of a mentor are coach, trainer, supervisor, preceptor (Murray, 2001; Vance & Olson, 1998). Coaches and trainers focus on developing specific work goals. Supervisors and preceptors have the responsibility to evaluate and discipline. Mentors do not take on these roles. A mentor's role is not to have power over the mentee, but rather the mentor and the mentee must stimulate each other (Huang & Lynch, 1995).

The mentor should have the desire to take on the role and believe in the value of mentoring. When possible, the mentor should be chosen by

171

the mentee rather than assigned. Mentoring is not successful when the mentor is given this added expectation as part of his or her workload without choice (Shea, 1997). Institutions may consider pre-selecting potential mentors based on their abilities and prepare them specifically for the uniqueness of the role. New parish nurses may then select from the prepared mentors, one they consider most fitting. It has been valuable to have mentors who themselves have previously been mentored.

No single method for mentoring in every relationship exists; however, most effective mentors possess **many** of the following characteristics.

Ability to Listen

Shea (1997) identifies listening as the premier art of mentoring. A mentor must listen with heart and spirit for the needs, strengths, and deficiencies the new parish nurse brings to the practice. Listening takes time and cannot be done when the mentor limits conversations with the parish nurse to short formal meetings that consist primarily of questioning the parish nurse about performance. Listening requires that a mentor speak less than a mentee in their conversations as opposed to a mentor filling the time with advice or instructions. Listening is enhanced by observing the nonverbal behaviors of the parish nurse. Negative behaviors and deficiencies are more easily heard and sometimes seen in this time of attentive listening than from reports or direct questions.

Ability to Guide Rather than Control

A mentor is effective neither by taking charge of the mentee's work nor by trying to clone the mentee into a standard model. A mentor is to assist a parish nurse become what he or she aspires to be using his or her distinctive gifts. The parish nurse benefits and grows when guided through difficulties. He or she learns to solve the problems of the practice. The mentor who criticizes or rescues rather than offering alternative ideas or who does not give objective feedback with sensitivity and support distorts the mentoring process. Mentors should not use power, nor have a need to control or encourage dependence in their mentees. Mentorship should focus on a process of becoming and not that of

being shaped or cloned (Morton-Cooper & Palmer, 1993).

Ability to Challenge and Foster the Dreams of the Parish Nurse

New parish nurses need assistance in setting realistic goals when the unfamiliarity of the new role and eagerness for success overshadow real-world limitations. The mentor fosters the parish nurse's self-confidence by helping him or her create achievable goals; however, the mentor does not need to accept *only* safe goals. The mentor must challenge the parish nurse to bring his or her unique vision and skills to the faith community for the nurse to feel successful. This goal requires the mentor to ignite the nurse's enthusiasm, be comfortable with the new ideas of the parish nurse, and have the maturity to foster them within the boundaries of the practice.

Ability to Create a Trusting, Compassionate Relationship

The mentor must be viewed as a confidential, caring, and loyal person who has faith in the parish nurse's ability. A mentor's credibility and humility are essential in the relationship. These traits foster an honest, open exchange between the two and allow the parish nurse to share struggles, frustrations, and failures, knowing they will be held in confidence and viewed compassionately by the mentor without judgment. A respected mentor who can appropriately use humor will find this adds an element of comfort to the relationship.

Ability to Advocate

In an institutional setting, a novice employee develops more confidence and skill if a mentor is also her advocate in the institution's network and culture. The unspoken customs and taboos in every workplace are best navigated when a mentor guides the new parish nurse through or around them and facilitates connectedness with new peers. Additionally the mentor is able to promote and encourage the parish nurse's participation in subgroups of the institution, appropriate community activities, and professional organizations.

Ability to Model Spirituality

The spiritual expression and dimension of the mentor should be a model for the mentee. This underscores the previously mentioned need to pre-select mentors who live out their spirituality. The human resource department of the institution must be aware that although discussing spirituality may be considered off-limits for some employees, the spirituality of parish nurses and those selected as mentors is central and necessary to the practice and therefore is not in conflict with personnel policies. For many new parish nurses, application of spiritual issues in the practice may be foreign and even discomforting. A spiritually mature mentor who models spiritual conversations and behaviors gently teaches the mentee acceptance of a spiritual focus in the practice and supports personal, spiritual growth (see Chapter 26).

Preparing mentors who possess these desired characteristics will predict the quality of the parish nurse and the resulting practice. Mentoring is a demanding role that requires dedication, time, and commitment. Morton-Cooper and Palmer (1993) believe this role also requires good judgment, the respect of others, a network of contacts, personal charisma, and the desire to invest time and share personal experiences. When mentoring is an added responsibility to a usual workload, a mentor should receive additional monetary compensation or other benefits. This demonstrates an institution's investment in the role of mentoring for the benefit of parish nurses.

Benefits of Mentoring

The mentor, the mentee, and the institution will all achieve benefits from an effective mentoring process. The mentor will gain a sense of pride in having an influence on the growth and development of the parish nurse. Mentoring provides a means of leaving a legacy to the profession. Being a mentor can confer on one the status of achievement and recognition among peers.

New ideas and questions that a mentee brings to the relationship can be a stimulus for the mentor's growth and for identifying gaps in one's own knowledge. The value the institution places on the mentoring process ensures that the mentor views the role as one deserving of his or her time and energy.

A parish nurse mentee benefits from the mentoring process by having the security and guidance of an experienced advisor to be eased into the new role and new environment. A survey of 500 clinical nurse specialists revealed that those who had a mentoring relationship indicated a significantly higher level of satisfaction than those who did not. The mentor's purpose "is to remind us that we can indeed survive the terror of the coming journey by moving through not around our fear" (Vance & Olson, 1998, p. 11). Instead of experiencing the trauma and problems that result from errors in learning situations, the parish nurse who is mentored has the benefit of the experienced mentor who is able to anticipate negative consequences before they occur and suggest steps to avoid them. A mentee's deficiencies can be detected by an objective mentor and sensitive suggestions offered to overcome them before they become a liability.

Mentees can be brought into areas of professional growth that they would not consider or areas that would not be open to them without the presence of a mentor. A mentor may take on a mentee as a collaborator in research. A mentee may be encouraged to publish or present at a professional conference by a mentor who offers assistance or support for their projects and ideas.

Institutions with parish nurse programs benefit from the mentoring process. This is especially true if they experience low turnover, high morale, and no oppressive political infrastructure (Morton-Cooper & Palmer, 1993). Hackensack University Medical Center credits its national recognition of quality to its mentoring process. Institutions that offer mentoring, done in a humanistic style, find it benefits the recruitment of new employees and promotes their productivity. The resulting outcome is a win-win situation: success for the institution's programs and satisfaction for the employee (Vance & Olson, 1998).

Strategies for Effective Mentoring

My personal experience as a mentor to a large number of parish nurses over the years demonstrated to me that becoming a parish nurse is a transforming process and requires mentoring that is supportive and sensitive to all dimensions of the nurse's life. I found that strategies needed to focus on the whole person. This ensured a relationship that contained healing properties and promoted wholeness and the uniqueness of each parish nurse. "When people feel strong and resilient—physically, mentally, emotionally and spiritually—they perform better with more passion for longer" (Loehr & Schwartz, 2001, p. 128). Following are suggestions based on my mentoring experiences in both institutional and educational parish nurse programs.

Mentoring the Physical Dimension

New parish nurses tend to put the needs of others first and this can result in ignoring their personal needs. New parish nurses that I have mentored report they have stopped their daily running or exercises in order to have more time for what they perceive are the multiple needs of their clients. This savior model in which they believe they are the only ones that can solve the client's problems is common. Using the analogy of the airlines gives them a broader perspective. Flight attendants, when explaining the need to use facemasks, tell passengers to put their own mask on before attempting to help others. Mentors can urge their parish nurses to find some form of physical activity that they enjoy and to enter the time this activity requires into their appointment book. This gives it the same importance as an appointment with a client or others.

Nutrition and dietary information is a common request parish nurses get from clients. When parish nurses have a weight problem, they have confessed that responding to this topic can be stressful. The mentor can provide an option other parish nurses with a similar problem have used. These nurses have shared their need for improved nutrition with the clients and together have participated in successful weight loss programs.

Mentoring the Emotional Dimension

The mentor needs to be aware of the stresses in the mentee's life apart from the professional role. "We can't separate our professional lives from our private lives; if our private lives suffer, they will affect our professional lives and vice versa" (Stoddard, 2003, p. 23). This is the point that most clearly illustrates the difference between

mentoring and preceptorship or training and must be understood by the mentor, the mentee, and the institution's administration and human resources department. Glanz (2002) urges institutions to realize they have employed a whole person, not just filled a position, and this expands the traditional view of orientation or training.

Many times in my role as mentor it was the personal life of the mentee that needed to be heard and understood. As the parish nurse develops in the role, the family will notice the change. As one nurse told me, "My husband said I'm different than I used to be." Family system theories predict that the change in one member will affect change in the other members. It may be appropriate for the mentor to meet the family and discuss this new role the parish nurse is taking on, with new hours, new challenges, and new demands that differ from previous nursing positions. Parish nurses are usually unaware how this new role will change them and consequently their families. It has been helpful for me as the mentor to discuss and to prepare them for this as they initiate their practice.

A heavily charged emotional issue that mentors need to address before problems occur is sexuality. Parish nurses of both genders have encountered a relationship in which sexual overtones or advances occurred. This is to be expected as the male or female parish nurse is easily seen as an appealing, loving, and accepting recipient for sexual advances from staff or clients. Although some nurses are quick to identify this, others require the objective guidance of an observant mentor. Listening to not only the verbal but also intuitively sensing an unspoken anxiety, I was able to put into words what a parish nurse could not. With tears and a sigh of relief she was able to relate the sexual advances her clergy person was making toward her. She acknowledged that she was naïve, inexperienced, and somewhat flattered when it first started. Now it was becoming uncomfortable and she found the trusting, understanding, and confidentiality of the mentor to be her support. In partnership, we were able to devise strategies to counteract the unwanted advances. She had to be made aware of her part in the situation and take responsibility for initiating new confronting behaviors that were ultimately successful. Without this help, she felt she would have had to leave her position. Reports from other parish nurses make it apparent that situations such as this are not rare. Mentors need to not only probe gently for the nurse to discuss the issue but also to be open to the potential for it and discuss appropriate behaviors before these situations occur.

The church is a new environment for nursing practice, and the parish nurse is usually unprepared for the politics that exist. I have worked with parish nurses who were naively manipulated and emotionally abused by the behaviors and tacit expectations of church leaders and clergy. The mentor is a more objective observer of the practice and more aware of these political systems. I have found this to be especially true when parish nurses practice in their own congregations. Members who are older or still view them solely as a friend may not accept them as professionals. Knowing which members hold the true power in the congregation is a necessity, and the mentor, though not fully aware of the specific situation and personalities, is usually able to guide the parish nurse through this quagmire that has caused the demise of the parish nurse program in some churches.

A novice parish nurse brings to the practice an expectation that is not always reality. Nurses are accustomed to quickly take on the responsibilities of a new position and to have their positions clearly understood by the staff and their clients. This is seldom true in a new parish nurse setting. Emotionally they feel they must accomplish more than is possible in their first few months. When members are slow to come to them, the staff is not accepting of them, and the clergy are not clear on how they are to function, the parish nurse begins to feel disappointed and inadequate. The mentor's role is to listen to these struggles and give perspective to their expectations. Setting realistic goals before beginning a practice is paramount in order for the parish nurse to feel successful. One nurse who had not yet begun a practice in a church asked me how she would be able to see "all my patients" if she had to spend time networking with staff and community resources. She mistakenly assumed that her appointment book would immediately fill with clients, a most unrealistic expectation for parish nurses. The mentor's response is to clarify that the goal of

the first 6 months is to learn the environment, the community, and the church's politics and to help the members correctly understand the role and its limitations. The mentor can advise that attending church committee meetings, worship services, church social events, and staff meetings are more realistic and acceptable goals. This is an emotionally fragile time for new parish nurses, and I was most aware of it when I agreed to meet a parish nurse the first morning she began at the church. Her previous experience had been in intensive care. She sat in an empty office, behind a bare desk with hands tightly folded and a forced smile and said, "What should I do now?"

One of the most effective strategies when mentoring new parish nurses is to connect them with other practicing parish nurses. "I look forward to the meetings every month and feel terrible if I have to miss one." This is a common response from parish nurses who belong to a formal or informal group. This is the place where they can share their successes and failures with peers who have been in similar settings with similar experiences. Strong professional and emotional bonds develop. Tears and laughter are released. The mentor may need to monitor the group, ensuring that it is functioning as a healthy support system. Supervisors, administrators, dominant personalities, or mentors should not control the group.

Mentoring the Mental Dimension

Parish nursing is an advanced practice role and as such demands mental processing that requires much energy. The mentor will often see the negative result of this in the expressions and body language of the parish nurse. The nurse is often guilty of spending more time with the work than is mentally healthy. The mentor's role is to help parish nurses understand that this is affecting his or her work and that the work will be more effective with more balance in their day. Parish nurses usually require strong encouragement to put opportunities for leisure and play into their appointment book. As a mentor I have had to ask what specific activities not related to work a parish nurse mentee had planned for a specific day. The answer would usually be some family responsibility or chore such as "grocery shopping" or "the wash" or "taking my mother to the doctor." It was difficult to convince the nurse that going on a family picnic or having a social lunch with a friend was a valuable use of time and contributed to good mental health. I have had parish nurses keep a log for one week, noting the instances when they engaged in true leisure activity. Rarely did they identify more than 1 to 2 hours a week, and some had no activities that could be classified as true leisure. There is a commonly held myth that nurses must always put the needs of others first. Mentors must show parish nurses the harm this myth can cause them. A strong model for taking time for one's self comes from Christian scripture, when Jesus left the crowds and went off alone.

There may be a reverse need when one is mentoring the mental dimension. The parish nurse can on occasion lack the mental stimulation necessary to be an effective practitioner. The mentor's role is to guide this nurse to resources that may be mentally stimulating. These may provide greater challenge and new knowledge and stimulate creative ideas. The mentor might recommend attendance at seminars, introduce the mentee to research or to unfamiliar publications, or suggest opportunities to work with community action groups. There might also be an opportunity to pair the mentee with a more experienced parish nurse for a specific time period. Care needs to be taken that the mentee not view these suggestions as additional requirements or expectations placed on the nurse. Rather seeds from which the parish nurse might grow need to be planted and allowed to emerge.

Mentoring the Spiritual Dimension

Stoddard (2003) believes that to be an effective mentor, the spiritual dimension of the mentee must be addressed. "You cannot succeed at mentoring the whole person without taking into account the spiritual dimension of the individual's life" (Stoddard, 2003, p. 157). A client's spiritual needs are often central to care in the parish nurse's practice. This requires parish nurses to have a mature relationship with God and an understanding of their personal spiritual life and to acknowledge the central role a person's spirit has in healing and wellness. A novice parish nurse approached me after a conference on spirituality

and excitedly told me how much she was enjoying her new role. I was pleased to hear this until she said, "except I don't get this spirituality part." Nurses who accept a role as a parish nurse without this awareness are not truly practicing within the scope of the specialty and are in great need of a mentor to help their spiritual development. The mentor should consider suggesting the mentee spend time with another parish nurse who can model spiritual care giving with actual clients. Giving spiritual care is rarely taught in nursing schools and is rarely modeled in institutional nursing units. Learning is most effective when a behavior is modeled. The parish nurse without role models may be very uneasy about praying or discussing spiritual matters. One parish nurse admitted to me that after 3 months of seeing a client, the client finally had to ask her, "Mary, aren't you ever going to pray with me?"

The mentor can support the introduction of spiritual interventions by offering very simple suggestions. Using printed prayers at first is usually easier than praying as part of a conversation. A tool to give new parish nurses can be an appropriate book of prayers. Parish nurses not used to praying with others or aloud will be especially concerned about "doing it right." "I can't talk in King James," said a new parish nurse who felt her words had to sound like scripture. The mentor can also use each meeting with the mentee to model prayer and how it is experienced. In all mentoring relationships, the mentor and the mentee always recommend intercessory prayer for each other and for the clients. This is not only empirically effective but is also based on the research of the effects of intercessory prayer.

Although parish nurses spend time in the church on Sundays, they may not be actively worshiping, even while attending the worship service. The parish nurse may have the feeling of being on the job/on the clock. The mentor should monitor how parish nurses are meeting their needs for worship and their personal relationship with God. This can require that the nurses worship in a setting other than the church in which they practice and perhaps attend study groups or social functions in other churches. The professional identity of parish nurses has at times interfered with and even limited their own opportunities for spiritual growth. Many conferences and seminars on spiritual topics are offered by religious denominations that can be helpful to the development of the parish nurse's spiritual insight and awareness.

If the mentor is part of a parish nurse support group or regularly attends the same institution's required meetings, the mentor can initially lead devotions at these events. Eventually the parish nurses can assume this responsibility. When there are support meetings, having a chaplain or spiritual leader present to help the parish nurses focus on the spiritual element in their presentation of case studies or questions of care is very helpful for facilitating individual spiritual development. Some mentors with successful parish nurse programs highly recommend parish nurses to routinely meet one-on-one with a chaplain to review their own spiritual development and the spiritual needs of his or her clients. Mentors may also give their mentees information about the practice of spiritual direction and assist in identifying appropriate resources for this process. Parish nurses who have worked with spiritual directors have found them beneficial. "He (the spiritual director) doesn't tell me what to do, but helps me see what God wants me to do with the problems I'm having."

Mentoring Strategies for All Encounters

Several strategies can ensure that the mentor does not take on the mode of supervisor or administrator. Stoddard (2003) warns that what is called mentoring often tends to be based on a position rather than a helping relationship. Supervisors often meet with those for whom they are responsible in the office or environment of the supervisor. The mentor of the parish nurse should arrange to have the meetings in the church where the nurse practices. This provides the mentor with the opportunity to directly observe how the nurse has impacted the church setting. Parish nurses may report that they have an office or designated area. The mentor can assess the appropriateness of the office site that may reflect the importance the church is giving the parish nurse's position. Is the office in an inaccessible site or hidden in unused rooms closed off from common areas? Is the parish nurse required to share space with another staff person? This may

severely restrict the confidentiality the nurse must maintain in the practice. The activities of the other staff person may take over the space or the time the nurse needs. Parish nurses have had to share space with secretaries, lay religious directors, Sunday school rooms, unvisited upstairs storage areas and/or closets. The mentor can be of help to these parish nurses by working with the church and nurse to find appropriate space. A clearly identified and visible room that affords privacy and accessibility increases the parish nurse's ability to connect with the members and increases the parish nurse's sense of value in and worth to the congregation.

In the church setting the mentor should try to meet and converse with other staff, especially the church secretary. This will add to the mentor's understanding of the personalities with whom the parish nurse is working and also provide insight into the regard and the relationship that the staff have for the parish nurse. In observing the church setting, the mentor is able to see visual signs of the parish nurse's presence. Is health information displayed in an appropriate place; is the nurse's bulletin board attractive and in an area of traffic; are articles well written in the weekly or monthly church publications? Is there a ready store of educational resources to offer clients, and are the resources accessible so that clients can select for themselves? These are features that are often not mentioned in written or verbal reports the parish nurse may submit, thus the mentor may be unaware of the situation and therefore unable to suggest methods to improve the practice.

The mentor should meet with a parish nurse in an informal space, without the physical barrier of a desk between them. The verbal and nonverbal exchange between the two will take on a different flavor, more supportive of a mentoring relationship. The use of a clipboard or forms by the mentor will tend to reflect a supervisory relationship and should not be used during the meeting.

The amount of time the mentor meets in person with the parish nurse is determined by the needs of the parish nurse: usually more time at the beginning of the practice, then weekly, and then monthly. The parish nurse should feel comfortable contacting the mentor more frequently as needed; however, the mentor should be able to set sensitive boundaries to the frequency of the contact. The mentor should be concerned if a parish nurse tells the mentor there is no need to meet. This may mean that the mentor is too restrictive or judgmental or possibly even too inexperienced with the practice of parish nursing to be credible. The parish nurse may view the mentor as less than helpful. I have been told by a parish nurse that she did not call her mentor because "I know more than she does about the practice."

The length of the mentoring process is not predetermined. It occurs when there is mutual agreement between the mentor and the mentee, as opposed to an institution's time commitment. There is always the potential that the mentee does not want to be weaned from the mentor, but the role of the mentor is to prepare for this throughout the mentoring process. "I think I need some more material to read," said one aspiring parish nurse. My response, however, was to say, "No, you need to call this number; they are looking for a parish nurse." The mentor must also guard against delaying the termination of the relationship, because of positive rewards perceived from the control and status of the mentoring position. Both parties need to be assured that while their relationship may no longer be termed mentoring, the experiences they have shared will usually have created a connection that is positive and maybe ongoing. This is not, however, a requirement for mentors nor mentees.

Conclusion

Effective mentoring is a whole person relationship that focuses on changing people from the inside out, not outside in (Stoddard, 2003). It is an honor for a person to be selected as a mentor, and the mentor must be committed to fulfilling the role. The mentor must avoid supervising, judging, managing or formally evaluating. The mentor must be able to set boundaries, respect confidentiality, instill trust, encourage growth, challenge with sensitivity, and care unconditionally. This requires time, maturity, and a humble desire to restore nursing to its original meaning—the care of the spirit.

REFERENCES

Glanz, B. (2000). *Handle with care: motivating and retaining employees.* New York: McGraw Hill.

Huang, C. & Lynch, J. (1995). *Mentoring: the Tao of giving and receiving wisdom.* New York: Harper Collins.

Loehr, J. & Schwartz, T. (2001). The making of a corporate athlete. *Harvard Business Review,* 79(1) pp 120-128, 176.

Morton-Cooper, A. & Palmer, A. (1993). *Mentoring and preceptorship.* London: Blackwell Scientific Publications.

Murray, M. (2001). *Beyond the myth and magic of mentoring.* San Francisco: Jossey-Bass.

Sellner, E. (1990). *Mentoring: the art of spiritual kinship.* Notre Dame, IN: Ave Maria Press.

Shea, G. (1997). *Mentoring: a practical guide.* Menlo Park, CA: Crisp Publications.

Stoddard, D. (2003). *The heart of mentoring.* Colorado Springs, CO: Nav Press.

Vance, C. & Olson, R. (1998). *The mentoring connection in nursing.* New York: Springer Publishing.

Encouraging the Heart of Parish Nurse Ministry: The Sabbatical Renewal Leave

Carol S. Tippe

A journey of sabbath time is about to begin...
Will I let go enough to let it take hold?
Or will I struggle with expectations and control and lose the
moments to be?
A journey of sabbath time is about to begin...
Will I trust in God's rhythm?
Will I trust others to continue the day to day?

The plan will take shape, you know,
but only in the listening
and the letting go.
— Carol Tippe

Encouraging regular sabbath rest and spiritual growth for the practicing parish nurse is an essential role of the parish nurse coordinator. The specialty of parish nursing will blossom if each practitioner takes time to value sabbath rest, spiritual growth, and visioning for the specialty in his or her daily practice. I wrote the above verses about 2 months before taking my first extended 4-month sabbatical leave from the ministry of parish nursing practice. It was an essential journey of sabbath time away from caregiving and into the restful, hopeful heart of God that gave me energy to continue professional parish nursing practice. In August of 1989, I became the first half-time paid parish nurse for St. Mark's United Methodist Church in Iowa City, Iowa, after 2 years of study by a grass-roots committee of the congregation. The church, growing and thriving in this urban academic community surrounded by rural Iowa, dedicated itself to being the first church in town to have a parish nurse program. The parish nurse program was integrated into the life of the congregation and expanded to a three-fourths–time position. I had been the parish nurse for the St. Mark's United Methodist congregation of 850 members, average age of 37, for 10 years at the time of my sabbatical. In 1998, after 2 years of study by our Staff Parish Relations Committee, a sabbatical leave policy for lay professional staff was adopted (see Appendix 16A). I was the first of the lay professional staff members to take advantage of the policy. The entire sabbatical leave was a time of spiritual growth full of many learning and stretching opportunities for the entire congregation!

The coordinator of a parish nurse program that values the spiritual journey of the parish nurse in practice and works to establish a pattern of regular spiritual renewal for each professional becomes an encourager and supporter of the heart of healthy parish nurse ministry in a congregation.

Parish nurse ministry in a congregation thrives when it finds its heart and health in God—and not just in many acts of kindness and caring. The coordinator of a healthy parish nurse program will be a role model for spiritual renewal practice, practicing what she preaches, by taking regular sabbath time and setting an overriding tone of regular spiritual renewal for the health of the entire program.

I have learned some lessons in forging sabbatical territory for parish nursing! I hope that by sharing these insights, I can assist other congregations to seriously consider sabbatical time for their parish nurses! If we could build an expectation of regular rest and renewal into the ministry of parish nursing practice, perhaps we could keep both nurse and congregation focused on God's work of love in our communities!

Planning and Communication for a Sabbatical Leave

Planning for a sabbatical is a slow, deliberate and prayerful process. It takes time for the spirit of valuing sabbath time to sink into the life of the congregation. It is a learning process on the part of the entire congregation—in worship, in stewardship, in committees, in leadership council meetings, and in staff meetings. Two of the best books on the planning of a sabbatical leave in a congregation are *Sabbatical Planning for Clergy and Congregations* by A. R. Bullock (1987) and *Journeying Toward Renewal: A Spiritual Companion for Pastoral Sabbaticals* by Melissa Sevier (2002). At St. Mark's, the writing of the sabbatical leave policy took approximately 2 years of study and committee work. Bullock (1987) and Sevier (2002), both of the Alban Institute, recommend at least 6 to 12 months of planning time before an actual time of sabbatical leave so that all the details of coverage may be planned. A congregation should go into the actual time of sabbatical knowing that the health ministry will be growing and changing because of this deliberate process of prayer and planning.

Communication of the sabbatical leave policy, plans for the first sabbatical leave, and detailed reassurances for the congregation are of utmost importance. A congregation, with all its layers of formal and informal communication, has to be well informed all along the process. The letters explaining the process and financing of the sabbatical leave were sent to congregational members and included in newsletters and bulletins during the planning period (see Appendixes 16B, 16C, 16D, and 16E). All members of the congregation need to have full details of the plans for transition and coverage of health ministry responsibilities in the day-to-day life of the congregation. Each member needs to know about the need for financial support of a sabbatical leave fund. The St. Mark's United Methodist congregation gave approximately $10,000 to gifts and memorials for the sabbatical leave fund to pay for planned expenses, salary, and benefits for the interim parish nurse. Sometimes denominational funds can be tapped for sabbatical support. The Louisville Institute offers grants for pastoral leave to both pastors and lay church staff. More information about the Louisville Institute and its Sabbatical Grants for Pastoral Leaders program may be obtained by accessing its website (www.louisville-institute.org) or by phone at (502) 992-5431. Grants are possible for both pastors and other religious leaders in congregations. I applied for one of their grants but did not receive one at the time of my sabbatical. However, the detailed process of applying helped in the clarification of my early plans for my sabbatical time and also lent credibility to the idea of sabbatical leave for members of the planning committee of our local congregation. Common questions about the sabbatical needed to be clearly addressed and readdressed by the Staff Parish Relations Committee, the church leadership, the staff, and the pastor specifically throughout the planning and implementation process.

The congregation needed to understand that sabbatical time is an intentional and planned time for spiritual growth, study, and sabbath rest. In our academic community of Iowa City, Iowa, the congregation needed to know that the traditional academic sabbatical as release time for research and travel was *not* the model! The emphasis for the time was the need for personal discernment, prayer, visioning, and rest in God. Some conferences would be attended, and some writing would occur, but the result of the sabbatical leave was not a well-researched paper but a well-rested and spiritually renewed person ready to vision future practice grounded in God's love and hope. This countercultural goal of rest and renewal instead of increased productivity was one of the liberating—but difficult to swallow—lessons for the congregation!

The more the congregation participated fully in the sabbatical leave process, the more growth happened in God's vision through this discernment process. Congregational prayer for the parish nurse and interim parish nurse, discernment questions for the health ministry, health ministry committee members, and volunteers expanded God's loving vision for the program overall. Appendix 16E lists some of the questions we asked the congregation to pray about during the sabbatical time. Every congregation will have a unique approach to this question-and-answer time, as unique as God's vision for that congregation's ministry.

The success of sabbatical depends largely on the pastors' and other church staff's support. The pastor's obvious support of the sabbatical in meetings and worship will lead the spiritual growth and renewal of the experience. One of the gifts of the sabbatical is the growth that happens in staff, committee, interim parish nurse, and lay support to cover the varied roles of the parish nurse while he or she is gone. New gifts may be discovered, and new directions for ministry may develop. Temporary replacement of the parish nurse by paid or volunteer persons offers new perspective in the staff role and may be a time for examining directions of the health ministry overall. It may also be an opportunity for the congregation to see the valuable role of the parish nurse separately from the personality and gifts of one particular person as parish nurse.

It is an affirming, worshipful act of God's hope for abundant living to actually recognize and celebrate the sabbatical transition inside a worship service. A specific responsive reading was written by our senior pastor to recognize and affirm sacred sabbatical as a part of Sunday worship (see Appendix 16F). It is highly encouraging that congregations integrate this value of sabbatical into worship life. An excellent resource for weaving sabbatical into worship is *Sabbath: Restoring the Sacred Rhythm of Rest* by Wayne Muller (1999). This book reaffirms the need for sabbath rest in all our lives and was the basis for a sermon series as our congregation explored the concepts of sabbath rest and renewal. I wrote the following poem in my journal to celebrate being

surrounded by a community of believers praying for my sabbatical time:

A Community of Believers

with me, within me,
even when alone.
A Promise never to leave;
that nothing can separate us
from Love in God.
Let me feel surrounded in comfort and community,
when I need to hide in You.
Let me feel surrounded in prayer,
upheld in hope and healing.
Let me surrender and let go into Your arms
of Grace –
in a spirit of trust,
in a spirit of peace,
in a spirit of hope.

Personal Challenges during a Sabbatical Leave

Learning to be Still

As a parish nurse and coordinator, I have found it difficult to rest, to move from doing to being in my life. Often each day seems full of urgent and important tasks to be done. I have to STOP regularly to recenter my ministry in God and find renewal for my faith so that I reach out with God's love and not my own agenda of doing! You can count on it taking 2 to 3 weeks of sabbatical time to begin to name the pile of distractions, grief, and unfinished business of a health ministry. Know this ahead of time! Bullock (1987) recommends planning a vacation period at the beginning of sabbatical time away and at the end to allow for transition time. A poem I wrote gives voice to my doing/being struggle during sabbatical time away:

Rest in Me

Quiet yourself – body, mind, and spirit
But how??
The foot taps…
The mind whirls…
The concerns continue…
The distractions pile…
Find space to seek the warmth.
Find space to swing in silence.
Find space to listen,
To dreams and visions,

To God's heart within you.
To Wisdom as She teaches you quietly.
It will be a great life-changing adventure!

Spiritual Direction and Reading

Having a spiritual director to meet with during the sabbatical time (and afterward!) is extremely helpful. This allows a transition into your own sabbatical journey with more ease. It gives you someone to listen to your own story with an ear for God's questions! I met with Ron DelBene (1995), an Episcopal priest and spiritual director in Birmingham, Alabama, for three 3-day sessions during my sabbatical. After years of helping people with sabbatical leave planning, Ron recommended this meeting schedule of beginning, middle, and ending spiritual direction. I selected Ron as my spiritual director for my sabbatical time because his writing about breath prayer and storytelling had been very important to me in my parish nurse practice. I had heard him speak in Iowa about grief and grieving and admired his spiritual storytelling from afar. It was a true gift of my sabbatical time to spend one-on-one time with Ron listening to my story of 10 years of parish nursing and my own life story. Even with my first spiritual direction appointment, I was able to hear dreams and visions. Sabbatical time is often a time alone, and even a lonely time, after having a daily parish nurse practice that is full to the brim with people and their concerns. Having a spiritual director helped me to name the renewal time and listen to my own needs for healing.

During a sabbatical time, finding devotional materials and readings that give a voice to the sabbatical discernment process is important. An established routine for devotional time must fit prayerfully with the changing vision of the quest of sabbath time. During my sabbatical, I spent time in reading and journal reflection each day. Two books of poetry, Chris Glaser's book *The Communion of Life* (1999) and Edwina Gateley's book *A Mystical Heart* (1998), were read each day and inspired personal poems in my journal. Other books had been on my list to read for months, and some were specifically chosen after naming themes for sabbatical learning and healing. I compiled a selected bibliography of readings that I would be delighted to share with readers upon request. Wayne Muller's (1996, 1999) writings on sabbatical rest were read in the planning stages of the sabbatical time and shared with the congregation. My sabbatical allowed more time than had ever been available to spend quietly listening to God. Spending a majority of sabbatical time at home requires the creation of a sacred space—physically, emotionally, and spiritually. Having a planned list of reading can frame the sabbatical time but allow for spontaneity and new learning, as God is directing this time. Visioning continues as an important ingredient to the time away from normal routine! One of the best pieces of advice that I received before my sabbatical was to *leave room for God* and not to fill up every waking moment with conferences and goals for the day.

The Need for Routine

The need for some of everyday life to remain stable in this sea of changing emotions, places, and relationships became very important during the sabbatical journey. Planning to attend one other church in the community for the majority of Sunday services and continuing to meet with a support group were essential for my continued growth. Continuing to meet with a discernment group in the community that had been a regular part of my schedule for the previous 2 years provided important support and reflection for which I was very grateful. At the same time, I felt significant grief at the temporary loss of very supportive daily contact with church staff colleagues and of church functions that remained so integrated into my daily life. The plan for the parish nurse on sabbatical time not to be available by phone or at church was very specifically addressed during the planning of the time away. This avoidance of personal contact with the congregation needs to be respected. Part of this was accomplished by having an interim, paid parish nurse in place and turning over the daily care to her competence. Time to grieve this loss of daily contact with the congregation and colleagues needs to be given. I needed time to grieve significant losses over the 10 years of compassionate caregiving, time to reflect on my grief, and time to remember what gifts I had received from the ministry of parish nursing practice!

One group to prepare for the difference of sabbatical time is the nurse's family and close friends. The rhythm of the days of sabbatical is so different that family and friends need to anticipate the change of routine and attention. Depending on the sabbatical plan, travel away from home may require childcare or eldercare planning. My family appreciated my increased availability for family time. My teenage girls also loved trying out some of the spiritual growth exercises with me, such as walking the labyrinths, journaling, and making collages. It was an opportunity to show them, as well, that renewal time is a valued part of any profession.

I found that having sabbatical time away for 4 months made me long for a regular daily routine of more time for prayer, retreat, and spiritual renewal. Planning short retreat moments and carving out time to listen to God more fully each day became a healthy priority. Needing to remember to "Be still and know that I am God" with a heart for God's hope after the sabbatical experience renewed my commitment to practice sabbath moments. This is reiterated in the following poem written during my sabbatical:

> With sighs too deep for words, God speaks to us
> Of need for healing time;
> "Be still and know that I am God."
> On this journey,
> Can I be still??
> Can I surrender doing for being?
> Can I love through prayer and silence?
> Can I leave behind busyness and take God's hand?

The Need for Creative Expression

Finally, a sabbatical allows for experimentation with creative expression of God's love. Use of the arts, nature, literature, poetry, and music allows the exploration of feelings associated with change and grief. I have found writing poetry to be an important reflective journaling exercise throughout my parish nurse ministry. I started writing poetry to explore the feelings of caring for beloved congregational members for whom I had cared over the years. I have also written poetry for congregational newsletter articles about the spiritual journey of health ministries' caregiving. Poetry has given me a creative outlet for sharing the spiritual journey of being a parish nurse. Recording of dreams and listening for God's call in the dream story has also assisted in this daily spiritual exploration. Sabbatical urges creativity in expressing the depth of your love for God. It strips away excuses, time commitments, and busyness and allows openness and vulnerability to find a voice for spiritual growth. I tried journaling, creative collage expressions, photography, and dream recording as I journeyed through the sabbatical time. New eyes, ears, and heart developed with exposure and practice during sabbatical exploration. The heart remembers once again that God is at the center of this ministry and at the center of all creative acts of love.

Reentering Congregational Life after Sabbatical Time

After 4 months away from the regular routine of parish nursing, I reentered the work of health ministry with renewed energy and new visions for programming. I had the advantage of having a nurse in my position half-time while I was gone for the sabbatical leave, so I did not return to a pile of unfinished business. The nurse that had taken my position returned to her member status with the congregation but had left behind her own gifts, talents, and expertise in her short time in the role. The congregation affirmed the fact that the parish nurse ministry needed to continue while I spent time on sabbatical. It reinforced the notion that the work of the ministry of parish nursing practice is an important ongoing ministry, not just a particular person doing nursing in our congregation.

The congregation received reports of my learning and renewal at their administrative council meetings and at the health and wholeness committee meetings. We established a Befrienders Lay Visitation ministry program as a result of training that happened during the sabbatical. We also reevaluated working styles within the ministry team and encouraged renewal time for other staff. Overall, the experience was extremely positive for the congregation and for me.

One particular outgrowth of the sabbatical time was a new vision for sabbatical time away for evaluation of best practices, for renewal of ministry energy, and for evaluation of future directions of the ministry of parish nursing practice in the local congregation. The concluding pages of this paper are a reflection of these sabbatical lessons extended to the practice of regular renewal and evaluation of practice for the entire specialty of parish nursing. The plan that follows is this author's reflection on how to incorporate regular sabbatical leave and evaluation into the ministry of parish nursing practice over time in a congregation. If we do not stop to reflect and vision, the practice of parish nursing will continue to just meet urgent crisis problems. The health of this specialty depends on regular self-care, renewal, and visioning by each parish nurse.

Sabbath Time: A Reflection on an Opportunity to Value Regular, Deliberative Visioning for the Ministry of Parish Nursing Practice

One overriding conclusion of my sabbatical experience was that the specialty of parish nursing needs to incorporate spiritual growth and renewal experiences into its expected professional evaluation procedures. Taking time out from constant caregiving to evaluate best practices in the specialty and to set goals and visions for the future practice in the local faith community must be a priority of the specialty of parish nursing. Renewal and sabbath rest at the programmatic level facilitated by the coordinator of a parish nurse program allows for growth and best practices to be shared and celebrated as God's ministry and love in action. Renewal time for the program honoring the interactive relational ongoing process between God, the person or persons cared for, the parish nurse, and other spiritual care team members, allows for breathing space and reflective time by all involved. Time apart from ministry for the group process of evaluating excellence in spiritual care celebrates God at work and *not* the comparison of one parish nurse's practice to another's unique practice. Time for group evaluation of best practices would showcase this unique ministry in each setting by developing a flexible, creative, and personalized process for the evaluation of each parish nurse.

The Process of Evaluating the Ministry of Parish Nursing Practice

The specialty of parish nursing should empha-size regular spiritual growth and renewal for its professional nurses and incorporate spiritual

growth and renewal into every program or regional level periodic evaluation process. I suggest that parish nurse programs and individual parish nurses spend deliberate sabbatical time at least every 5 years to evaluate best practices in parish nursing and visions for the future of the specialty. Parish nursing should refocus some of the specialty's energies into the development of a system for recognizing, encouraging, and sharing experiences of excellence in professional parish nurse practice. I specifically hope we can develop regional or statewide centers for excellence in parish nurse practice that could support ongoing renewal and periodic evaluation of the spiritual care and spiritual growth of parish nurses. The following distinct characteristics of the ministry of parish nursing practice must be remembered as any evaluation process is developed for parish nursing practice:

- The goal of any process developed is centered on God's work done through very human parish nurses. If we truly believe that it is God's work done by God-gifted parish nurses, the process should recognize the spiritual growth and renewal of the parish nurse as essential to the excellent spiritual care provided by the parish nurse.

- Much of what is provided as spiritual care by parish nurses is difficult to quantify. Outcomes of spiritual interventions are an interactive relational ongoing process between God, the person or persons cared for, the parish nurse, and other spiritual care team members. Any evaluation process should recognize and utilize this relational understanding.

- If we truly celebrate God at work through the practice of this professional specialty, the process of evaluating excellence in spiritual care celebrates God at work and *not* the comparison of one parish nurse's practice to another's practice. The process should not be based on human rewards or comparisons.

- Nursing theories that include caring and identify spiritual diagnoses and interventions are just beginning to be more fully understood and appreciated within the profession of nursing. The process of evaluation of excellence in spiritual care by parish nurses should assist in the growth of this understanding.

- Spiritual caregiving by the parish nurse is centered on advocacy for healing and whole person well-being. It is a unique, dynamic, and spiritually transforming process with each person. The evaluation of excellence should showcase this uniqueness by developing a flexible, creative, and personalized process for each parish nurse.

Several related professional fields of practice lend some helpful information to the development of a process for evaluating excellence in parish nursing. The American Holistic Nurses Association, Healing Touch International, Chaplaincy Certification, and the National Board for Professional Teaching Standards have models for standards, certification, professional portfolio development, and peer review. Box 16-1 lists the websites for these and other organizations. Parish nursing can gain valuable professional insights from these models for visioning, evaluation, and renewal.

Insights on Visioning and Evaluating Parish Nursing Practice

Some of the learning gained from my sabbatical leave follows:

1. *The importance of developing and sharing a professional portfolio of best practices in peer groups.* This practice can identify strengths of the profession and its practitioners and can build a body of knowledge for the specialty's interventions. It can also facilitate the sharing of stories of practice and encourage creativity.
2. *The importance of planned regular regional retreats for personal and group visioning.* Naming directions for the specialty as a group, program, or region facilitates the vision and honors the process and time spent as essential to quality practice of the specialty.

Having regional centers for peer review of the ministry of parish nursing practice could help peers to organize, encourage, and recognize excellence in practice.

3. *The importance of peer review and spiritual insight.* The specialty of parish nursing can be very independent and isolating. Group insight and telling of stories is essential to the spiritual renewal of the specialty.
4. *The importance of mentoring and spiritual guidance.* Individuals practicing the profession of parish nursing need the insights of mentors, spiritual guides, and other peers to keep their practice of parish nursing fresh, creative, and centered on God's ministry within the faith community.
5. *The importance of writing narrative statements of faith development and stories of parish nurse practice.* Spiritual growth and renewal requires intensive study, reflection, and journaling. Writing the stories of faith development preserves the stories for future study and insight. With attention to confidentiality and permission, stories should be shared in congregations when possible, in support groups of parish nurses, and in book and magazine article form to illustrate the practice of the specialty of parish nursing. National conferences for parish nursing and health ministries such as the annual Westberg Symposium, sponsored by the International Parish Nurse Resource Center, and the annual Health Ministries Conference could be places for sharing the important stories and reflections on the ministry of parish nursing practice.
6. *The importance of verbatim writing and sharing in group process.* Skill in client

---

BOX 16-1   Websites of Professional Organizations Related to Parish Nursing

American Holistic Nurses Association: www.ahna.org; (800) 278-2462
Healing Touch International: www.healingtouch.net; (303) 989-7982
National Association of Catholic Chaplains: www.nacc.org; (414) 483-4898
Association for Clinical Pastoral Education: www.acpe.edu
Association of Professional Chaplains: www.professionalchaplains.org; (847) 240-1014
National Board for Professional Teaching Standards: www.nbpts.org
Louisville Institute: www.louisville-institute.org

interaction and sharing lessons learned from evaluation of that interaction provide insight into the therapeutic use of self as a professional in ministry.

A Model for Incorporating Sabbath Time, Spiritually Based Evaluation, and Best Practices in the Ministry of Parish Nursing Practice

Every 5 years of professional practice, each parish nurse would compile a professional portfolio of spiritual care expertise. The materials for this portfolio would be collected in the ongoing daily practice of the parish nurse, but separate time would be needed for compilation and practice reflection. He or she would submit this portfolio to a regional or state peer review team for commentary and evaluation. He or she would have a professional sabbatical renewal leave of at least 3 months for professional compilation of the portfolio, spiritual direction, renewal, and rest. The portfolio would include evidence of the key characteristics of exemplary spiritual care in written reflection and case studies collected during daily practice, possible videos of group and individual interventions, letters of endorsement and recommendation, journal entries, and other creative submissions of individual and group spiritual care. Three months after submission of the portfolio, the parish nurse would meet with the peer review team in person for open dialogue of lessons learned, dreams for the improvement of spiritual care practice, and insights for personal spiritual growth.

Key components in compiling a sabbatical portfolio include:

1. Background information on parish nurse and faith community
   - Basic education in parish nursing
   - Submission of continuing education courses
   - Basic nursing educational background
   - Clinical Pastoral Education completed
   - Other spiritual care education or specialty education completed
   - Completion of certification exam in parish nursing when available
   - Current position description and description of the faith community

2. Evidence of ongoing commitment to personal spiritual growth while practicing as a parish nurse
   - Spiritual autobiography and updates
   - Personal spiritual assessment
   - Mentor relationship development
   - Retreat plan and evidence and/or continuing education
   - Spiritual reading bibliography and commentary
   - Spiritual guidance by spiritual director or peer group
   - Journaling on proposed spiritual questions
     What are you learning about yourself?
     In what ways are you searching inwardly?
     What do you not know?
     What are you clinging to that you thought you knew?
     What stories are you thankful for?
     How are you continuing to search for your heart and practice?
     How do you get 'full' so that you can continue to give to others?
     What dreams or visions do you have for yourself?
     What stories of mystery and miracle have you lived?
     In what ways are you serving the health ministry with creativity, imagination, and love?

3. Evidence of the relational nature of spiritual care: God, person, parish nurse, supportive family members, other spiritual care team
   - Full case studies submitted with ministerial reflection and faith reflection
   - Full use of nursing process: assessment, diagnosis, interventions, evaluation
   - One verbatim dialogue—written or video
   - Letters of support from within the faith community and denomination
   - Regular attendance at parish nurse support group and church staff support meetings
   - Evidence of collaborative team spiritual care from:
     pastor and other staff
     lay ministers
     other agency collaboration
   - Evidence of both group and individual spiritual care

4. Celebrations of God at work through the ministry of parish nursing in your faith community: stories, video, worship experiences, programming that integrates spiritual care
5. Documentation of the use of specific spiritual interventions for spiritual care roles of advocacy, comforter, companion, and resource guide
   • Prayer and rituals
   • Integrative active listening
   • Presence
   • Worship
   • Retreat
   • Reading/writing
   • Music
   • Encouragement of spiritual reflection
   • Whole-person care
   • Other developing interventions
6. Identification of areas for continued growth
   • Visions for the ongoing parish nurse practice
   • Identification of needs for specific continuing education/ retreat/sabbatical renewal

Why Commit to the Process of Visioning and Renewal?

With the integration of a periodic deliberate renewal and reflection process, the specialty of parish nursing will take time to regularly evaluate and learn from the practice of specific parish nurses.

Parish nurses will value their own spiritual growth as essential to quality spiritual care provided in their faith communities.

Individuals, groups, and faith communities will benefit from improved spiritual care provided by rested, reflective parish nurses.

Most important, God's work of love and care will be done in the world!

Conclusion

One final poem written at the end of my sabbatical leave expresses the renewal of God's love and hopeful vision for future health ministry:

Breath of God,
Ruah,
Indwelling Spirit,
Presence of Grace and Love;
Breathe on me and fill me with new visions.
Visions of courage,
Hope,
Mutual ministry,
Servanthood,
Leadership,
Wholism,
Collegiality,
Community.
Breath of God,
Ruah,
Indwelling Spirit,
Presence of Grace and Love.

REFERENCES

Bullock, A.R. (1987). Sabbatical planning for clergy and congregations. Bethesda, MD: The Alban Institute.
DelBene, R. (1995). Hunger of the heart: a call to spiritual growth. Nashville: Upper Room Books.
Gateley, E. (1998). A mystical heart. New York: Crossroad Publishing.
Glaser, C. (1999). Communion of life: meditations for the new millennium. Louisville, KY: Westminster John Knox Press.
Morgan, R. (1996). Remembering your story, realizing your faith: a guide for spiritual autobiography. Nashville: Upper Room Books.

Muller, W. (1996). How then shall we live?: four simple questions that reveal the beauty and meaning of our lives. New York: Bantam Books.
Muller, W. (1999). Sabbath: restoring the sacred rhythm of rest. New York: Bantam Books.
Sevier, M.B. (2002). Journeying toward renewal: a spiritual companion for pastoral sabbaticals. Bethesda, MD: The Alban Institute.

APPENDIX 16A

Lay Professional/Program Staff Sabbatical Leave Policy

The following sabbatical leave policy applies to program staff members of St. Mark's UMC who have been employed at St. Mark's for a minimum of 5 years continuous service under the following conditions:

One sabbatical leave may be granted for up to 12 months.

The content and purpose of the leave is to be related to the staff person's work responsibilities, to expand or enhance person's ability to perform ministry and the ministry of the church. Leave may be granted without or with pay (full or partial) depending on the availability of funds in the "sabbatical leave fund" established by St. Mark's and administered by the Staff Parish Relations Committee.

Request for sabbatical leave is made by the staff person in writing to the SPRC, preferably 9 months before the leave begins.

A Sabbatical Leave subcommittee of the SPRC will be established to meet with staff persons exploring leave possibilities. This subcommittee will assist the staff person and ministry areas that work with the staff person in working out the details of the leave for presentation to the SPRC. The SPRC will make a recommendation to the Administrative Council concerning the leave. A decision on the leave typically will be made 6 months before the leave is to begin.

The SPRC is responsible for ensuring the staffing of the church during the leave. Leave may or may not be granted depending upon the availability of adequate staffing for the church. After the first leave additional sabbatical leaves may be granted, one sabbatical leave for every additional 5 years of service.

Only one staff member of St. Mark's shall be on sabbatical leave at any one time.

All parties are referred to the following resources for sabbatical leaves: *The Discipline of the United Methodist Church*; the policies of the Iowa Annual Conference of the United Methodist Church; and *Sabbatical Planning for Clergy and Congregations* or subsequent edition by A. Richard Bullock, published by the Alban Institute.

This policy does not apply to clergy under appointment by the United Methodist Church. Policies regarding clergy sabbatical leave are established by the Iowa Annual Conference of the United Methodist Church and *The Discipline of the United Methodist Church*.

Reprinted with permission of St. Mark's United Methodist Church, Iowa City, Iowa.

APPENDIX 16B

First Congregational Letter: SPRC Announces First Sabbatical Leave

Brothers and Sisters in Christ,

During the past year, the Administrative Council has adopted a Sabbatical Leave Policy recommended by the Staff Parish Relations Committee (SPRC), in acknowledgment of the longevity of the staff serving our congregation at St. Mark's and in a sincere sense of partnership with the staff in maintaining their spiritual health and well-being over the long term. The sabbatical leave is important for the future growth of ministries at St. Mark's. We have been fortunate to attract and keep such a productive staff. This will provide another opportunity for the congregation to acknowledge our staff's essential work for the church.

In accordance with the Sabbatical Leave Policy, and after ten years of highly dedicated service, Carol Tippe has now planned a sabbatical with the approval of and in close consultation with the SPRC. A fully paid sabbatical is scheduled for March 15 to July 15, 2000, for which Carol has developed a positive program of rest, spiritual renewal, and service as well as study in the areas of servant leadership, gifts for ministry, and directions for health ministry. SPRC is convinced that Carol will not only attend to her own renewal but also return with spiritual gifts to enhance the ministry of St. Marks.

SPRC has determined that the best approach to maintaining the health and wholeness programming at St. Mark's in Carol's absence is to 1) solicit volunteers from the Health and Wholeness Committee, Worship Committee, lay leaders, and other volunteers for a number of large and small activities; and 2) hire a temporary professional nurse with extended training in counseling and experience in hospital visitation to provide 15 hours' service per week on a flexible schedule. This temporary paid position is interim only.

We are fortunate to have identified Karen Kuntz, a member of St. Mark's since 1990, who has agreed to accept this temporary position. Karen has a Doctor of Nursing (ND) degree from Case Western Reserve University (1988) and is a Certified Clinical Specialist in Adult Psychiatric Mental Health Nursing. She has worked as a staff nurse in adult psychiatric nursing since 1988, at University Hospitals and Clinics in Iowa City since 1990. For the last 2 years she has also worked part-time in a temporary position with the Psychiatric Nursing Consult—Liaison Service seeing medical patients. She has completed a parish nurse class over the ICN (a course Carol Tippe helped to develop). She has also been involved with the Health and Wholeness Committee at St. Mark's for several years and is the current chair. Karen will be compensated at $14.50 per hour plus standard benefits, for a total package of approximately $4241 over the 4 months.

The plan for funding of sabbatical leaves is handled on a case-by-case basis. SPRC has recommended and Administrative Council has approved Carol's sabbatical at full salary. The interim parish nurse costs will be funded from the Thompson Gift. With the recent announcement that Carol's sabbatical did not receive funding from the grant applied for, we are still exploring ways to fund Carol's estimated out-of-pocket expenses of $5,000.

To help cover these costs and build up the fund for the future, the congregation is invited to give to the Sabbatical Leave fund as the spirit moves you.

For further information, feel free to contact any member of the SPRC.

Reprinted with permission of St. Mark's United Methodist Church, Iowa City, Iowa.

Second Congregational Letter: Questions and Answers About Sabbatical for Parish Nurse

February 9, 2000

Dear Friends in Christ,

Several repeated questions about the sabbatical leave for our parish nurse, Carol Tippe, have come to the attention of the committees of Health & Wholeness and Staff-Parish Relations. We thank everyone for their questions and support of the sabbatical leave program. On the back of this page is the financial report of the leave. Please continue to direct your questions to the SPRC, Health & Wholeness, Carol Tippe, and/or Pastor Harlan. Printed below are the five most often asked questions and answers.

When does your vacation start? Sabbatical time is not vacation, but a time for spiritual growth, study, and sabbath rest. She will be traveling to conferences (see back page), completing study, and spending time in prayer and journaling for her benefit and for the benefit of the church. The sabbatical time is four months: March 15 to July 15, 2000.

What is the difference between sabbatical and a study leave or leave of absence? St. Mark's UMC's sabbatical leave program is an intentional and planned time of spiritual growth, study, and sabbath rest. This makes it quite different from the traditional academic leave or continuing education. The SPRC has worked with Carol to design the Sabbath program, emphasizing the need for discernment for Carol as a parish nurse and the future needs of the health ministries program of St. Mark's. Much of what is planned fits into the visioning process for the church. The study includes mentoring, information, and new approaches from various leaders and ministry settings that will benefit both Carol and St. Mark's UMC.

How is the transition being planned for the four months' coverage of health ministries by Karen Kuntz and the Health & Wholeness Committee? Karen is already orienting with Carol for 20 hours from now to March 15. She will be visiting families with Carol and doing some hospital visitation with Carol. As in any pastoral care ministry, it will be necessary for anyone who desires care from Karen as the parish nurse to contact her. Good pastoral care ethics dictates that information not be passed from one caregiver to another without the involvement of the parishioner.

Can we contact Carol while she is on sabbatical leave? Carol will not be available for any visits or by phone during her sabbatical leave. Karen will be available for office hours on Tuesdays, Thursdays, and Sundays and by phone for concerns and emergencies. Pastor Harlan and Karen will maintain the team approach to pastoral care needs, counseling, and visitation. Access to pastoral care can be done as it always has been: by calling the parish office.

How can the congregation participate in the sabbatical leave? Sabbatical leave is a time of learning for both the staff member on leave *and* the congregation. Congregational prayer for both Carol and the congregation; study; discernment; discussion; volunteering to assist in care giving; and when you are in need of pastoral care, speaking that clearly to either Pastor Harlan and/or Karen are all good ways to support the time of sabbatical. For instance, only Mercy Hospital has a program to call the church when someone is in the hospital, but it is not their priority to do so. Their first priority is to make the necessary treatment. It is really the responsibility of the person in the hospital and/or family or friends to contact the church. Jesus was met by many people requiring care, yet in every case it was the responsibility of the person needing care to make that need known to Jesus.

There may be many more questions about the sabbatical leave, simply because this is the first time that St. Mark's has done this. When and if you have any questions, please contact the SPRC, Health & Wholeness Committee, Pastor Harlan, and/or the parish office with your questions.

Grace & Peace,

The Staff Parish Relations Committee (SPRC); The Health & Wholeness Committee;
Pastor Harlan Gillespie; Carol Tippe, Parish Nurse; Karen Kuntz, Interim Parish Nurse

APPENDIX 16D

Parish Nurse Sabbatical Leave: Financial Report

Planned Expenses

Sabbatical Program, March 15 through July 15, 2000	$ 5,100.00
Amounts listed include tuition, fees, transportation to and from the event, room & board.	
Spiritual Direction with Ron DelBene, Birmingham, AL	1,800.00
Spiritual Life of Spiritual Leaders, Shalem Institute, Bethesda, MD	800.00
Health Ministries Association National Meeting, Houston, TX	800.00
The Interconnected Web/Church of the Savior	1,000.00
Be Frienders Basic Foundation Training, St. Paul, MN	600.00
Prairie Woods Retreat Center/Retreat-Study Days	100.00
Salary/Benefits for Interim Parish Nurse	4,946.00
Based upon 20 hrs of transition & 15 hrs./week 03/15 through -7/15	
Salary	4,097.00
FICA	314.00
Accountable Reimbursement Plan for work related expenses	500.00
Worker's Compensation	35.00
III. Total	$10,046.00

Income

All income listed has been received to date.

Congregational Giving to the Parish Nurse Sabbatical Leave	$ 2,330.00
Peterson Memorial Fund	3,840.00
Thompson Gift	3,876.00
Total	$10,046.00

   Those persons wishing to contribute to the sabbatical leave for Carol Tippe may do so by making an offering to St. Mark's UMC with the memo "Parish Nurse Sabbatical." These contributions to the Parish Nurse Sabbatical offerings will offset the Peterson Memorial and Thompson Gift. This "offset" money from the Peterson and Thompson funds will go into the Sabbatical Leave Fund for future staff sabbaticals. Persons who wish to give to the Sabbatical Leave Fund for future staff sabbaticals may do so at any time making an offering to St. Mark's with the memo "Sabbatical Leave Fund."

Reprinted with permission of St. Mark's United Methodist Church, Iowa City, Iowa.

APPENDIX 16E

Questions for Congregational Exploration: March 2000 Newsletter Article

"I came that you may have life and have it abundantly. " -John 10b

This week Carol begins her sabbatical time away form St. Mark's. On Wednesday, March 15, Karen and a team of lay persons will be taking over the health ministry program.

In the next 4 months, we invite you to join in this time of reflection and renewal of our Health Ministries at St. Mark's. We invite you to 'live the questions' together that will guide us to a new vision for health ministry outreach. Consider the following questions and give the Health and Wholeness Committee or Karen Kuntz, Interim Parish Nurse, your insights.

- What are the strengths of our health ministry at St. Mark's and how can we build on those strengths?
- What is God calling us to do in our Journey toward Wholeness together in this community?
- What vision and dreams do you have for St. Mark's Health Ministry? What needs do you see around you that we could address together?
- What one new program or support group would you like to see start in the fall?
- In what ways could we strengthen lay ministry involvement in the health ministry outreach to members and beyond?
- What opportunities for healing services and prayer should be offered regularly?
- How would you like to join the work of health ministry with your God-given skills and gifts?

Reprinted with permission of St. Mark's United Methodist Church, Iowa City, Iowa.

APPENDIX 16F

Worship Dedication and Blessing for Parish Nurse Sabbatical
March 6, 2000 Service of Recognition and Affirmation of Sacred Sabbatical

RECOGNITION & AFFIRMATION OF SACRED SABBATICAL

Many times Jesus went away for prayer and renewal. Separated from the crowds, alone, or with a few disciples, there was the intentional time and place for being with God. Today we affirm such a sacred sabbatical for Carol Tippe as our parish nurse. Sacred sabbatical time is not a luxury, but a necessity. We pray God's blessings upon you, Carol, as you seek God's guidance, reflect upon God's call in your life, and as you are renewed in the grace and love of God. We covenant to pray for you during this time and to support you as we also learn, renew, and reflect upon our ministry of health and wholeness.

While the time of sacred sabbatical is to be a time of change for both Carol and us as a congregation, it is also a time of learning and renewal of God's constant and unchanging love for us and for others. We also seek a sacred sabbatical by covenanting with one another to learn something new about our call to ministry of health and wholeness, to support Karen Kuntz as our interim parish nurse, to seek her expertise, and to journey with her as we journey together in a partnership of ministry in Jesus' name.

Let us pray. Gracious God from whom all sacred calls of ministry come, be with us all as we seek a sacred sabbatical. Bless Carol. Bless Karen. Bless us all. Renew us. Transform us. Cause us to grow in love, seeking the health and the wholeness that you have made for all humanity in Jesus Christ. And thereby may we always seek to bless all humanity in your healing and wholeness. Amen.

Written by Rev. Harlan Gillespie, Pastor of St. Mark's United Methodist Church, Iowa City, Iowa. Reprinted with permission of the author.

Distance Delivery of Parish Nurse Education

Cynthia Z. Gustafson

17

The age of distance delivery for nursing education is here (Segal-Isaacson, 2002). A new litany of teaching methods has arrived including terms such as web-based courses, synchronous and asynchronous online discussion boards, Internet journal discussions, and e-mail for nursing scholarship (Chaffin & Maddux, 2004). These innovations in technology have expanded the capacity of educational institutions to reach far beyond their own geographic areas to provide learning opportunities (Brown, Kirkpatrick & Wrisley, 2003).

Web courses are revolutionary in providing education to students who live at a distance or who cannot attend class at a prescribed time (Kiehl, 2004). Many nursing programs are meeting the needs of nursing students with online technology and reporting positive results for students and educators (Zucker & Asselin, 2003). This migration to distance delivery in parish nurse preparation is evolving more slowly. Opportunities for learners to access parish nurse education, especially basic preparation via distance delivery, are limited.

The majority of educational preparation programs in parish nursing are delivered face-to-face via lecture, discussion, and small group sharing. These programs include time for students to share in the process of spiritual formation with important activities such as prayer and worship. If parish nurses are being asked in their practice to lead worship, provide prayer and grow spiritually through community life, how can these skills be acquired in a preparation course that is completed alone in front of a computer or video screen?

It can be done. A handful of distance delivery programs for basic parish nursing education are available. These web-based programs include online discussions and feedback or interactive video conferencing that is similar to live classroom interaction. Allen College in Iowa, Saint Louis University School of Nursing, and the University of Southern Indiana School of Nursing and Health Professions all have online basic parish nurse preparation courses available. The Parish Nurse Center at Carroll College in Montana uses a combination of distance delivery and face-to-face interaction with the use of a statewide interactive videoconferencing network. The challenge for these programs is to build a sense of a present community in spite of distance delivery.

Online Courses: Advantages and Challenges

Basic Course Design

An online course in basic parish nurse preparation is delivered in a series of classes and over a designated time frame much like a traditional course—but without being in the physical classroom. If the parish nurse preparation course is affiliated with a college or university (as most are) the online course is then available for a student throughout a semester such as a 15-week time period. During this time period, the student can access or "attend" the class at any hour or day of the week via their personal computer. Students in online nursing education classes report that it is a "real treat not to attend class every week and to attend at their own convenience—even in bathrobe and slippers" (Thiele, 2003, p. 365).

For example, Saint Louis University offers a basic parish nurse preparation course each semester and, because of demand, also in a summer semester (L'Ecuyer, 2004). A student wishing to enroll registers before the start of the semester and receives detailed information on the technology and instructions needed to access the course as well as tips on how to take an online course. Students for this course are directed to web-based resources describing what it takes to be successful as an online student.

Examples of the types of tips given to the learner include being open-minded about sharing personal experiences; being able to communicate through writing; being self-motivated and self-disciplined, and being able to accept critical thinking and decision making as part of the learning process. All of these skills are especially helpful for basic parish nurse preparation in making the most of an online course that will develop a sense of present community.

Learners for the Saint Louis University course then can access the basic content of the preparation course through the use of audio lectures prepared by expert faculty accompanied with handouts and specific readings. Other online courses use specific textbook assignments to deliver the course content, and new technology in online nursing education provides for the use video streaming to enhance content presentation (Smith-Stoner & Willer, 2003). Each week a new lecture is offered on the website. Students are encouraged to set aside sufficient time each week as they would a scheduled class to access the material. Because the student can listen to the lecture or read materials at his or her convenience, an online course is flexible. If the student is busy during one of the weeks, she or he can access course content later.

However, this methodology has a downside. The course coordinator of the Allen College (Waterloo, Iowa) basic preparation course reports that an online course is not for procrastinators nor for those who cannot fit the time into their schedule to complete a course (Weepie, 2004). An online course instructor must emphasize to the student the good practice of time on task. To help promote this practice, instructors can use the following teaching tools for the students: weekly timelines in the online syllabus, a current course calendar, reminders posted on discussion boards of upcoming due dates, help for students in how to prioritize web "surfing," and clear expectations of frequency and quality of class discussion times (Koeckeritz, Malkiewicz, & Henderson, 2002).

Building Community Through Online Discussion

In addition to delivery of content, online courses rely heavily on students and faculty discussions as a way to acquire knowledge, share knowledge, and demonstrate course outcomes. Online discussions can be done as asynchronous communication or when participants do not need to be logged on simultaneously in the form of e-mail or a discussion board (Wills, Strommel, & Simmons, 2001). Students can log on to a bulletin board or forum at anytime and "check the latest comments, think it over, and respond by adding their own thoughts" (Chaffin et al, 2004). Another method is synchronous communication, in which faculty and students communicate at the same time like in a real classroom or online in a real-time chat room (Wills et al, 2001). This involves accommodating everyone's schedules and may not be as easily supported by all members' hardware or software (Chaffin et al, 2004).

Discussion can be much richer in the online venue than in the traditional classroom. For parish nurse preparation, students from online courses can be connected throughout the country and potentially throughout the world. "Virtual learning communities can be formed in the online environment" (Koeckeritz et al, 2002).

Learning can be both academic and social for the discussion groups, especially in small groups (Koeckeritz et al, 2002). Through the class-threaded discussion, the group can discuss an assignment, develop a response, and post input (Koeckeritz et al, 2002). In an online discussion, every member gets the opportunity to respond, whereas in the classroom environment a person's preference or personality or a limited timeframe might not allow responses from each group member (Wilhelm, Rodehorst, Young, Jenson, & Stepans, 2003). "These discussions provide opportunities for peers to connect, share information, and collaborate on coursework" (Buckley, 2003, p. 367).

Online discussions can go to a deeper level through the use of different pedagogical methods that could be used with parish nurse preparation or continuing education courses for parish nurses. McGrath (2002) describes the use of problem-based learning (PBL) for an online course with nurse practitioners. This methodology provided the nurses an opportunity to explore a complex case study with real-life patient encounters. The students work through discussion and rationale about how to handle the situations with the faculty acting as facilitators, not dispensers of facts. Process is important to this model and allows students to reveal their own thinking and decision making (McGrath, 2002). This technique is particularly appropriate for adult learners, such as parish nurse students who want to integrate their own knowledge into their practice. It would be a rich method for drawing out a student's spiritual beliefs and how those beliefs can interface with actions.

Another tool for developing critical competence in an applied discipline such as nursing practice is reflective journaling (Kessler & Lund, 2004). This teaching tool helps students "develop awareness of how they employ clinical decision-making skills" (Kessler et al, 2004, p. 21). In this method, the journal is a place to evaluate and record thought processes and actions in clinical experiences; one goal is improved self-efficacy (Kessler et al, 2004). Unlike PBL, reflective journaling is not done in the context of the larger online discussion but as a personal discussion between student and faculty member. Faculty members can provide feedback, guidance, and support to the student through secured responses (Kessler et al, 2004). This methodology would be especially helpful to a course in parish nursing beyond basic preparation, such as a mentoring relationship between a novice parish nurse and an experienced parish nurse.

The online courses in parish nurse preparation also provide students an opportunity to complete structured assignments on the role of parish nursing. These assignments are a means for the student to begin the work of this ministry in their faith community. This enhances the online experience, as the student now needs to interact face-to-face with those who he or she intends to serve. These assignments relate to the basic content of the preparation course and serve as a means for hands-on learning. For example, a student begins the process of assessing the health needs of the community through a variety of methods. As the student begins this assignment, the virtual class community offers a support group of the other students and faculty readily available to lend support and guidance and a sharing of ideas.

Online courses can use methodologies to enhance the sense of present community without ever meeting face-to-face. Adding a personal touch may be as simple as an exchange of pictures on a website, a brief biographical statement from each learner, a sincere welcome from the instructor, and timely frequent feedback (Koeckeritz et al, 2002). Lack of these simple tips can result in a common complaint from students related to online discussions: lack of immediate feedback from the instructor (Wills et al, 2001) as well as a desire for more feedback related to clinical expertise (Wilhelm et al, 2003).

Technology: Bane and Blessing

Another disadvantage related by students and faculty about online courses is the actual interface with the technology (Wills et al, 2001). Students can become very frustrated if they do not have technical support available (Frith & Kee, 2003). A student who is not proficient with the computer faces a large learning curve (Cragg, Humbert, & Doucette, 2004). This might be especially true with students seeking parish nurse preparation. Many of these students are retired nurses coming back to serve in a meaningful way during retirement years, and it can take some time and effort to get the skills needed to participate in an online course, whereas the young learner who has grown up with the technology may feel more comfortable.

Cragg et al. (2004, p. 20) describes the development of a "toolbox" for nursing students to improve computer skills and practice exercises for those needing extra help prior to the onset of the course. These tools range from paper-based materials to the basics of computer technology and include a face-to-face orientation session if appropriate. Web-based materials are used after the learner has mastered access, CD-ROMs for the software needed, and human support via the telephone (Cragg et al, 2004). These made for a smooth and positive transition into this new learning environment and also provided ongoing support.

The parish nurse preparation courses available online are associated with colleges and universities that can maximize this type of technical support and expertise. Saint Louis University and University of Southern Indiana place their parish nurse courses within the context of the continuing education departments of the university, where support staff facilitate the implementation of the course and address the technological issues. This is an important consideration for parish nurse educators developing online courses.

Faculty Preparation and Good Pedagogy

Not only do students have anxiety related to online courses, faculty do as well. It can be a daunting task for a seasoned classroom teacher to move to a new platform. Again, this could be especially true for faculty teaching parish nurse preparation, because many have had long careers in nursing education. What would be the first step to acclimating to this methodology? Dauffenbach, Murphy, and Zellner (2004) describe their college's approach: all new online faculty must participate as students in an online course before becoming instructors. The results of this work were positive for most faculty participating in this orientation; most were navigating the program with ease by the end and understood students' needs during online instruction. "Everyone recognized there is a learning curve with something new and there most be adequate support present from the beginning to give individuals a can-do attitude" (Dauffenbach et al, 2004, p. 73).

A second theme associated with the work of Dauffenbach et al (2004) was the time commitment needed to participate in online learning. This theme of time commitment for the instructor is reoccurring in the literature describing faculty reaction and especially the time commitment

needed to prepare the course (Christianson, Tiene & Luft, 2002; Wills et al, 2001). Significant time is needed both to develop an online course and to implement it the first time.

Not all professors are daunted by teaching online courses. Donnelly (2002) concludes that after teaching six online courses, she believes that "online learning leads to outcomes that equal or surpass traditional course formats" (p. 13). She gives the following suggestions for "teachers and students willing to take the cyber-learning plunge" (Donnelly, 2002, p. 13). She recommends that online teachers should: plot out the entire course in detail the semester before putting it online, master the software used for delivery of content and virtual classroom interactions, prepare for numerous e-mails from students, give prompt and thorough feedback, and be open to the idea of maintaining relationships with online students that persist far past the course completion (Donnelly, 2002). This last suggestion is especially relevant for parish nurse online courses because mutual deep relationships can form between instructor and student in the rich spiritual environment of the faith community.

For parish nurse educators willing to get started in the realm of online education, help in the nursing education literature abounds (O'Neil, Fisher & Newbold, 2004). Barker (2002) presents a case study approach to instructional design in web-based courses. She reveals that the natural tendency for faculty is to focus on the course content, but "rather the question should be, how will the students learn?" (Barker, 2002, p. 185). This question allows for the faculty to act as coaches, supporters, mentors, guides, and evaluators, and these roles are very appropriate roles for parish nurse educators, whether online or face-to-face. This is part of the process piece in the preparation of parish nurses.

Barker (2002) suggests that online courses be designed in modules that comprise an overview, performance objectives, a major content summary, readings, exercises, study journal exercises, assignments, and class discussion forums. Each part is explained in detail to the students as they work through the course. This approach allows for a visualization of the overall course content put into manageable parts for development and implementation. Barker (2002) also stresses the importance of classic principles of adult learning as developed by Malcolm Knowles in the context of mutuality and collaboration—two more principles relevant to parish nursing instruction and the need for building a present community.

Students report that the online learning environment is flexible, convenient, and accessible to many resources and that asynchronous discussions and chats are effective (Ali, Hodson-Carlton, & Ryan, 2004). What is the one factor that most predicts student satisfaction with online education? DeBourgh (2003) finds that good pedagogy is the key to student satisfaction. It is the quality and effectiveness of the instructor and the instruction, not the technology that is associated with student satisfaction (DeBourgh, 2003).

"Chickering and Gamson's (1991) *Seven Principles for Good Practice in Undergraduate Education* have been widely circulated and applied to college campuses throughout the United States and Canada" (Koeckeritz et al, 2002, p. 283). The application of these principles for online education in nursing gives insight to course design and implementation (Koeckeritz et al, 2002). These principles can also serve as a guide for developing distance education to parish nursing education.

1. *Good practice encourages student-faculty contact.* Faculty must be present to students, whether in the face-to-face classroom or the virtual classroom. Warmth and welcoming from the instructor is important to establishing the community of learners.
2. *Good practice encourages cooperation among students.* Discussion is vital to learning, especially for parish nurses. Ideas, beliefs, disappointments, triumphs, in ministry formation need to be shared, and much of parish nurse education is about forming skills for ministry in faith communities. This practice can be done via distance education.
3. *Good practice encourages active learning.* As adult learners, parish nurse students need active learning experiences to be able to apply their knowledge to work in the faith community. Active learning is found in the online course through threaded discussions, case study interpretations, and applications of projects to the faith community.
4. *Good practice gives feedback.* Prompt feedback is a must in the classroom, whether it is the interactive videoconference classroom or the

secure reflective journaling e-mail. The "old-fashioned technology" of the telephone is another way to make connections.

5. *Good practice emphasizes time on task.* Course calendars and specific deadlines can help learners to manage their time. Online work can overburden the student with time commitments; this problem must be addressed to allow for a satisfying experience.
6. *Good practice communicates high expectations.* Parish nurse courses are often held as continuing education events, and students are not given grades upon completion. Many do provide a certificate of completion; therefore, expectations about what constitutes completion of the course need to be clear in the distance delivery environment.
7. *Good practice respects diverse talents and ways of learning.* Parish nurse educators using distance-learning modalities need to be aware of their students' particular learning styles. Good descriptions given upfront of what skills are needed to be a successful learner in a distance delivery course are a good way to make sure this type of course is appropriate for a particular parish nurse.

Distance Delivery via Interactive Video Conferencing

Another method of distance education is the use of an interactive video conferencing network or system. This method is used by the Parish Nurse Center at Carroll College in Montana. Because Montana covers such a large geographical area, this method decreases travel time for participants and affords an opportunity to be "live" across the state without being in one location (Gustafson, 1999a, 1999b). In Montana the statewide interactive videoconferencing system METNET is used because it allows for the greatest statewide access through regional education centers such as universities and community colleges. This system also interfaces with the state's telemedicine networks that are located at many of the rural hospitals. This combination allows students to connect from border to border without travel. In Montana, that is a distance of over 600 miles. It is all done through use of an Integrated Services Digital Network (ISDN) line, using telephone connections.

This distance technology is much like a "live classroom." Presenters can come to a podium and deliver real-time lectures and have real-time interaction such as a question/answer session. Students are provided in advance the needed handouts to use at their locations. Faculty and students learn to adapt to the slight delay in the technology as sometimes the picture comes before words. The system is as good as the on-site operators or technicians who run the camera and sound. If the technician is in tune with the presenter and students, good interaction can occur as a presenter in one location can have a close-up camera angle to answer a question with a student that is also shown in a close camera angle at a remote sight.

Introductions of students at each site are a must. This practice allows for connection for the whole group. Class lists are helpful, and following class schedules with specific agendas detailing time and speaker make for positive feedback. A course coordinator at each remote location enhances the personal feel for students. These coordinators or hosts welcome and greet the participants as they arrive, answer questions pertaining to the local site, and work with the technician to make operations run smoothly. Distance education outcomes can be enhanced with the use of a course coordinator (Schulz, 2002).

The preparation course at Carroll College Parish Nurse Center is not completely delivered via distance. Half of the course content is delivered with this methodology, and then students complete the last half of the preparation time during an on-campus retreat that features more interactive group sessions related to case studies, prayer, and worship. When students arrive on campus and meet the other students whom they have seen only over the television screen, they comment that they still feel as if they know each other! This combination of distance learning and face-to-face interaction is meeting the needs for the state. Allen College also uses a combination of online and face-to-face; all students in the online course are invited to an Iowa statewide opening and closing ceremony.

Cost is one distinct disadvantage of the ISDN line technology. Active for over 20 years, this technology remains costly (Sackett, Campbell-Heider, & Blyth, 2004). The cost of using the METNET system in Montana for delivery of 16 hours of instruction to six sites accounts for at least half of the total operating budget of the course. Cost of interactive videoconferencing systems was one of the reasons that the Iowa network of parish nurse educators went to online preparation through Allen College in Waterloo. New modalities delivering interactive distance conferencing, such as internet protocol (IP), are available. Sackett et al (2004) provide an excellent discussion of the use of IP for a nurse practitioner teaching session, relating that the goal of IP is "seamless conferencing over the Internet" and that it can be accomplished with reduced costs (Sackett et al, 2004, p. 106).

Conclusion

In addition to basic parish nurse preparation, many parish nurse learners are seeking distance education in theology and ministry to enhance their practice. A wealth of opportunities allow students to explore online courses in these areas. North Park Theological Seminary in Chicago has been a leader in offering online courses towards a certificate in health ministry. Fisher's Net, an e-learning community network for theological studies, is another forum that has offered online courses specifically for parish nurses, such as Prayer for Parish Nurses. The format as described for online courses of content delivery via reading assignments and reflection time on discussion boards as well as journaling are all used for these types of courses.

"Technology has generated new challenges for education and the information age, including access to all groups, providing for meaningful critical reflection about significant information, and promoting a sense of community" (Wilhelm et al, 2003, p. 318). Although this statement is being applied to general nursing education in this context, it can also be applied to parish nurse education.

Parish nurse education must be accessible to all groups, and distance delivery can help to meet that access need. Parish nurse education is about challenging learners to use critical reflection to explore deep meaning from ministry interactions, and online modalities can meet this challenge. Parish nursing education is also about promoting a sense of community: a community of learners and teachers, and to relate learning to the context of ministry practice in the faith community.

The challenge is for distance delivery in parish nurse education to enhance student acquisition of ministry skills and build a sense of community. These processes and sense of community are flourishing in the live classroom and the virtual classroom. They can continue to be enriched as parish nurse educators use creativity and openness as keys to the ongoing development of quality distance education in parish nurse education.

REFERENCES

Ali, N., Hodson-Carlton, K., & Ryan, M. (2004). Students' perceptions of online learning. *Nurse Educator*, 29: 111-115.

Barker, A. (2002). A case study in instructional design for Web-based courses. *Nursing Education Perspectives*, 23:183-186.

Brown, S., Kirkpatrick, M. & Wrisley, C. (2003). Evaluative parameters of a web-based nursing leadership course from the learner's perspective. *Journal of Nursing Education*, 42:134-137.

Buckley, K. (2003). Evaluation of classroom-based, Web-enhanced, and Web-based distance learning nutrition courses for undergraduate nursing. *Journal of Nursing Education*, 42: 367-370.

Chaffin, A. & Maddux, C. (2004). Internet teaching methods for use in baccalaureate nursing education. *CIN: Computers, Informatics, Nursing*, 22: 132-142.

Chickering, A. & Gamson, Z. (1991). *Applying the seven principles of good practice in undergraduate education: new directions for teaching and learning.* San Francisco: Jossey-Bass.

Christianson, L., Tiene, D., & Luft, P. (2002). Web-based teaching in undergraduate nursing programs. *Nurse Educator*, 27: 276-282.

Cragg, C., Humbert, J., & Doucette, S. (2004). A toolbox of technical supports for nurses new to Web learning. *CIN: Computers, Informatics, Nursing*, 22: 19-25.

Dauffenbach, V., Murphy, L., & Zellner, K. (2004). Distance education experiential learning activity for novice faculty. *Nurse Educator*, 29: 71-74.

DeBourgh, G. (2003). Predictors of student satisfaction in distance-delivered graduate nursing courses: what matters most? *Journal of Professional Nursing*, 19: 149-163.

Donnelly, G. (2002). On-line learning: Take the cyber plunge. *Nursing*, 32(1):13.

Frith, K. & Kee, C. (2003). The effect of communication on nursing student outcomes in a Web-based course. *Journal of Nursing Education*, 42: 350-358.

Gustafson, C. (1999a). Distance learning parish nurse preparation model for Montana. *Perspectives in Parish Nursing*, Spring/Summer: 4-5.

Gustafson, C. (1999b). Parish nursing in Montana: statewide preparation via distance learning. *Pulse: Montana Nurses' Association*, April/May/June.

Kessler, P. & Lund, C. (2004). Reflective journaling: developing an online journal for distance education. *Nurse Educator*, 29: 20-24.

Kiehl, E. (2004). The traveling classroom. *Nurse Educator*, 29: 49-51.

Koeckertz, J., Malkiewicz, J., & Henderson, A. (2002). The seven principles of good practice: applications for online education in nursing. *Nurse Educator*, 27: 283-287.

L'Ecuyer, K. (2004) (personal communication, 16 June, 2004).

McGrath, D. (2002). Teaching on the front lines: using the Internet and Problem-Based Learning to enhance the classroom teaching. *Holistic Nursing Practice*, 16:5-13.

O'Neil, C., Fisher, C., & Newbold, S. (2004). *Developing an online course: best practices for nurse educators.* New York: Springer Publishing Company.

Sackett, K., Campbell-Heider, N., & Blyth, J. (2004). The evolution and evaluation of videoconferencing technology for graduate nursing education. *CIN: Computers, Informatics, Nursing*, 22: 101-106.

Segal-Isaacson, A. (2002). Distance learning: Technology puts continuing education within reach. *Nursing, 32,* (1), 14-16.

Schulz, P. (2002). The role of the course coordinator in a distance education course. *Nurse Educator*, 27: 217-221.

Smith-Stoner, M. & Willer, A. (2003). Video streaming in nursing education: Bringing life to online education. *Nurse Educator*, 28: 66-70.

Thiele, J. (2003). Learning patterns of online students. *Journal of Nursing Education,* 42: 364-366.

Weepie, A. (2004) (personal communication, 16 June, 2004).

Wilhelm, S., Rodehorst, K, Young, S., Jensen, L. & Stepans, M. (2003). Students' perceptions of the effectiveness of an asynchronous on-line seminar. *Journal of Professional Nursing*, 19: 313-319.

Wills, C., Stommel, M., & Simmons, M. (2001). Implementing a completely web-based nursing research course: instructional design, process, and evaluation considerations. *Journal of Nursing Education*, 40: 359-362.

Zucker, D. & Asselin, M. (2003). Migrating to the web: the transformation of a traditional RN to BS program. *Journal of Continuing Education in Nursing*, 34(2): 86-89.

Challenges to Parish Nurse Education

Mary Ann McDermott
Phyllis Ann Solari-Twadell

18

What are the challenges that face parish nurse education in this new millennium? They are not unlike those that face education and nursing education today. In recent times many academic institutions renounced or seemingly chose to distance their religious denominational sponsorship in order to move into the mainstream of academe. We are privileged, however, to be working with teachers, students, and administrators who overtly profess a spiritual motivation to their endeavors. It was refreshing to read, in this section, chapters that addressed efforts to strengthen content and processes—some familiar and some brand new—that offer the opportunity to facilitate wholeness of parish nurses for the future.

Following the themes for challenges outlined in Chapter 9 on challenges to the ministry, we have reordered them here to reflect our own perspective on priorities for parish nurse education.

The Challenge of Mindset

The distancing of academic institutions from their religious roots has had repercussions on nursing schools' curricula as well. Many of the parish nurses in practice today as well as the coordinators and educators were initially prepared in hospital diploma schools of nursing sponsored by religious orders and/or denominations. There was an implicit, if not always explicit, expectation that students would recognize and address the care of the human spirit in their patients. As nursing education moved into academic institutions, both public and private, this expectation was not usually clearly articulated. We have seen great variability across the country in implementing core content on spirituality in undergraduate and graduate program curricula. Future nurses will come to the ministry of parish nursing practice with a different educational foundation in spiritual care. Some will have a very solid foundation; some will view parish nursing as a component of the practice of complimentary alternative medicine (CAM). Some nurses will approach the practice as a site of care for community health nursing.

The decision to move the basic preparation for parish nursing and the coordinator curricula from healthcare institutions to the academic mainstream was a deliberate one, as Chapter 11 pointed out. The granting of continuing education units (CEUs) for the curricula offerings still predominates; however, the location of the curricula in the college/university setting increases its visibility to a wide range of educators. Processes for approval of course offerings, the necessity of having teachers who have peer-reviewed faculty appointments, publication in course catalogues and in the schedule, the ensuing discussion of appropriate content at faculty meetings—all of these measures increase the opportunity to tell the story of parish nursing to a broad audience. The integration of spiritual care into the entire nursing program, changes the mindset of our colleagues on the faculty. The idea that nursing is a vocation, a calling, becomes once again part of the language more easily spoken in our profession.

The identified faculty member responsible for the parish nursing curricula often becomes, ready or not, an acknowledged spiritual leader within the faculty. Usually, parish nurse educators in the college or university have not been engaged in parish nursing practice to any great extent. Initially this faculty person was identified as a point person, a liaison, someone known to be sympathetic to parish nursing and who held the credentials to sponsor the course in the institution. Required to take the basic parish nurse course before attending the educator preparation, the faculty member may or may not be an individual who recognizes the need for spiritual formation for self. This is usually identified as an essential requisite for the growth and development of the nurse engaged directly in the ministry. Chapters 4 and 14, Spiritual Formation and Learning to Pray, respectively, are not only essential reading for the parish nurse but also for the educator. This involves a change in mindset. The educator needs to be both knowledgeable about and practiced in the different ways of integrating prayer into the care for oneself as well as others. In Chapter 12, Cross states that we are not all expected to follow her path of attaining dual graduate degrees in order to demonstrate dual competencies, but what are the implications? What is appropriate for the parish nurse educator? The educator, by virtue of her position, is a person of influence within the parish nurse community, the professional nursing community, and the academic community. The model of spiritual leadership in Chapter 26 provides the parish nurse educator a language for thinking about her own capacities that are already present or need to be developed to effectively exert her influence in this area.

In Chapter 10, McDermott spoke briefly to the benefits of a parish nurse educator community. The International Parish Nursing Resource Center has provided a structure for networking the parish nurse educators. Technology facilitates this opportunity; however, some educators need to reflect on the value and worth of connecting with this community on a more regular basis. Beyond simple networking, the sharing of best practices, and doing curricular updating and revision, this community can provide collegial and spiritual support to its members.

A shift in mindset is desirable, we believe, for parish nurse educators in coming to acknowledge and value the significance of process as well as content in the curricula. This is not always an easy matter. Process elements are viewed as time-consuming and requiring creativity. We find writing and justifying the objectives for these activities difficult. Yet the process components of the basic parish nurse curriculum are distinguishing characteristics of this educational offering. Covering—or rather, uncovering—content by didactic presentations is engrained in all of us. It is how most of us were taught. The lecture is time-efficient yet inappropriate as the sole teaching/learning strategy for parish nursing. As Gustafson points out, it takes even more imagination to incorporate process elements in the distance-learning mode of delivering the program/s. Of course the whole idea of distance learning is a challenge to some of us, both as teachers and learners. The lack of readiness of parish nurse educators to implement quality programs through this technology is apparent, as is the reluctance of some nurses "of a certain age" to immerse themselves in a new way of learning.

Two areas included in this section are less familiar to us. Matheus points out the benefits and reciprocal nature of mentoring in parish nursing in Chapter 15. Matheus provided *that* mentoring on a personal level to a number of parish nurses in this country. However, few programs have elected to provide this as a complement to their basic programs on any formal basis. To be sure, some informal mentoring is occurring. We lack, however, the widespread tradition of mentoring within our society for women and consequently have had little experience of it in our profession. Parish nurse educators could do much to change the tradition! The other area that is unfamiliar to us, both in our society and in nursing, is the idea of extended sabbath. In Chapter 16, Tippe points out that this sabbatical is not to be likened to the academic sabbatical, which expects tangible outcomes like publications or completed research. Yet the periodic time for a sabbatical does have a history and tradition for clergy. Might parish nurse educators assist those in the ministry of parish nursing practice to be articulate spokespersons for ensuring this time for their personal renewal and revisioning?

The Challenge of Infrastructure and Resources

No infrastructure has been well developed as the underlying base or foundation, especially for an organization or system to provide support for parish nursing education. Positioning educational programming within educational institutions in collaboration with healthcare institutions, systems, and/or regional parish nursing networks has both strengths and limitations.

The International Parish Nurse Resource Center continues to bring educators together to develop curricula and to learn. The Center is not a professional nursing membership organization. *The Scope and Standards of Practice for Parish Nursing* were independently developed and recently revised by the Health Ministries Organization, a membership organization for not only parish nurses but also for all who are interested in health ministries. The American Nurses Association acknowledged the Health Ministry Association as the organization representing the specialty of parish nursing in 1997. Meeting the challenge of bringing these two organizations into alignment to work together so that curricula are developed that reflect the *Standards of Practice* is urgent. In many ways, parish nursing is ahead of other advanced practice and specialty nursing organizations in efforts to standardize core curricula. Quite often, institutions around the country have faculty who independently develop their own curricula. Years/decades later, as credentialing and certification are viewed as desirable, attempts are made to come together in agreement around essential content. Subsequently, a great deal of compromise is required to bring all these factions together to support core curricula. Parish nursing curricula were developed and continue to be updated and revised through a national consensus model. The model is based on research, and its development was supported by two faith-based universities. Although faculty can certainly add material and time to their offerings, the core content (endorsed) has been agreed on from the beginning.

The development of a process for certification in parish nursing has been discussed as the next logical progression in the maturation of this specialty. This is an expensive undertaking and one that is best done in collaboration with an organization that has a strong history in developing these processes. The International Parish Nurse Resource Center,

having the standardized core curriculum, has recently been in discussion with the American Nurses Association Credentialing Center regarding the development of a *Certificate in Parish Nursing*. It will be important to follow this development and see if this responds to the need for parish nurses to document their expertise in the ministry of parish nursing practice. If this certificate is developed it will be important that the current standardized core curriculum now disseminated through the International Parish Nurse Resource center is revised to reflect the most current research in parish nursing.

Both a relevant infrastructure and adequate resources will be necessary for a large-scale evidence-based curricular revision. Will the Deaconess Foundation support the International Parish Nurse Resource Center in initiating and funding this process? What will the role of the Health Ministries Association be? How should/could denominations at a corporate level interact with this process? How should/will academic institutions and their faculty participate? What will the curricular framework look like? How should standardized nursing language and *The Scope and Standards of Practice* be reflected in the curricula? Will a distance-learning format be designed for the curricula as an integral part of the revision? How will revised curricula be distributed? How will educators become familiar with and be prepared to teach both the process elements and the content? How will research be incorporated into the revision process?

Although efforts to remedy the situation have been made, poor geographical distribution of parish nurse curricula persists. A few states still lack any local programming and depend on institutions in neighboring states to bring their offerings on-site. Some congregations incur the expense of sending interested nurses out of state for the basic preparation. Perhaps the International Parish Nurse Resource Center could identify institutions and individuals in these underserved areas? Other areas of the country have the opposite problem. Programming overlap exists in many major cities. Several universities offer parish nursing preparation during the same time period. Parish nurse educators and their administrators lack the will to plan collaboratively rather than competitively for local programming. In these times of scarce resources, could these individuals promote a collaborative model infrastructure to other institutional leaders? The International Parish Nurse Resource Center has never wanted to be—and we certainly are not advocating they be—the gatekeeper that determines which institution's faculty will receive the curricula and be prepared to teach the curricula. This decision should be made locally. One example of local efforts to coordinate parish nurse educational offerings is the Wisconsin Parish Nurse Educators. This group is closely linked to the Wisconsin Parish Nurse Coalition, which is a special interest group of the Wisconsin Nurses Association. This parish nurse educator group convenes on a regular basis to dialogue, problem solve, and share best practices in parish nurse education.

Both infrastructure and resources for parish nursing education are in short supply in congregations, as well as in healthcare and educational institutions. For example, little national support for competency-based curricula and performance evaluation currently exists. Parish nurses, coordinators, and educators are not being widely encouraged to enroll in credit-bearing coursework for spiritual formation or to develop dual competencies, and the lack of tuition benefits for enrollment of this sort institutionalizes this problem. A research study of parish nurses currently practicing in the United States reported that 54% (n = 623) of the respondents have no funding for continuing education through their parish nurse positions. Of those that had funding (46%, n = 534), 41% (n = 219) identified that the funding came from the congregation, whereas 14% (n = 75) reported that their funding for continuing education came through an agreement with a healthcare institution (Solari-Twadell, 2002). These deficits in infrastructure and resources also apply to challenges involved in the implementation of a sabbatical leave.

The Challenge of Inspiration and Vision

A lack of vision hinders and may even prohibit the long-term survival—and certainly the vitality—of a movement. Parish nurse education has a vision and mission that must be revisited and modified as needed on a regular basis. As the ministry of parish nursing practice grows and matures, the collective vision and mission for parish nursing

education must always complement and challenge the ministry of parish nursing practice. In this section parish nurse educators were urged to "teach who you are." In the next section in a chapter on spiritual leadership, all those involved in parish nursing are asked to develop and/or acknowledge their capacities so that they might engage in spiritual leadership. What would parish nursing education look like in the future if all coordinators and educators embodied spiritual leadership and, in turn, taught who they were?

As a tangible outcome of her sabbatical time, Tippe developed a vision for sharing best practices and for preparing a portfolio of practice as an evaluative tool to assess the work of parish nurses. New ideas, like those coming from Tippe, from parish nurses that inspire us need to be communicated, fostered, and supported within the parish nurse educator community.

The Challenge of Clarity in Our Language and in All Our Communication

A number of terms used in our ministry of parish nursing practice continue to be ambiguous to the parish nursing community as well as the larger community. The challenge in the years ahead will be to clarify our terminology. For example, what does *dual competency/competencies* imply? How do you acquire them and demonstrate them? For what positions are nurses qualified when they gain this knowledge and new skills?

What are the implications of incorporating standardized language into the curricula? Will this attempt by national and international nursing leaders to clarify nursing language be perceived by parish nurses as burden or boon? A great deal of education, role modeling, support, and clarity of benefits for using standardized nursing vocabularies will need to be in place to make a smooth transition to a parish nurse community unfamiliar with the progress of this initiative over the last two decades. The influence of parish nurse educators in *translating* the value of this effort will be critical. This will be a challenge for many parish nurse educators who themselves are not knowledgeable on use of standardized nursing vocabularies. This new way of thinking and documenting seems beyond the everyday need of parish nurses who are already challenged to keep current on a myriad of diseases, medications, and technologies that those nurses with a narrower specialty do not encounter. However, as noted in Chapter 3, distinct advantages for parish nursing lie in the standardized nursing vocabularies to document the diagnosis, interventions, and outcomes.

Do all parish nurse educators believe that any registered nurse who uses the title *parish nurse* must have as a minimum a basic course preparation course to maintain that title? Fifteen years ago, Small (1990) described the parish nursing graduate program she had developed at Georgetown. Over the intervening years, during colloquia and in publications, other educators have advocated for master's preparation for this role (Magilvy & Brown, 1997). How will the parish nursing movement respond to the concept that parish nursing is an advanced nursing specialty, as indicated by having a defined scope and standards of practice document? Should a process be initiated to take first steps in advancing toward a certification designation for the parish nurse? If so, how should/would that process be financed? Will sufficient numbers of parish nurses, many of whom are volunteers, be interested in sitting for and willing to pay for such a credential? What will happen to others who choose not to engage in that process?

Parish nurse educators need to communicate more frequently with one another to establish a thriving parish nurse educator community. Also important is clear communication regarding the ministry and preparation for that ministry with colleagues in their schools of nursing and universities as well as to the faith communities and to denominational leadership. Often more comfortable with speaking, parish nurse educators need to write about the ministry in respected nursing and religious publications. Writing for magazines that are appealing to a broader public, while not counting for promotion and tenure, will serve the movement well. If you do not have the time to write or identify writing among your own gifts, encourage writing among the coordinators and parish nurses with whom you interact.

Clearly these and a number of other challenges for parish nursing education lie ahead, but as noted earlier, "Make room for the Holy Spirit!"

REFERENCES

Magilvy, J.K. & Brown, N.J. (1997). Parish nursing: advanced practice nursing model for healthier communities. *Advanced Practice Nursing Quarterly,* 2(4): 62-72.

Small, N. (1990). Curriculum development for parish nursing. In Solari-Twadell, P.A. & McDermott, M.A. (Eds.). *Parish nursing: promoting whole person health within faith communities.* Thousand Oaks, CA: Sage.

Solari-Twadell, P.A. (2002). The differentiation of the ministry of parish nursing practice within congregations. *Dissertation Abstracts International* 63(06), 569A, UMI No. 3056442.

UNIT III

Administration
of the Ministry
of Parish
Nursing Practice

Administration of Parish Nursing: Describing the Roles

19

Lisa M. Zerull
Phyllis Ann Solari-Twadell

The administration of parish nursing programs, networks, and services today is most often fulfilled by a nurse who holds the title of parish nurse coordinator (PNC). The PNC is defined as a liaison between an institution, parish nurse, pastor and/or congregation for the purpose of developing, supporting, and maintaining the ministry of parish nursing practice. The institution can be defined as a hospital, healthcare system, home care agency, community coalition, public health department, hospice, long-term care facility, health maintenance organization, school of nursing, or community agency (Solari-Twadell, 1999b, p. 5). The PNC combines the knowledge of parish nursing and management with that of spiritual leadership to guide nurses in the ministry of parish nursing practice with the goal of improving the overall health status of the congregation (Schweitzer, Norberg, & Larson, 2002). The PNC collaborates with other community services, parish nurse coordinators, possible funding sources, and local government. This chapter discusses: the role of the PNC; suggested preparation for the role; position titles; recommended qualities of leadership for this role; responsibilities associated with the role; and expectations of the PNC position. This chapter also will explore the role of the PNC as administrator. Clarification of this unique leadership role is needed to ensure the development of quality relationships among stakeholders and constituents

in order that the continuation of the ministry of parish nursing practice is assured and service to congregation members through the parish nurse is accessible.

Historical Overview and Development of the Parish Nurse Coordinator Role

With the visionary wisdom of Dr. Granger Westberg, there was no doubt that he had creative ideas regarding how parish nurses could reach out with a whole person perspective to those that they served. In Peterson's book entitled *Granger Westberg Verbatim: A Vision for Faith and Health* (1982), Westberg stated, "we are a part of a movement in history much greater than ourselves and greater even, than the entire healthcare institution: a movement of the Spirit, renewing and revitalizing human life" (p. 18). In his many writings on health ministry, Reverend Westberg briefly talked about the role of the parish nurse coordinator. One can assume that he would be pleased how the role of the parish nurse coordinator has emerged to support the ministry of parish nursing practice to evolve while carrying forth his vision of whole person health.

The PNC role emerged in the late 1980s as a response to the need for parish nurses in the community to have a designated leader who could coordinate, provide opportunities for continuing education, and offer direction to the parish nurse while representing the sponsoring healthcare institution. As with any professional nursing role, continuing education needs to be focused on professional networking, skill development, systems thinking, enhancement of knowledge, and the impact of the political environment to remain abreast of their area of practice. Parish nurses also require ongoing education in spirituality, personal spiritual growth and development, prevention, and health promotion, as well as changes in care of particular disease processes. Remaining current with information pertinent to various age groups and cultures enhances the parish nurse's ability to address the whole person needs of parishioners in this evolving ministry. Most often the access to continuing education, spiritual formation, and healthcare resources was made available through the position that emerged from sponsoring healthcare organizations. The title given to this position was the parish nurse coordinator (PNC).

During 1997 and 1998 two curricula were developed and endorsed through the work of the International Parish Nurse Resource Center (McDermott et al, 1998; McDermott et al, 1999). The first curriculum was designed as a basic preparation for the beginning parish nurse. The second curriculum was specifically designed for PNCs. This curriculum includes content focused on valuing the mission of parish nursing; spiritual/transformational leadership; working with different religious traditions; self-care for the parish nurse coordinator; planning for the ongoing development of the parish nurse—personally, professionally, and spiritually—nurturing ongoing spiritual formation for themselves and the parish nurses within the programs they manage; and human resource and fiscal management. Completion of this course is recommended for anyone considering serving as a PNC. Colleges and universities throughout the United States offer both educational programs with nurse participants receiving a certificate of completion. PNCs who have taken the parish nurse coordinator educational program positively evaluate the content, noting its articulation of the rationale, background, knowledge, and tools to manage parish nurses. Thus this program is highly recommended for all PNCs.

In April, 2000, parish nurse educators representing multiple academic institutions once again convened to revise the initial core curricula for the preparation of both parish nurses and PNCs. As the role of the parish nurse evolves and health ministries mature, the need to continually revise the content for preparing PNCs for their position remains.

Coordinator Role and Responsibilities Defined

Several studies have investigated the role of the PNC (Solari-Twadell, 1999a; Schweitzer et al, 2002; Rethermeyer, 2004). These studies generally have found varying levels of nursing management experience, educational preparation, levels of responsibility, and diversity of functions for those in the role of the PNC. Their titles and job descriptions differ, as do their reporting relationships. Some report to hospitals or other community healthcare organizations (e.g., long-term care facilities, health departments, or community organizations); some are employed by specific denominations; still others are supported by a single congregation or by a collaborative group of congregations that unite and support regional networks of parish nurses.

One study of a convenience sample of 66 PNCs reported the responsibilities of the PNC to include the following (Schweitzer et al, 2002):

- Evaluate the performance of the parish nurse
- Establish both formal and informal agreements with congregations
- Evaluate the participation of the faith community
- Educate the parish nurses in conjunction with colleges/universities
- Provide for continuing education for the parish nurse
- Participate as faculty in parish nurse preparation curricula

These findings do not reflect other recommended functions of the parish nurse coordinator such as: participation in selection of the parish nurse, development of policies and procedures for the ministry of parish nursing practice, development and management of a program budget, long-range strategic planning, development and monitoring of a documentation system for the parish nurses, and development of regular reports on the activities and outcomes of the parish nurse program.

The PNC function can be formed by a variety of influences contributing to the diversity in the responsibilities of this position. The individual's experience, education, values, and spirituality can naturally shape the position as well as the PNC's understanding and experience of the parish nurse role and its relationship to existing health ministries within a congregation. A second influence on the PNC role is the mission, vision, strategic plan, and resources of the sponsoring organization. Third, the organizational framework of the ministry of parish nursing practice has a strong impact since some PNCs function out of an institution or agency, whereas others function out of a community-based network or specific congregation (Solari-Twadell, 1999b). The organizational framework of the organization sponsoring the parish nurse program may also dictate the financial support for the program, the salary of the coordinator, and the full-time equivalency dedicated for the position. For example, is the parish nurse coordinator position full-time, half-time or quarter-time? Fourth, the age of the program will influence the time the coordinator spends with designated facets of the role. A new program will mandate that the PNC is spending a majority of time in the community, establishing relationships and introducing the program. A longstanding ministry of parish nursing practice will be more focused on maintaining relationships and evaluation strategies. And last, the geographic area, needs of the congregations, and number of parish nurses within a parish nurse program, service, or network can also shape the responsibilities, activities, and priorities of the PNC.

PNCs must be highly motivated internally because part of their responsibility in working with the parish nurse is to motivate them to do the best in serving the members of their congregation. Parish nursing can be a stressful position because the nurse serving as a parish nurse is often working in isolation, without the direct support of other colleagues. Without the support of a PNC, the parish nurse may get over committed, assume responsibilities beyond the scope of the role and/or personal competencies. By getting caught in any of these situations the nurse is putting herself or himself in jeopardy of compromise, ultimately undermining any personal credibility and/or the credibility of the ministry of parish nursing practice. In the evaluation of one parish nurse coalition in Northwest Virginia that consists of paid and unpaid parish nurses, it was noted that the best PNC is someone who serves as a role

model, is deeply spiritual and intentional about his or her spiritual growth, and is attuned to the needs of the parish nurses through ongoing one-to-one and network support.

Through interviewing a collective group of PNCs from around the country Solari-Twadell (1999a) found four distinct management roles in parish nursing. All of these roles were titled *parish nurse coordinator;* however, their functions demonstrated different levels of responsibility and accountability. The first role identified from these interviews was *director*. The profile of this role is related to a larger institution, primarily a healthcare organization, and includes responsibility for administrative functions related to parish nurses who are also paid employees of that organization. The second role is *manager.* The manager is often employed by an organization and is primarily responsible for the promotion and establishment of congregations in initiating unpaid (i.e., volunteer) parish nurse programs. This position is a helpful resource for the congregation and parish nurses, facilitating unpaid parish nurses to network regularly. The third role was a *coordinator* within the congregation. When three or more parish nurses within one congregation work together as a team, one nurse often coordinates the work of the group. This nurse takes responsibility for making assignments and keeping track of documentation and records and generally ensures that the parish nurse ministry and the congregation's overall health ministry function well. Another type of coordination position in parish nursing can occur within a religious denomination. Some denominations have selected a nurse to bring together parish nurses from the same denomination for the purposeof setting policy for health ministry within the specific denominational structure. Most of the positions that have been described are paid. Unpaid parish nurse coordinator positions often function within a single congregation. Some of the positions at the denominational level also may be unpaid. Survey findings revealed that many different titles are held by those given the responsibility of managing a parish nurse program, service, or network. Some of these titles are *coordinators, managers, supervisors, directors,* or *administrators,* each having differing definitions of their respective roles.

While each of the previously described positions that use the title PNC has distinct differences, the position descriptions using these titles may have similar objectives. The influence of setting and role function of the PNC position will dictate different skill sets. For example, the tasks of an institutionally based PNC involving the administration of parish nurse employees paid by an institution will differ greatly from those of PNCs who provide resource support for unpaid parish nurses primarily directed by their congregation's governing body. A PNC employed by a public health department may have a greater focus on deploying community support services such as staff to provide immunizations or health screenings in collaboration with parish nurses from multiple congregations. PNCs employed by a denomination may have the primary task of coordinating parish nurses from a region or state, nationally or internationally for primarily educational purposes. Within a congregation, a PNC is expected to develop a cohesive parish nurse team by delegating tasks and ensuring consistency in ministry to the congregation.

Common to each PNC is his or her accountability to multiple entities or organizations. In 1998, the American Nurses Association (ANA) officially recognized parish nursing as a specialty in nursing and in 1998 approved the parish nurse scope and standards for practice (ANA, 1998). Each state Board of Nursing dictates its standards for nursing practice for licensure throughout the designated state. The PNC is responsible for addressing both the scope and standards for parish nursing practice and the regulations of their State Board in creating policies and procedures that adhere to these requirements. PNCs employed by hospital institutions accredited by the Joint Commission for the Accreditation of Healthcare Organizations (JCAHO) are responsible for ensuring adherence to those standards pertaining to the ministry of parish nursing practice—namely, those standards addressing continuum of care and the assessment of and provision for spiritual needs of clients.

The PNC is also accountable to the institution she or he may be representing. This may include the submission of regular written reports that document the work of the parish nurses providing justification for continued financial support of the PNC position and the institutions ongoing support of the ministry of parish nursing practice. Education partners from local colleges or universities would also anticipate a strong relationship with the PNC. This relationship involves collaborative development of ongoing basic preparation and continuing education programs for the parish nurse in order to maintain the competency of the parish nurse along with the overall quality of the parish nurse program, service, or network.

Congregations that have integrated parish nurses into the life of their communities often rely on the regional network and the PNC for providing education and opportunities for spiritual growth and development for the parish nurse. This creates an accountability from the regional PNC to the congregations in supporting and sustaining the parish nurse ministries through encouraging competent parish nurses (see Chapter 13). The last entity to whom the PNC has accountability is the greater community. Individuals who come from the greater community to access services offered by the parish nurse through a local congregation are looking for well educated, competent parish nurse professionals to assist them in achieving individualized levels of whole person wellness.

Each PNC position has unique aspects associated with it due to the different geographical settings, local economics, constituents and numbers, as well as diversity, of congregations. Therefore this role may have similarity in function while at the same time consist of different complexities in the role due to variables previously noted. Given the comprehensiveness of the PNC role it is important to emphasize the PNC as *administrator*. The parish nurse administrator has the following three primary areas of responsibility:

1. Administration of the parish nurse network including strategic planning, budget creation, and fiscal accountability;
2. Actualization of the sponsoring institution/ agency mission, vision, and goals; and
3. Growth and development of the ministry of parish nurse practice to the greater community or geographic region.

These three foci of the administration of a ministry of parish nursing practice can apply to any setting and role defined for the PNC. The complexity of these foci emphasize the need for a formal preparation for the PNC, sufficient time designated for the accomplishment of the objectives of the position, dedication of resources for accomplishing the objectives of the ministry of parish nursing practice, and clarity about the responsibilities and accountabilities of the PNC role.

In planning the development of a PNC position the importance and complexity of these three foci demand thoughtful consideration. The following are steps in that process which must be addressed:

- Understanding of the ministry of parish nursing practice and requirements noted in the scope and standards for parish nursing practice
- Consideration of how the development of this role is related to the strategic plan of the organization
- Clear understanding of the geographic, demographic and denominational diversity and how these may impact the work of the PNC
- Development of the job description, including: a minimum skill set, clear objectives and responsibilities that are commensurate with the time and remuneration allotted to the position (see Appendixes 19-A and B)
- Dedicated resources for program development that will extend over at least a 5-year period
- Provision for basic preparation of the PNC and attendance at regular continuing education programs directed to this work

Considerations in Defining the Parish Nurse Coordinator Role

As in many appointed management roles in nursing, a nurse is given a title of coordinator on Friday and is expected to perform the duties of the position the following Monday—almost a guarantee of failure or, at the very least, a slow start. Other considerations—such as education, infrastructure, and reporting relationship; timelines for program development; and workload—are necessary in defining and supporting the PNC role. In addition to thoughtful review of geographic setting, current congregational relationships and the compatibility of the mission of the institution with the philosophy of parish nursing should be considered during the development of the parish nurse management position.

Formal educational preparation for the PNC role is essential to performance success. This education should include participation in the Basic Preparation Course for Parish Nurse Coordinators offered through the International Parish Nurse Resource Center. In addition, most healthcare institutions offer leadership development or management courses to support new managers in their roles. Books, conferences, and journal articles are also helpful tools for preparation and ongoing development. Less formal yet perhaps most needed are mutually agreed-upon mentoring opportunities with other more experienced managers. This provides for the provision of ongoing feedback promoting the "sustained practice, reflection, and dialogue that fosters the acquisition of new knowledge and skills" (Dufour & Eaker, 1998, p. 265).

Within each sponsoring organization an infrastructure impacts the PNC from an operational and decision-making standpoint. This infrastructure includes the following:

- *Governance/management structure*: Reporting relationships, organizational hierarchy and culture, leadership style
- *Strategic planning*: Mission, vision, goals, overarching objectives on a defined timeline
- *Human resources*: Personnel management, including job descriptions, interview guidelines, contractual agreements
- *Fiscal management*: Budget administration; grant management
- *Marketing*: Written and/or automated materials to elicit interest in parish nursing; notification of educational and network events
- *Public relations:* Communication with internal and external groups in written and verbal form
- *Information management*: Technology support, documentation, individual parish nurse and summative network monthly and annual statistics and outcomes
- *Quality/performance improvement*: Performance standards and outcomes measurement
- *Legal*: Adherence to the nurse practice act and other regulatory groups, statutes, and laws
- *Pastoral and spiritual care*: Activities and/or events planned to offer spiritual support and continuing pastoral education (CPE)
- *Support services/partnerships*: Other community persons, groups, or organizations working together to support the parish nurse network; grant partnerships

- *Community relations*: External relationship development with organizations in the community

A thorough understanding of each component within the infrastructure of an organization is critical to the success of the PNC and the integration of the ministry of parish nursing practice into the life of the sponsoring agency as well as the sponsoring faith community.

Questions to consider when considering assuming a position of parish nurse management include the following. What is the history or traditions of the parish nurse program? What is the time dedicated for the position? Full-time? Half-time? To whom does the PNC position report? What is the size of the program, service, network? What are the needs of the congregations and parish nurses in the program, service, network? Which faith traditions are represented in the program, service, and network and in the regional community? What is the culture of the community? What are the financial support and resources available to support the ongoing development of the ministry of parish nursing practice? How is the ministry of parish nursing practice integrated into the strategic plan of the sponsoring agency? What resources are available for continuing education of the coordinator and parish nurses? How is the ongoing spiritual formation of the coordinator and parish nurses provided for? Finally, what do the governing institution and any existing parish nurse advisory groups expect?

With dwindling reimbursement available to sponsoring healthcare institutions, many PNCs are part-time employees who work approximately 20 hours per week. As parish nurse networks grow, especially with unpaid models, budget constraints often limit ability to increase paid hours. The savvy PNC must prioritize tasks, delegating where possible, and continue to report the stories and outcomes achieved through parish nursing. With the multitude of considerations required for defining the role of the PNC, the wide variation in practice is no surprise.

Barriers to the Parish Nurse Coordinator Role

Without thoughtful preparation and careful attention to defining the PNC role, barriers will exist impacting parish nurse program development, performance, and outcomes. The first set of barriers may exist in relationship to the sponsoring institution. Budget constraints may allow only for a part- time position, yet the sponsoring institution might expect full-time work. The parish nurse manager will be challenged to prioritize and delegate, giving special attention to those tasks that ensure the integrity of the parish nurse program. The PNC position may be vulnerable to ongoing financial constraints of the sponsoring institution or soft funding provided through grants. With limited funding available either through the sponsoring institution or from grant support, the PNC must have a good understanding of the strategic plans for the sponsoring institution and must at every opportunity show the value of supporting the ongoing growth and development of the parish nurse ministry.

A second set of barriers may be directly tied to the role itself. First, if the role or the expectations from the institution, parish nurses, or clergy are unclear, measuring success is difficult; job dissatisfaction can result. Accountability to one or more entities (i.e., multiple sponsoring institutions, area congregations, etc.) may impede job performance; the parish nurse network could suffer as a result. Perhaps the PNC is inexperienced or uneducated in parish nursing and therefore does not fully understand the scope of the role and the needs of the parish nurse network or how to attend to them. Without intentionally seeking opportunities for personal development, the PNC may be an ineffective leader, unable to develop sufficient relationships and more likely to experience burnout.

A third set of barriers focuses on relationships. PNCs must understand the value of relationships and the highly relational nature of their work as well as how these relationships contribute to the ultimate success of the ministry of parish nursing practice. Unless the PNC establishes whole person based relationships with parish nurses within the network, the parish nurse may feel disconnected, fail to comply with their job descriptions, neglect his or her accountability, and ultimately lose passion for the ministry. Without relationships with congregational leaders, the PNC may inaccurately evaluate the ministry or long-term support required by the sponsoring institution. Failure of the coordinator to create the necessary relationships to support all three areas of development for the network (personal, professional, and spiritual) may limit the skills, knowledge, and possibilities of ministry for each parish nurse.

Relationship development with different departments and significant leaders within the institution can impact the development of the ministry of parish nursing practice. Failure to establish relationships with significant people within the sponsoring organization may lead to lack of knowledge of expertise available to support the ongoing development or resourcing of the parish nurse network. It is important to keep those individuals internal to the institution as informed as the external community regarding new developments or changes in the ministry of parish nursing practice within local congregations and the parish nurse network. After all, some members of the local congregations are employees of the sponsoring institution. If employees of the sponsoring institution are informed, they may be some of the strongest advocates for the ministry of parish nursing practice in their congregation and consequently within the sponsoring institution.

Relationships are also important with other agencies in the community. If the PNC is well networked with other community agencies she or he may then have recommendations for the parish nurses on where the parish nurse can access resources for intended programs for the congregation. This knowledge, which is developed through relationships, can help the nurse avoid scarcity of resources. The PNC may also be a source for multiple agencies to collaborate with several congregations in accomplishing an objective that is identified by the local health department. The PNC can be the natural conduit for public health resources to be made available for congregations in the community. This will enhance the connectedness for all and often times eliminate duplicity of programs using the few resources available for the maximum good. The highly relational nature of the PNC demands a person who is outgoing, has excellent communication skills, and values the importance of developing and sustaining relationships.

A fourth set of barriers may present from within the institution. Even if the institution professes a desire to coordinate a parish nurse program, the institution may not understand sufficiently the ministry of parish nursing practice. In this case, it may not dedicate the necessary funds to the creation, maintenance, and long-term sustenance

of such a program. This lack of understanding and underresourcing may also include inadequate reporting relationships within the organization. For example, it is much more effective for the PNC to report to a Senior Vice President of Mission Services than the Director of Pastoral Care. Another factor that can undermine the management of the ministry of parish nursing practice is the PNC's inability to develop and manage her or his operational budget. Some PNCs have no information regarding the budgetary allotments dedicated to the operation of the ministry of parish nursing practice within their institutions. These institutional issues can continually frustrate the PNC who is trying to do the requested work with little or no budget, knowledge of the budget, infrastructure, or personal supervision.

The last set of barriers relates to community partners. Just as relationships with parish nurses are important, so too are collaborations between the PNC and multiple community partners (i.e., congregations, community agencies, etc.). Each partner can contribute much to a parish nurse network—through education, support for the ministry, goods and services, and creative ideas for growth and expansion of health ministries in a community. So much more can be accomplished when partners collaborate toward a common goal. Another important possible outcome of community partnerships is the direct or indirect financial support. Congregations and community organizations are often more willing to support the ministry of parish nursing practice when they have been involved in the planning for current and future activities of the ministry. In addition, available grant monies for faith-based initiatives often require evidence of community partnerships because of the documented value of relationships for sustaining programs.

Leadership and the Parish Nurse Coordinator

PNCs have the opportunity to *lead* rather than simply manage parish nurses within their network. Just as subtle differences define leaders and managers, behavior differs between the PNC and the parish nurse administrator. Porter-O'Grady (1999) states that nurses should "no longer prescribe to what a person does but see leader behavior as the result of a relationship between leaders and followers… allowing for the achievement of shared goals to which each party has committed" (p. 346). PNCs who are successful in leading their parish nurse networks possess the many gifts of spiritual leadership. They establish trusting relationships with a high degree of integrity and collaborate with their many community partners. A shared vision for developing and sustaining parish nursing can be clearly articulated when the PNC *leader* fully understands the benefit of *community*—coming together for a common purpose. In community, diversity of people and opinions are welcomed, encouraged, and celebrated. PNC *leaders* are creative, have nurtured self-awareness, and participate in their leadership style. They are quintessential learners; they have abundant energy and motivation. And finally, they intentionally take time for self-assessment, their own spiritual development, self-care, and periodic review of their own performance.

Common to many references on effective management are the definitions of leadership that can be applied to PNCs and their leadership style. Leadership styles include: 1) authoritarian; 2) facilitator; 3) manager; 4) collaborator; 5) paternalist/maternalist; 6) servant/partner; 7) visionary; and 8) spiritual. It can be argued that the best PNC *leader* combines each leadership style, depending upon what is needed at the time, for the ongoing development of parish nursing.

Ongoing Development of Parish Nurses

In planning for the ongoing development of the parish nurse, the PNC must consider each individual parish nurse and, to foster growth, must focus on his or her personal, professional, and spiritual needs. Just as parish nursing is founded on whole person care for its congregation, so too does the parish nurse manager minister to the body, mind, and spirit in his or her personal contact with parish nurses. Each parish nurse and congregational setting is unique. It is important for the PNC to remember that once you have met one parish nurse, you have met one parish nurse. Each ministry of parish nursing practice is based upon the nurse's knowledge, professional clinical experience (e.g., perinatal vs. medical surgical vs. pediatric), spiritual maturity, available resources, and time available for ministry. With this in mind, the PNC can work toward getting to know the

parish nurse by developing a strong relationship and trust with each parish nurse in her or his network. The following may assist in this effort:

- Who is this parish nurse? What are her or his strengths? What are her or his challenges in the parish nurse role? Opportunities for improvement?
- What is the nature of her or his "call" to the ministry of parish nursing practice?
- What is her or his level of spiritual maturity, and where are her or his spiritual growth needs?
- What aspects of the parish nurse role and/or services is she or he currently offering to her or his congregation (e.g., education, screening, referral and resources)?
- How is she or he supported within the organizational hierarchy of her or his congregation? Is she or he a member of the congregational staff?
- What are her or his special needs? Visions for the future?
- What are her or his expectations of you as the parish nurse administrator? Support needs?
- What are her or his ideas for the parish nurse regional network?

Personal Development of the Parish Nurse

The best way to get to know a parish nurse is to meet with the individual in her or his faith community on a regular, continual schedule throughout the year. It is important to take the time to hear the stories of her or his ministry and to mutually discern where the parish nurse feels challenged in her or his role or where continuing education or spiritual direction may provide opportunities for support and ongoing development. One parish nurse manager who coordinates a large network of parish nurses suggests that it is mandatory for the coordinator to project a loving, caring concern and interest for each parish nurse. This is important because parish nurses often overlook the need to take the time for self-care. Every parish nurse manager needs to foster the expectation with every parish nurse that there is an ongoing attention to spiritual, professional, and emotional maturity for each parish nurse. The parish nurse manager serves as a primary role model for these qualities. If a mutually receptive relationship exists, the parish nurse manager may mentor the parish nurse. Some of the mentoring behaviors may include the following:

Teaching	Modeling	Informing
Prescribing	Questioning	Supporting
Protecting	Promoting	Encouraging
Affirming	Inspiring	Challenging
Counseling	Listening	Probing
Clarifying	Advising	Befriending

Professional Development of the Parish Nurse

Providing professional development opportunities for parish nurses involves a variety of skills on the part of the PNC. First, the PNC needs to assess not only what the regional network of parish nurses is requesting but also what they may need in terms of continuing education. If there is a local educational institution the PNC should collaborate with the educator who coordinates the basic preparation course for parish nurses, perhaps even teaching several of the modules that focus on parish nurse practice, such as documentation or setting up a beginning parish nurse practice. Then, as the PNC gets to know each parish nurse in her or his program, service, or network, she or he can identify on an ongoing basis those topics of interests to the majority of the nurses. The following should be assessed for each parish nurse:

- Educational background
- Learning styles and readiness to learn
- Faith traditions and/or denomination
- Culture, both personal and the community served
- Previous experiences
- Factors influencing parish nurse professional and learning needs (e.g., *Scope and Standards of Parish Nursing*; Nurse State Practice Act; advancements in healthcare delivery)
- Spiritual maturity

Once the professional development needs of the parish nurses have been identified, the venue for education can be determined. For example, will the topic be best presented at a monthly network meeting? Or should a 1- to 3-day retreat be planned to best fulfill the educational needs of the parish nurses? Does the parish nurse need the experienced PNC to assist them plan an event such as a health fair? Should a book be purchased

and made available to each nurse in the network? These are just some of the many creative strategies for PNCs to meet the professional needs of their networks.

Professional development strategies are the following:

- Independent study packets or resources
- Continuing education opportunities or events
- Parish nurse resource library (e.g., books, videos, and movies)
- Ongoing evaluation and feedback
- Networking opportunities (e.g., monthly meetings and annual retreats)
- Publications, research, identifying best practices in parish nursing

Spiritual Development of the Parish Nurse

Spiritual development is notably the most challenging yet most foundational focus of the three development areas to which PNCs attend in working with the parish nurses. In developing a parish nurse network, the successful coordinator will intentionally assess the spiritual development of each nurse. What is her or his level of spiritual maturity, and what are her or his needs for spiritual growth? How does the nurse define God, her or his rituals of faith, and her or his own spirituality? How comfortable is the nurse with providing for the spiritual ministry of her or his parishioners (i.e., praying with people, assessing spirituality, etc.)? What support or resources does this nurse need? What steps has the nurse taken to enhance her or his own spiritual growth and development? Does the parish nurse have a spiritual director? Does the parish nurse have a personal plan for ongoing spiritual formation?

Some intentional strategies for PNCs to promote spiritual development of the parish nurses may include the following:

- Praying with each nurse and for the parish nurse network
- Providing printed materials (e.g., newsletters, sample bulletin boards, and reprintable reference information)
- Including devotions or worship in the agenda for every gathering of the network
- Planning retreats for renewal, education, and spiritual growth

- Finding ways to promote theological reflection and highlighting opportunities to promote the link between faith and health
- Identifying the resources in the area that may offer spiritual direction

The PNC is not the sole provider of spiritual support for parish nurses. Finding and using regional resources such as clergy, chaplains, congregations, denominations, spiritual directors, or experts in spirituality and religion bring a richness and diversity of information to the parish nurse network. The PNC is looked to as a primary role model and resource and should attend to periodic review of her or his own spiritual nurturing, including consideration of spiritual direction for themselves.

Parish Nurse Coordinator Support

Support for the PNC can come from the sponsoring organization or area community partners, including parish nurses, educational institutions, continuing education, professional parish nurse coordinator regional groups, the International Parish Nurse Resource Center, Health Ministries Association, other specialty nursing organizations and review of the current literature. Just as parish nurses benefit from a network of parish nurses for sharing and support, the PNC also benefits from interacting with other PNCs from networks within their region, state, denomination, nationally or even internationally. Coming together to network provides opportunities to share ideas and affirm the PNC role and responsibilities, often preventing some mistakes in coordinating a network. What is working well in specific parish nurse networks? How best would other PNCs address the same challenge? Learn to share successes, borrow good ideas, and reprint with permission. Learning from each other is not only helpful but results in the building of a strong professional support network.

At a gathering of PNCs during the 2004 Health Ministries Association annual conference, survey results regarding the education needs of PNCs were shared. The topics of most interest focused on leadership skills, outcome measurements, standards of practice, finance, collaboration, capacity building with the broader community, and meeting spiritual needs. These topics further reinforce the need for formal education to prepare PNCs

for their role, a clearly defined job description, and opportunities for continuing education and mentoring relationships.

Lessons Learned

Through trial and error, assistance from others, networking, and divine inspiration many successful institutional model parish nurse networks in collaboration with the local university and area congregations exist today. The following are some helpful suggestions for those nurses who are given the opportunity and blessing to become PNCs:

- Perform a self-assessment as you prepare for the position. What are your strengths and weaknesses? In what areas of the PNC position would you like grow? What is your plan for preparing or strengthening your PNC role?
- Complete a PNC preparation course as the foundation for your practice.
- Seek out mentors and education opportunities to learn new skills and fulfill the professional responsibilities of the position.
- Identify sponsoring institution requirements of administrative/management staff and ensure that your position also follows those requirements.
- Compare and contrast job descriptions of other PNCs when you are creating the description for your position.
- If you have never administered a parish nurse program, seek out experienced coordinators to learn the best from the best.
- Pray for personal guidance and continue to pray for the success of the parish nurse network.
- Consider getting a spiritual director
- Seek community partners that can work collaboratively with congregations supporting the ministry of parish nursing practice.
- Establish an advisory group consisting of clergy, representatives from an academic institution, and a health system. This triadic partnership is a highly collaborative model that not only delegates responsibilities but also keeps each of the three partners informed of activities working toward common goals.

- Understand the value of partnerships—most grant sources require collaborative partnerships. So much more can be accomplished together.
- Support congregational health ministries—experienced and successful parish nurse networks have found that it is critical because the parish nurse(s) will often experience burnout unless tasks are shared and a foundation of support from clergy, lay health promoters and other healthcare professionals exists.
- Create congregational contracts between the sponsoring network institution and each congregation in the network. Recognize that these contracts help to ensure compliance with standards for practice, documentation, and reporting of outcomes. These contracts are helpful in establishing compliance especially in unpaid models where there are differing levels of accountability within the group parish nurses.
- Complete at least quarterly and annual reports for the sponsoring institution taking into consideration the organizational mission vision and strategic plan. Be sure to include the stories of how parishioners have been touched by parish nurses.
- Understand the value of a simple written note of support. This is in addition to thoughtfully planned network meetings, retreats, and one-on-one time with each parish nurse.
- Prioritize and set boundaries for effective time management as well as fiscal and professional accountability.
- It is important to remember that when meeting a new parish nurse, pastor or congregation that this is a new opportunity for learning. If the new relationship is approached in the posture of a student, there is likely to be great learning, finding out what is needed to be known. If the new relationship is approached as if one already knows, in all likelihood little, if any, of what you need to know will be learned.
- Always work at expanding the network of peers made up of other PNCs. Every problem experienced by a PNC has probably been experienced before. Use that network

of PNCs to enrich your work and life as a whole.
- Welcome diversity as there is a richness in the difference; celebrate the special gifts of each child of God.

Conclusion

So many adventures, challenges, joys, and blessings await those who assume management of a parish nurse program, service, or network. This management position provides opportunities to interact with wonderful nurses, supportive clergy, congregation leadership, and committed community agencies as well as creative coordinators from around the world—all dedicated to promoting the health of whole persons in body, mind, and spirit. One only has to mention the words *parish nursing,* and the stage is set to hear some wonderful stories of parish nurse ministry making a difference in the lives of others. The most successful parish nurse managers are those who recognize and promote the gifts of their nurses, assisting them to grow in the special ministry that is parish nursing. To God be the glory and to Reverend Granger Westberg, sincere thanks for planting the original seeds for parish nursing: "In the future, the story of whole person healthcare will be carried forward by me and all the fine people who have given them-selves to this enterprise" (Peterson, p. 18). The ever evolving role of parish nurse management follows Westberg's vision with the responsibility of effectively administrating a network of parish nurses called to the ministry of parish nursing practice. In closing, the authors leave you with the following prayer for the parish nurse administrator.

Divine Spirit, we come to you in search of ways to be loving, good, and effective guides to your people we lead in your ministry of parish nursing practice. We see ourselves as your servants in this work and look for the special gifts you have given us for leadership. We pledge to be honest in discerning where we still are need of growth and to be attentive to those needs. Send your grace and bless the work we are doing and to all the people who are contributing to the success of your work. We acknowledge that it is only with your blessings that our ideas, plans, and goals succeed. We go in full confidence of your continual love and safekeeping. Amen.

REFERENCES

American Nurses Association. (1998). *Scope and standards of parish nursing practice*. (9806st). Washington, DC: Author.

DuFour, R. & Eaker, R. (1998) *Professional learning communities at work: best practices for enhancing student achievement*. Reston, VA: Association for Supervision and Curriculum Development.

McDermott, M.A., Solari-Twadell, P.A., & Matheus, R. (1998) Promoting quality education for the parish nurse and parish nurse coordinator. *Nursing and Health Care Perspectives*, January: 4-6.

McDermott, M.A., Solari-Twadell, P.A., & Matheus, R. (1999). Educational preparation. In Solari-Twadell, P.A. & McDermott, M.A. Parish nursing: Promoting whole person health within faith communities. Thousand Oaks, CA: Sage Publications.

Porter-O'Grady, T. In Wilson, C.K. & Porter-O'Grady, T. (1999). *Leading the revolution in health care: advancing systems, igniting performance* (2nd ed.). Gaithersburg, MD: Aspen Publishers, Inc.

Peterson, W.M. (Ed.). (1982). *Granger Westberg verbatim: a vision for faith & health*. St Louis: International Parish Nurse Resource Center.

Rethermeyer, A. (2004, July). Parish Nurse Coordinator Survey Results. *Symposium conducted at the meeting of the Parish Nurse Coordinator Network*, Seattle, WA: International Parish Nurse Resource Center.

Schweitzer, R., Norberg, M., & Larson, L. (2002). The parish nurse coordinator: a bridge to spiritual health care leadership for the future. *Journal of Holistic Nursing*, (20)3: 207-231.

Solari-Twadell, A. (1999a, Spring/Summer). Manager's memo. *Perspectives in parish nursing practice*, Advocate HealthCare, 6.

Solari–Twadell, P.A. (1999b). The emerging practice of parish nursing. In Solari-Twadell, P.A. & McDermott, M.A. Parish nursing: Promoting whole person health within faith communities. Thousand Oaks, CA: Sage Publications.

APPENDIX 19A

Job Description

JOB TITLE: PARISH NURSE COORDINATOR
DEPARTMENT: MISSION AND MINISTRY
REPORTS TO: VICE PRESIDENT

Qualifications

- Minimum: baccalaureate in nursing. Master's degree preferred.
- Current RN licensure in the state, as applicable.
- Demonstrated skills in planning, budgeting, marketing, organizing, and managing professions/specialties in complex functions and processes.
- Minimum: 5 years of clinical (preferably in community health) and 2 years of management experience.
- Understanding of the ministry of parish nursing practice.

Special Skills or Capacities

This position requires a person who is creative and open-minded with experience in program development and improving care processes. The person should exhibit leadership capacities and a positive attitude, possess excellent written and verbal communication skills, and have the ability to work collaboratively with a variety of community partners (e.g., congregations). He or she should display a professional demeanor and be able to prioritize workloads. Previous experience working in a congregation is preferred. The person should exhibit spiritual maturity.

15% *ADMINISTRATIVE/ORGANIZATIONAL*

Develops a system for evaluation and quality.

Responsible for interpreting and communicating objectives/strategic plans with parish nurses.

Coordinates the collection, collation, and analysis of data and outcomes for programs/activities.

Ensures compliance with regulations and standards that apply to parish nursing, including policies/procedures, performance improvement, and other documentation.

Contributes to the performance improvement process.

Administrates budget for assigned cost center in a fiscally responsible manner.

Participates in the formal evaluation of the parish nurse.

15% *LEADERSHIP*

Exhibits leadership skills in designing, revising, and expanding the ministry of parish nursing practice.

Identifies opportunities for the provision of community-needed services not provided by the healthcare institution.

Serves as a positive role model in community, customer, and employee relations.

Identifies personal and professional goals and evaluates achievement.

20% *NETWORK GROWTH*

Continues to develop and strengthen partnerships with regional community organizations (e.g., interfaith congregations, universities, schools of nursing, health departments, etc.).

Creates and distributes information (e.g., pamphlets, displays, newsletters, articles, and presentations) to elicit interest in the ministry of parish nursing practice.

Participates as adjunct faculty for community-based programs.

Continued

Job Description—cont'd

10%   EDUCATION/PRESENTATION

Accountable for identifying learning needs, spiritual growth, and resources to respond to these needs.

Ensures that area parish nurses receive continuing education for professional, personal, and spiritual growth.

Provides presentations to persons and/or groups within the healthcare institution and the greater community on topics of interest and parish nursing.

Contributes to community events as appropriate (i.e., planning, organizing, participating and/or evaluating).

Develops, implements, and evaluates a system for the development of parish nurse competencies.

Completes required inservices on schedule.

Effective Date:
Revision Date:
Review Date:

Parish Nurse Coordinator Responsibilities

Complete basic and parish nurse coordinator education.
The parish nurse coordinator position provides the following:

ADMINISTRATION/ORGANIZATION

- Participate in the annual evaluation of the parish nurses.
- Formalize agreements/covenants with participating network congregations.
- Refine documentation forms and reporting process from participating network congregations.
- Develop policies and procedures to serve as guidelines for parish nurse in individual congregations.
- Manage budget (operating, capital, program budgets) for parish nurse network.
- Contribute to special projects for the health system and in collaboration with other parish nurse coordinators (e.g., create documentation forms; develop outcomes reporting mechanisms).
- Complete annual report of regional parish nurse network activities, including statistics and outcomes.
- Explore grant opportunities to offset program expenses and allow for expansion of outreach.
- Manage grants received.
- Evaluate and monitor quality of the parish nurse network.
- Provide intentional support to parish nurses (personal, professional, and spiritual).
- Develop a referral network of parish nurses to serve the needs of complex patients in our community to reinforce prescribed regimens of care, encourage advance directives, and to refer back to appropriate point of access for care delivery.
- Participate in the development of the annual operating budget for the parish nurse network.

LEADERSHIP

- Serve as a resource for area parish nurses, interested nurses, clergy, and congregations.
- Meet on a regular basis with parish nurses to determine level of activity and need for support.
- Create orientation notebook for parish nurses joining the regional parish nurse network.
- Provide spiritual support and renewal to regional parish nurse network.
- Represent the health system and the regional parish nurse network with other state parish nurse networks.
- Coordinate bimonthly network meetings—engage speaker, plan meeting, send invitations, fill out paperwork for contact hours/ CEUs.
- Coordinate annual parish nurse retreat—plan, organize, implement, and evaluate retreat.
- Strengthen communication and collaborative relationships with regional clergy and hospital chaplains/pastoral care.
- Develop and chair an advisory board consisting of designated internal and community representatives.
- Serve as a role model for area parish nurses.
- Seek continuing education for personal, professional, and spiritual growth.
- Attend to self-care.
- Identify personal and professional goals and evaluate achievement.

Parish Nurse Coordinator Responsibilities—cont'd

EDUCATION/PRESENTATION

- Teach pertinent modules in both the basic parish nurse preparation course and the parish nurse coordinator preparation course offered through the local university.
- In collaboration with the local university, create congregational health ministry education and wellness outreach specific to congregations without an RN.
- Develop, implement, and evaluate a system for parish nurse competency.

NETWORK GROWTH

- Create parish nurse packets with specific information describing regional parish nurse network.
- Create a parish nurse website and resource links.
- Sell parish nurse items (e.g., logo shirt, hat, tote bags) to offset program expenses.
- Market and elicit additional interest in and support of parish nursing in the primary, secondary, and tertiary service areas of the health system.
- Reply via e-mail, phone, or postal mail to requests from parish nurses, nurses, clergy, and congregations for resource information.
- Give presentations to clergy, nurses, health ministry groups, and to governing bodies within a congregation.
- Write, edit, and produce a quarterly parish nurse newsletter.

Quality of the Ministry of Parish Nursing Practice in an Outcomes Environment

20

Lisa Burkhart

Phyllis Ann Solari-Twadell

Parish nursing is in the unique position of bridging two worlds—the world of healthcare and the world of faith communities. Those individuals whose lives have been touched by parish nurses clearly understand the importance of the ministry of parish nursing practice. However, parish nursing is a relatively new nursing specialty, and although it has grown significantly over the years through a grassroots movement, it is neither well integrated into the continuum of care, nor is it fully funded. Parish nursing has the potential to fill a great need in our country, particularly in addressing the needs outlined in *Healthy People 2010*, by providing health promotion and disease prevention care, as well as improving access to healthcare and decreasing health disparities (United States Department of Health and Human Services, 2000).

There may not be a hospital in every town, but there is a faith community in every town. Why then is parish nursing struggling to be funded? In the current healthcare environment, those who fund—be they the health system, the congregation, or foundations—require documentation of both the quality and value of the services rendered. The question "What is it that parish nurses do that is value added?" needs to be answered. To facilitate the growth of parish nurse practice, it is critical to develop a ministry that reflects both quality and value.

A foundational contribution that will support the ministry is an administrative and financial infrastructure that will contribute to the sustainability of the ministry. This infrastructure must include a system to collect relevant outcome data that can be used to demonstrate value and quality. This chapter presents a review of the literature and elements that are relevant to the development of quality parish nurse programs and variables that can measure the impact of the ministry of parish nursing practice as well as the quality and value of the ministry.

Nursing, Parish Nursing, and Quality

Parish nursing literature has a dearth of information regarding value, quality, and outcomes of the services rendered through the ministry of parish nursing practice (Lloyd & Ludwig-Beymer, 1999; Ludwig-Beymer, Welsch, & Micek, 1998; American Nurses Association, 1998). However, these concepts have been studied and researched in healthcare and nursing over the years. Research in identifying and measuring health-related outcomes has a long history, beginning with Florence Nightingale in the 1860s during the Crimean War (Nightingale, 1994). In more modern times, significant development of quality research occurred in the 1960s, particularly in relation to physician care, using Donabedian's model of quality (1966). In this model, quality is defined by the healthcare entity—be it a hospital or a nursing specialty—in terms of assessment areas related to structure, process, and outcome indicators.

In 1995, the American Nurses Association (ANA), using Donabedian's model, sponsored a meta-analysis of nursing literature to determine

227

the structure, process, and outcome indicators of nursing quality in acute care. This work resulted in a *Nursing Care Report Card for Acute Care* (ANA, 1995). In this report, structure was defined as staffing patterns that affect quality and quantity of care. Process was defined as measures related to how care is delivered. Outcomes were defined as "indicators [that] focus on how patients, and their conditions, are affected by their interaction with nursing staff" (ANA, 1995, p. viii).

In 2000, the ANA published quality indicators for the community setting. These quality indicators included: utilization of services; patient satisfaction; patient risk reduction; increase in protective factors related to caregivers; level of functioning, ADL/IADL; level of functioning, psychosocial functioning; changes in symptom severity; and strength of the therapeutic alliance between the nurse, patient, and family (ANA, 2000).

Structure/Input Quality Indicators

Research pertaining to the identification of quality indicators for the ministry of parish nursing practice has not been well documented in the parish nurse literature. In one study, Solari-Twadell (2002) surveyed 2330 parish nurses to measure the importance of 37 factors that are important to the parish nurse fulfilling the role. These factors were derived from the parish nursing literature and the researcher's experience. Over half (54%) of the sample responded. The data resulted in a ranking of the 37 factors, as shown in Table 20-1. The research was based on Deming's theory that defines quality through the eyes of the user. Deming (1986) stated "quality can be defined only in terms of the agent. Who is the judge of quality? A product may get high marks in the judgement of the customer, on one scale, and low marks on another" (Deming, 1986, p. 168). For example, the pastor may believe that the parish nurse is presenting a diversity of educational programs for the members of the congregation, yet the participants of the educational programs are not evaluating the content of the programs as being "very good." Using Deming's model, the 37 factors are inputs to the system.

The findings of this study indicate that the presence or absence of these 37 factors differentiates the nature of the ministry of parish nursing practice. For example, parish nurses who are paid are more likely to serve higher-income families, work in larger congregations located in larger cities, have more support from their pastors, and have a health cabinet in place. Parish nurses in paid models also tend to have a relationship with a health system, have policies and procedures in place, participate in an evaluation process, and have access to nursing supervision. These parish nurses also tend to be more interested in taking a certification exam in parish nursing, if one were available. Conversely, those parish nurses in unpaid models worked fewer hours weekly and had less structure or support (Solari-Twadell, 2002).

Parish nurse coordinators and other administrators interested in developing or improving the infrastructure for a ministry of parish nursing practice are encouraged to further explore these input factors. For example, are resources available for the parish nurse to attend the basic preparation in parish nursing or continuing education programs? Is there a strong relationship and alliance between the parish nurse and the pastor? Is there a plan for the ongoing spiritual formation of the parish nurse? Are the resources available to support this plan? Is there an opportunity for the parish nurse to network with other parish nurses? Is there a health cabinet or committee that can support the work of the parish nurse? Are there competencies identified for the parish nurses?

Process Quality Indicators

Donabedian's (1985) theory includes the use of process indicators. Process indicators relate to how care is delivered. Parish nurses and congregational/health system supporting committees and staff determine how the ministry of parish nursing practice is implemented. The majority of available parish nurse process data includes demographic statistics describing clients served and parish nurse interventions. Chapter 3, Appendix 3H identifies a combined set of 30 interventions that parish nurses use several times a day, daily, weekly, and monthly (Solari-Twadell, 2002). Table 8-1 in Chapter 8 includes the required elements in a parish nurse documentation system. The parish nurse most likely will collect the ongoing process statistical data for

TABLE 20-1   Ranking and Relative Percentages of Factors Identified as Being Important to Parish Nurses in Fulfilling their Role

Input Factor	Input Category	Frequency Very Important (n=1161)	Relative % Very Important (n=1161)	Relative % Important (n=1161)	Relative % Unimportant (n=1161)
1. Participation in Basic Preparation	Support	966	84%	14%	2%
2. Personal Religious Belief	Parish Nurse	965	84%	12%	4%
3. Support from Pastor	Support	833	76%	18%	6%
4. Networking	Support	749	65%	27%	8%
5. Spiritual Direction	Support	673	58%	28%	14%
6. Length of Time in Nursing	Parish Nurse	645	56%	38%	16%
7. Continuing Education	Support	622	54%	36%	10%
8. Volunteers	Resource	549	48%	28%	24%
9. Current Person to Whom She or He Reports	Organizational Framework	521	45%	37%	18%
10. Health Cabinet	Resource	496	43%	31%	26%
11. Additional Staff	Congregation	400	35%	41%	24%
12. Religious Denomination Served	Congregation	391	34%	32%	34%
13. Length of Time in Parish Nursing	Parish Nurse	327	28%	53%	19%
14. Regular Reports	Organizational Framework	326	28%	41%	31%
15. Length of Time in Role	Parish Nurse	317	28%	48%	24%
16. Line Item on Budget	Resource	317	28%	35%	37%
17. Written Policies and Procedures	Organizational Framework	310	27%	35%	38%
18. Written Job Description	Organizational Framework	299	26%	37%	37%
19. Being Paid	Organizational Framework	253	22%	17%	61%
20. Current Position Title	Organizational Framework	246	21%	42%	37%
21. Documentation System	Organizational Framework	242	21%	42%	37%
22. Access to Nursing Supervisor	Support	237	21%	22%	57%
23. Certification	Parish Nurse	239	21%	32%	47%
24. Size of Congregation	Congregation	236	21%	40%	39%
25. Geographic Location	Congregation	234	20%	38%	42%
26. Orientation	Support	214	19%	19%	62%
27. Relationship with Healthcare System	Organizational Framework	199	17%	15%	68%

(From Solari-Twadell, P.A. (2002). The differentiation of the ministry of parish nursing practice within congregations. *Dissertation Abstracts International*, 63(06), 569A. UMI No. 3056442.)

Continued

TABLE 20-1 Ranking and Relative Percentages of Factors Identified as Being Important to Parish Nurses in Fulfilling their Role—cont'd

Input Factor	Input Category	Frequency Very Important (n=1161)	Relative % Very Important (n=1161)	Relative % Important (n=1161)	Relative % Unimportant (n=1161)
28. Relationship with Physician	Support	160	13%	20%	67%
29. Formal Evaluation	Organizational Framework	150	14%	27%	59%
30. Selection Process	Organizational Framework	136	12%	23%	65%
31. Friend of the Center	Parish Nurse	97	9%	20%	71%
32. Membership HMA	Parish Nurse	90	8%	17%	75%
33. Use of Standardized Language	Organizational Framework	78	7%	20%	73%
34. Personal Ethnicity	Parish Nurse	75	7%	18%	75%
35. Ethnicity of Congregation	Congregation	74	6%	18%	76%
36. Membership Specialty Organization	Parish Nurse	64	6%	15%	79%
37. Membership ANA	Parish Nurse	47	4%	13%	83%

summary reports. Data derived from documentation can be tabulated and aggregated to communicate specific aspects of the ministry of parish nursing practice to the congregation and/or health system. This statistical data can relate to the number of one-on-one interactions, the nature of the interactions, the number of group programs, and number of individuals who attend the group programs and is important in identifying the value added services provided by the parish nurse. Figure 20-1 is an example of a statistical report that can be derived from the Integration documentation system (Burkhart, 2002b). Chapter 8 presents the documentation system in more detail. As part of the parish nurse documentation system, individual parish nurse reports can be tabulated into a database to reflect monthly, quarterly, or annual parish nurse activities. These reports are helpful in communicating the nature of ongoing work per church, hospital region, or the health system region.

Quality Outcome Indicators

A few studies identify outcomes or client needs relevant to parish nursing practice. The outcome indicators identified in the parish nurse literature are summarized in Table 20-2. Parish nurse coordinators/managers are encouraged to evaluate the usefulness of measuring these possible outcome indicators.

Weis, Matheus, and Schank (1997) analyzed monthly parish nurse reports and interviewed 11 parish nurses in 11 faith communities in a culturally diverse large metropolitan area. Results indicated that parish nurses address nine Healthy People 2000 objectives, which are listed in Table 20-2. Matteson, Reilly, & Moseley (2000) surveyed homebound elderly who belonged to a church to measure functional needs and quality of life. Results indicated that this elderly population had relatively high functioning and quality of life, and that level of functioning was directly

Parish Nurse Program Report

2001	August	Burkhart

Individual Interactions:			N	%			N	%
		New client	2	33.3	Age:	0 - 12	0	0
Number:	6	Previously seen	4	66.7		13 - 17	0	0
		Male	1	83.3		18 - 30	0	0
Hours:	5.5	Female	5	16.7		31 - 50	3	50
		Parishioner	5	83.3		51 - 60	1	16.6
		Non-parishioner	1	16.7		66 - 80	2	33.3
						Over 80	0	0
		Location				Unknown	0	0
		Church	2	33				
		Nurse office	1	17	**Ethnic Heritage**			
		Visit to HCP	0	0		Caucasian	6	100
		Hospital	0	0		Black	0	0
		Home visit	1	17		Hispanic	0	0
		Nursing home	0	0		Asian/Oriental	0	0
		Phone	2	33		Native American	0	0
		Mail	0	0		Middle Eastern	0	0
		Pantry	0	0		Far East	0	0
		Other	0	0		Multi-cultural	0	0
						Other	0	0
						Unknown	0	0

Parish Nurse Program Report

2001	August	Burkhart

Individual Interactions	Interdisciplinary Collaboration	N	% of Total Interactions	Interventions	N	% of Total
	Medical Categories			Physiological: Basic	0	0
	Cardiac/Vascular	2	33.3	Physiological: Complex	0	0
	Respiratory	0	0	Behavior/Cognitive	0	0
	Renal/Urinary	0	0	Communication enhancement	0	0
	GI/Hepatic/Biliary	0	0	Coping/Spiritual/Religious	5	83
	Metabolic/Immune	0	0	Client education	5	83
	Neurological/Sensory	0	0	Psychological comfort	1	17
	Muscular/Skeletal	0	0	Safety	2	33
	Reproductive	0	0	Family	1	17
	Drug Interactions	0	0	Health system	2	33
	Psychological	3	50	*Source of Referral*		*% of New Clients*
	Spiritual and/or Religious	3	50	Client	2	100
				Parishioner	0	0
	Health Patterns (Concerns/Diagnoses)			Non-parishioner	0	0
	Health promotion	2	33	Pastoral staff	0	0
	Nutrition	0	0	Physician	0	0
	Elimination	0	0	Other health provider	0	0
	Activity/Rest	1	17	Media	0	0
	Perception/Cognition	3	50	Parish nurse	0	0
	Self/Perception	0	0	Family	0	0
	Role/Relationship	1	17	*Referral to:*		*% of Total*
	Sexuality/Reproductive	0	0	Pastoral staff	0	0
	Coping/Stress	2	33	Physician	1	17
	Life principles	2	33	Other health provider	0	0
	Safety/Protection	0	0	Church resource	0	0
	Comfort	1	17	Community resource	0	0
	Growth/Development	0	0	TOTAL SYSTEM REFERRALS	1	17

Figure 20-1   Statistical Report (From Burkhart L. (2002). Integration: a documentation system reporting whole person care. Evanston, IL: Author. [Available for purchase through the International Parish Nurse Resource Center, Deaconess Foundation.])

Continued

2001	August	Burkhart

Group Activities		Screenings	Number	Participants	Abnormal	New	Meetings	# Times	Hrs
Total		Blood Pressure	2	65	9	1	Pastor/Staff	4	4
Participants:	65	Cholesterol	0	0	0	0	Health and Wellness	0	0
		Glucose	0	0	0	0	Other Church Committee	0	0
Time (hours):		Lice	0	0	0	0	Community/Liaison/Networking	1	1
		Health	0	0	0	0	System/Liaison/Networking	0	0
Plan	6	Hearing/Vision	0	0	0	0	Parish Nurse	1	6
		Ht/Wt	0	0	0	0	Other	0	0
Program	4	Other	0	0	0	0	Attendance at Church Functions		
		Group Programs		Number	Participants		Worship Services	0	0
		Education		0	0		Healing Services	0	0
		Support		0	0		Funerals	1	2
		Spiritual		0	0		Wakes	1	1
		Environmental/Safety		0	0		Fellowship	0	0
		Community Outreach		0	0		Other	0	0
		Other		0	0		Office Work		
		Visual/Written Programs					Report Writing		0
		Newsletter/Bulletin		1			Resource Development		2
SUBTOTAL		Health Display		1			Documentation		1.25
HOURS:	10	Continuing Education					Other		0
		Professional Development		0			Volunteer Coordination		2
		Programs Attended		1			TOTAL HOURS		29.25
							Paid		20
							Unpaid		9.25

Figure 20-1, cont'd Statistical Report (From Burkhart L. [2002]. Integration: a documentation system reporting whole person care. Evanston, IL: Author. [Available for purchase through the International Parish Nurse Resource Center, Deaconess Foundation.])

TABLE 20-2 Outcome Indicators in the Parish Nursing Literature

Source	Outcome Indicators
Weis, Matheus, & Schank, 1997	Blood pressure knowledge and control Overweight prevalence and weight loss practices Vigorous physical activity Breast self-exam and mammogram Home fire safety Stress management Reduce heart disease and stroke Reduce child abuse Maintain ADLs 65+
Baldwin, Humbles, Armmer, & Cramer, 2001	Screening Education Health promotion/disease prevention Disease processes/living with disease Ambulatory care for low-income Direct service provision Referrals for direct service provision Risk reduction program Exercise Weight loss Individual health counseling

From Burkhart, L. (2002a). NOC in Parish Nursing: Reliability, Validity, and Utility in a Community-based setting, Presentation at *NANDA, NIC, NOC 2002: Developing, Linking and Integrating Nursing Language and Informatics*, Chicago, 12 April 2002.

TABLE 20-2   Outcome Indicators in the Parish Nursing Literature—cont'd

Source	Outcome Indicators
Swinney, Anson-Wonkka, Maki, & Corneau, 2001	Smoking cessation Adequate sleep/rest Care coordination/life integration Alcohol consumption Spousal and child abuse Teen education Risk-taking behaviors Self-esteem Peer pressure Elderly education Alcohol consumption Transportation Health advocacy Finances Extended care Living wills Prescription drugs Childcare coordination Delivery of meals to elderly and sick Visiting families in crisis Promote family integrity Respite care Grief support
Matteson, Reilly, & Moseley, 2000	Level of functioning Quality of life
Burkhart, 2002a; Moorhead, Johnson, & Maas, 2004	Spiritual well-being Acceptance of health status Health-promoting behaviors Health orientation Health-seeking behaviors Social involvement Caregiver well-being Caregiver-patient relationship
Burkhart, 2002b	Individual client health outcomes (NOCs) Parish nurse activities (i.e., one-on-one interactions, group programs, meetings, office work) Client satisfaction Impact on healthcare service use Referrals to other healthcare providers
Rethemeyer & Wehling, 2004	Role of the parish nurse Personal beliefs Role in the health ministry Care and services Educational programs Newsletter articles

related to quality of life, suggesting that those who belong to a faith community and have access to a parish nurse may experience a higher quality of life than others. Results, however, are limited because the researchers did not report sample data or specific numeric results. Baldwin, Humbles, Armmer, and Cramer (2001) surveyed a random sample of parishioners from five urban African-American churches in central Illinois to determine congregants' perceived needs, as listed in Table 20-2. Results indicated that respondents were more concerned with health habits than specific disease symptoms and felt that the parish nurse provides a vital role in health screenings and health education. In 2001, Swinney, Anson-Wonkka, Maki, and Corneau (2001) reported the results of a needs assessment for a large Catholic congregation. Although the majority of these respondents felt they were in good health, physical concerns included use of tobacco, adequate sleep/rest, and adequate care for general health problems. Psychological care included need for support and advice related to alcohol consumption, as well as spousal and child abuse. Follow-up focus group analysis indicated a need for teen education, particularly in relation to risk-taking behaviors, low self-esteem, and peer pressure. Senior citizen issues included alcohol consumption; transportation; health advocacy; and information about finances, extended care, living wills, and prescription drugs. Other concerns included childcare coordination, delivery of meals to elderly and sick, and visiting families in crisis. Preventive care included promoting family integrity, providing respite care, and grief support.

Burkhart (2002a) reported outcomes research that measured the reliability and validity of the Nursing Outcomes Classification (NOC), funded through the U.S. National Institute for Nursing Research (Moorhead, Johnson, & Maas, 2004). Parish nursing was one test group for the research. During the study, parish nurses chose which NOCs were appropriate to study in parish nursing. Results are listed in Table 20-2 (Burkhart, 2002a). Also in 2002, Burkhart published a parish nurse documentation system that integrated both client-specific and program outcome measurements. This work came out of a Kellogg-funded grant and was based on focus group research with parish nurses in the Chicagoland area as well as parish nurses who attended two Westberg Symposiums. The system also was piloted with two parish nurse programs (Burkhart, 2002b).

In 2004, the International Parish Nurse Resource Center, Deaconess Foundation, published a parish nurse ministry survey that included six elements. The survey measures clients' perspectives of their health, changed behavior, and satisfaction with parish nursing. The survey was developed by the authors and reviewed by a focus group of parish nurses. The concepts measured in the survey are not clearly defined, and no reliability or validity data is published. Rethemeyer and Wehling (2004) reported that the survey was implemented in the St. Louis area and presented general satisfaction with the parish nurse program. Numeric results listed the percent of respondents who felt the parish nurse impacted certain health behaviors (e.g., blood pressure checks, eating more healthily). However, whether these health behaviors were actualized is unclear. Several studies researched case management models located in a church (Trofino, Hughes, O'Brien, Mack, Marrinan, & Hay, 2000; Hughes, Trofino, O'Brien, Mack, & Marrinan, 2001). Although interesting, these models are not consistent with parish nursing as defined in the *Scope and Standards of Parish Nursing Practice* (ANA, 1998).

Outcomes are identified and measured for a reason. They identify what health-related services affect client health and can guide resource allocation and future care to maximize impact on client health (Donabedian, 1985; Moorhead, Johnson, & Maas, 2004). Outcome measurements can provide information that will reflect both the value and quality of parish nursing services rendered.

Table 20-2 provides a list of possible outcome indicators. However, this list can appear complicated when one is choosing outcome indicators for an individual program. A conceptual model can help parish nurse coordinators/managers decide what quality indicators are relevant to their programs. Research in parish nursing does not provide a conclusive outcome model for parish nurses. Therefore the authors developed a conceptual model, shown in Figure 20-2, derived from both parish nurse literature and nursing informatics.

Although parish nurses are in a unique position of providing a bridge between the health system

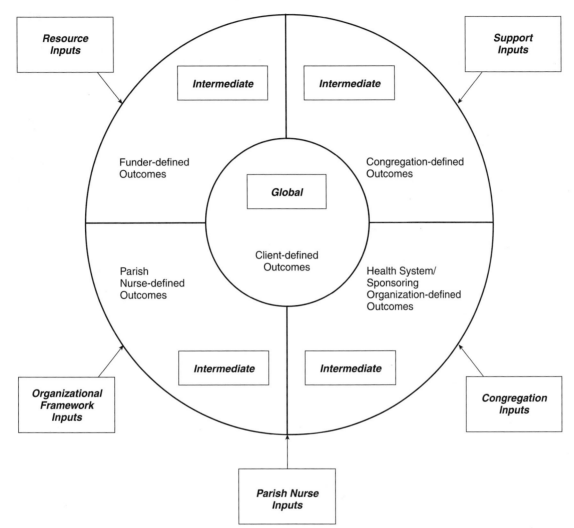

Figure 20-2   Outcomes Model for the Ministry of Parish Nursing Practice. (Developed by Lisa Burkhart and Phyllis Ann Solari-Twadell.)

and the faith community, this positioning can complicate outcome measurement. The healthcare institution and the congregation represent two distinct cultures that may recognize and value different outcomes and measurement strategies. In addition, each organization may have different stakeholders, or groups of individuals who have a vested interested in the ministry of parish nursing practice. Djupe, Lloyd, and Ludwig-Beymer (1994) identified five stakeholder groups invested in parish nursing services offered through Lutheran General Hospital: congregational leadership, health system leadership, funders, parish nurses, and parishioners/clients. Each stakeholder may have different goals in mind when supporting the parish nurse program/ministry. Whether an institution-based or congregation-based program, each stakeholder needs to articulate relevant outcomes from his or her perspective. The model takes into consideration stakeholders' perceptions.

Nursing informatics also provided structure in the development of this model. The Nursing

Outcomes Classification model, developed by Moorhead, Johnson, & Maas (2004), was adapted to parish nursing to assist in providing clarity and systematic understanding of different types of quality indicators, integrating input and outcome quality indicators.

Parish Nurse Quality Model

As shown in Figure 20-2, this adapted outcome model identifies three categories of measurements: inputs, intermediate outcomes, and global outcomes. Inputs affect outcomes. Solari-Twadell identified five primary categories of inputs: resources, support, organizational framework, congregation, and parish nurse–related indicators (Solari-Twadell, 2002). Specific inputs related to each of these input categories are noted in Table 20-1.

Stakeholders that are invested in the specific ministry of parish nursing practice identify intermediate outcome indicators. Stakeholders include congregational leadership, health system/ sponsoring organization leadership, those who fund the ministry of parish nursing practice, and parish nurses. Identified outcomes may differ based on the stakeholder. Specific outcome indicators can be derived from Table 20-2 or can be newly identified by the stakeholder. For example, congregational leadership may be interested in expanding church membership, promoting volunteerism, and improving spiritual health. Health systems may be interested in marketing health system services, increasing referrals to the health system, and fostering good will. Particularly, not-for-profit healthcare entities may need to justify that the parish nurse program provides a certain degree of community service. Many states require institutions to submit a Community Benefit Inventory for Social Accountability report to maintain not-for-profit status. In the 1990s, many health systems were challenged to justify their status (Coalition for Nonprofit Health Care, 1999). Parish nurse programs can help fulfill this requirement. Health system leadership needs to identify what information is needed to fulfill this requirement. Those who fund the ministry of parish nursing practice may have different goals. Many parish nurse programs are funded through grants. Grants are awarded based on federal,

state, or local healthcare initiatives. Many of these initiatives are based on the *Healthy People 2010* objectives, which is available online at www.healthypeople.gov (United States Department of Health and Human Services, 2000). Parish nurses may identify additional goals, including resource support, communication, and role clarity.

The ministry of parish nursing practice exists to promote whole person health for the clients served. The global outcomes noted in Figure 20-2 refer to client-defined indicators. These client-defined indicators may be determined by the client or collaboratively by both the client and the parish nurse. Clients may be interested in improved health (both actual and perceived) as well as satisfaction with the program.

Although each stakeholder may identify different goals, it is critical that after the goals are identified, members of each stakeholder group come together and agree upon the list of outcomes related to these goals. Djupe, Lloyd, and Ludwig-Beymer (1994) identified stakeholder alignment as critical to the sustainability of a parish nurse program.

Measuring Outcomes

Once outcomes are identified, they need to be measured. Measurement systems are contingent on the concept being measured. Many parish nurse outcomes only require tracking and tabulating (e.g., number of one-on-one interactions, client attendance at programs). Client satisfaction and health-related outcomes are more difficult to measure. Client satisfaction must be measured by the client—be it through qualitative stories or quantitative surveys. Qualitative stories are collected individually, whereas quantitative data represent aggregate data. Because parish nurses may impact parishioners indirectly through group programs, newsletters, or bulletin articles, it is best to survey the entire congregation to measure client satisfaction. Examples of client satisfaction surveys are available for purchase through the International Parish Nurse Resource Center. A sample survey is also included in the Integration documentation manual (Burkhart, 2002b), which is presented in Figure 20-3.

Health-related outcomes are more difficult to measure because health is measured in many

Client Satisfaction Survey

1. Have you made contact with the parish nurse?
   ❏ No
   ❏ Yes (please check which service and circle how satisfied you are with the service)

❏ I have read bulletin and/or newsletter articles on health topics written by the parish nurse.	Very Satisfied	Satisfied	Neutral	Dissatisfied	Very Dissatisfied
❏ I have participated in a screening activity, for example, blood pressure or cholesterol checks offered by the parish nurse.	Very Satisfied	Satisfied	Neutral	Dissatisfied	Very Dissatisfied
❏ I have attended a health education program that was coordinated or presented by the parish nurse.	Very Satisfied	Satisfied	Neutral	Dissatisfied	Very Dissatisfied
❏ I have attended a support group that was coordinated or facilitated by the parish nurse.	Very Satisfied	Satisfied	Neutral	Dissatisfied	Very Dissatisfied
❏ I have talked with the parish nurse about a personal matter such as medications, a new diagnosis, a relationship, or my overall health and well-being.	Very Satisfied	Satisfied	Neutral	Dissatisfied	Very Dissatisfied
❏ A member of my family has talked with the parish nurse about a personal matter such as medications, a new diagnosis, a relationship, or my overall health and well-being.	Very Satisfied	Satisfied	Neutral	Dissatisfied	Very Dissatisfied
❏ The parish nurse has referred me to a physician and/or a group or organization in the congregation or community where I could go for further assistance.	Very Satisfied	Satisfied	Neutral	Dissatisfied	Very Dissatisfied
❏ I have participated as a volunteer from this congregation who provides service to poor, homeless, shut-ins, or bereaved.	Very Satisfied	Satisfied	Neutral	Dissatisfied	Very Dissatisfied
❏ The parish nurse has helped me draw upon my spiritual strength in dealing with health issues.	Very Satisfied	Satisfied	Neutral	Dissatisfied	Very Dissatisfied

Comments:

Figure 20-3   Client Satisfaction Survey. (From Burkhart, L. [2002]. *Integration: A documentation system reporting whole person care.* Evanston, IL: Author. [Available for purchase through the International Parish Nurse Resource Center, Deaconess Foundation.])

Continued

Client Satisfaction Survey—cont'd

2. What is your opinion of the parish nurse program?
   o Excellent. It is a most valuable ministry of this congregation.
   o Good program. It is important to the congregation.
   o Adequate but needs improvement (please note how it could be improved).
   o Poor. Needs unmet (please note how this ministry could better meet the needs of this congregation).
   o Not needed (please explain).

   Comments:

3. In your opinion, how well do you see the ministry of parish nursing practice contributing to the well-being of the congregation?
   o Excellent
   o Good
   o Average
   o Fair
   o Poor

   Comments:

Thank you for completing this survey!

Figure 20-3, cont'd   Client Satisfaction Survey. (From Burkhart, L. [2002]. *Integration: A documentation system reporting whole person care.* Evanston, IL: Author. [Available for purchase through the International Parish Nurse Resource Center, Deaconess Foundation.])

different ways. There also can be multiple influences on the determination of health (U.S. Department of Health and Human Services, 2001). The University of Iowa Nursing Outcomes Classification (NOC) Team offers one strategy to measure a variety of health outcomes (Moorhead, Johnson, & Maas, 2004). NOC (2004) is a list of 330 different health-related outcome measurement tools. Examples of outcomes that may be relevant in parish nursing are listed in Table 20-3. Individual clients and/or the parish nurses can identify client-related specific NOC outcomes and measure them over time. As part of a federally funded grant by the National Institute of Nursing Research, parish nurses tested NOC's reliability and validity, particularly in relation to the spiritual and health promotion outcomes (Burkhart, 2002a, Burkhart, 2005). Specific reliability and validity data are included in the 2004 edition of NOC (Moorhead, Johnson, & Maas, 2004).

Research supports the use of NOC in measuring the spiritual dimension of care (Burkhart, 2004). When choosing specific outcome measurement tools, one must ensure the tool is accurate and reliable and is supported by research.

Conclusion

Parish nursing began as a grassroots movement. It grew in response to the recognition that faith communities are sources of whole person health. Health is maximized when physical, psychological, social, and spiritual health are integrated into care and when identification of illness patterns occurs in early stages of the illness. Parish nurses address whole person care, and because of their on-going relationship as part of the faith community, parish nurses can assist clients in preventing or identifying illness patterns early in the disease process.

TABLE 20-3   Parish Nursing–Related NOC Measurements

Type of Measurement	NOC Labels*
Physical Measurements	Vital signs
	Self-care—activities of daily living
	Self-care—instrumental activities of daily living
	Fluid balance
	Circulation status
	Nutritional status
	Weight control
	Diabetes self-management
	Cardiac disease self-management
	Asthma self-management
	Symptom control
	Pain control
Psychological Measurements	Coping
	Anxiety level
	Stress level
Social Measurements	Social support
	Social involvement
	Family coping
	Family integrity
	Family support during treatment
Spiritual Measurements	Spiritual health
	Hope
	Acceptance: health status
	Grief resolution
Environmental	Safe home environment
	Risk control
Client Satisfaction	Client satisfaction: access to care resources
	Client satisfaction: cultural needs fulfillment
	Client satisfaction: communication
	Client satisfaction: teaching

*The detailed NOC tool is available in Moorhead, S., Johnson, M., & Mass, M. (2004). *Iowa outcomes project: nursing outcomes classification (NOC)*. St. Louis: Mosby.

To promote quality in the ministry of parish nursing practice, each program must identify quality indicators. These indicators include relevant structural components, process variables, and outcome indicators. Structural components require ongoing support beginning at start-up and continuing throughout the lifecycle of the ministry. Program stakeholders also need to be identified and need to participate in supporting the program. This includes defining what process indicators

are necessary to communicate on-going parish nurse activities, resource needs, and expectations. These data can be collected through a documentation system and summarized monthly, quarterly, and/or annually. Finally, outcome indicators also need to be identified and a system put into place for ongoing measurement. This chapter provides a structure, the state of the art, and a challenge for those who are interested in demonstrating both the quality and value of the ministry of parish nursing practice in their setting. This information will be instrumental in documenting the essential services and significant results of those services. Once this information can be explicated, it will be a source of interest to those who fund efficient and effective strategies for preventing illness, early identification of disease, and healthcare coordination across the healthcare continuum. This can be accomplished by integrating physical, psychological, social, and spiritual care that follows clients throughout their lifetimes. The congregation can provide lifetime follow-up, given the individual's continual involvement and participation in his or her faith community. It is critical, however, that the community who envisioned this ministry participates in ensuring its quality and demonstrating its value.

REFERENCES

American Nurses Association. (1995). *Nursing report card for acute care*. Washington, DC: Author.

American Nurses Association. (1998). *Scope and standards of parish nursing practice*. (9806st). Washington DC: Author.

American Nurses Association. (2000). *Nursing quality indicators beyond acute care: measurement instruments*. Washington, DC: Author.

Baldwin, K.A., Humbles, P.L., Armmer, F.A., & Cramer, M. (2001). Perceived health needs of urban African American church congregates. *Public Health Nursing*, 18: 295-303.

Burkhart, L. (2002a). "NOC in Parish Nursing: Reliability, Validity, and Utility in a Community-based Setting," Presentation at *NANDA, NIC, NOC 2002: Developing, Linking and Integrating Nursing Language and Informatics*, Chicago, 12 April 2002.

Burkhart, L. (2002b). *Integration: A documentation system reporting whole person care*. Evanston, IL: Author. Available for purchase through the International Parish Nurse Resource Center, Deaconess Foundation.

Burkhart, L. (2005). A click away: documenting spiritual care. *The Journal of Christian Nursing, Winter.* 22(1): 6-13.

Coalition for Nonprofit Health Care (1999). Redefining the community benefit standard: State law approaches to ensure the social accountability of nonprofit health care organizations. Washington, DC: Author.

Deming, W.E. (1986). *Out of the crisis*. Cambridge, MA: Massachusetts Institute of Technology.

Djupe, A.M., Lloyd, R.C. and Ludwig-Beymer, P. (1994). *Alignment of key stakeholder groups,* Park Ridge, IL: Advocate Health Care, unpublished manuscript.

Donabedian, A. (1966). Evaluating the quality of medical care. *Milbank Memorial Fund Quarterly* 44 (3) 166-206.

Donabedian, A. (1985). *Explorations in quality assessment and monitoring, volume III: the methods and findings of quality assessment and monitoring, an illustrated analysis*. Ann Arbor, MI: Health Administration Press.

Hughes, C.B., Trofino, J., O'Brien, B.L., Mack, J., & Marrinan, M. (2001). Primary care parish nursing: Outcomes and implications. *Nursing Administration Quarterly*, 26(1): 45-59.

Lloyd, R. & Ludwig-Beymer, P. (1999). Listening to faith communities: Collaboration with those served. In Solari-Twadell, P.A. & McDermott, M.A. *Parish nursing: Promoting whole-person health within faith communities*. Thousand Oaks, CA: Sage.

Ludwig-Beymer, P., Welsch, C. & Tuzik Micek, W. (1998). Keeping people healthy: Parish nursing's role in CQI. *Journal of Christian Nursing*, 15(1): 28-31.

Matteson, M. A., Reilly, M., & Moseley, M. (2000). Needs assessment of homebound elders in a parish church: Implications for parish nursing. *Geriatric Nursing*, 21(3): 144-147.

Moorhead, S., Johnson, M., & Maas, M. (2004). *Iowa outcomes project: nursing outcomes classification (NOC)*. Philadelphia: Mosby.

Nightingale, F. (1994). *Suggestions for thought*. In M. Calabria, & J. Macrae (Eds.). Philadelphia: University of Pennsylvania Press.

Rethemeyer, A., & Wehling, B.A. (2004). How are we doing?: measuring the effectiveness of parish nursing. *Journal of Christian Nursing*, 21(2): 10-12.

Solari-Twadell, P.A. (2002). The differentiation of the ministry of parish nursing practice within congregations. *Dissertation Abstracts International*, 63(06): 569A. UMI No. 3056442.

Swinney, J., Anson-Wonkka, C., Maki, E., & Corneau, J. (2001). Community assessment: a church community and the parish nurse. *Public Health Nursing*, 18(4): 40-44.

Trofino, J., Hughes, C. B., O'Brien, B. L., Mack, J., Marrinan, M.A., & Hay, K.M. (2000). Primary care parish nursing: academic, service, and parish partnership. *Nursing Administration Quarterly*, 25(1): 59-74.

U.S. Department of Health and Human Services. (2000). *Healthy People 2010*. Washington, DC: Author.

Weis, D., Matheus, R., & Schank, M.J. (1997). Health care delivery in faith communities: the parish nurse model. *Public Health Nursing*, 14(6): 368-372.

Parish Nurse Coordinator: Working with Congregations and Clergy in Fostering the Ministry of Parish Nursing Practice

21

Joan M. Burke
Phyllis Ann Solari-Twadell

Reverend Granger Westberg would often speak of the parish nurses as "having one foot in the sciences and one foot in the humanities, one foot in the spiritual world and one in the physical one" (*Journal of Christian Nursing*, 1989, p. 26). Parish Nurse Coordinators (PNC) stand in these arenas and are also grounded in the healthcare institutions they serve as well as in the congregations that are the institution's partners or collaborators in offering the ministry of parish nursing practice. The implications for PNCs is that they must have the capacity to speak and interpret the language of the healthcare institution, as well as the language of the religious denominations represented by the congregational partners. In order for the relationship of these two partners to grow, each partner—meaning congregation and healthcare institution—must be able to reach out and be willing to modify their behavior, traditions and policies over time for the purpose of engaging the other. The parish nurse coordinator becomes the primary interpreter for both partners assisting in this process of engagement. Given the differences represented by the characteristics of these two organizations, this is not a simple responsibility (Appendix 21A). The healthcare institution and the local congregation in some ways are unlikely partners, given the differences between them. However, each can serve its constituency more effectively by developing partnerships that result in better care for the community.

The Benefits of a Partnership with a Healthcare Institution

Westberg approached Lutheran General Hospital regarding the concept of the parish nurse before he approached the six congregations about initiating such a ministry. In his wisdom he knew the benefits of supporting the ministry of parish nursing practice through a relationship between these two partners. Pape (2002) discusses some of the benefits of this arrangement in developing and sustaining the ministry of parish nursing practice in congregations. Pape describes three primary benefits provided to the congregation by healthcare institutions. They are resources, supervision, and support. Resources may not only be financial but can also include personnel that have expertise to share through educational programs offered in the congregation. Supervision not only consists of nursing skills but also ongoing spiritual development of the parish nurse. Support can include but not be limited to consultation on development and integration of the ministry of parish nursing practice into the life of the congregation and ongoing evaluation of the parish nurse. Pape (2002) states "contributions of the healthcare institutions need to continue for some time to bring stability and definition to the practice of parish nursing" (p. 203). Pape's point is well taken; congregations have relegated their mission in health to hospitals. Hospitals or healthcare systems today are not really about health. They are about acute care. Restoration takes place at home or in other settings in the community. The congregation that partners with a healthcare system to develop a ministry of parish nursing practice will benefit from the expertise of the professionals in healthcare, knowledge regarding professional requirements and registration, as well as being able to participate in the continuum of care offered through the healthcare system. In addition, nonprofit healthcare systems through their community benefit programs often have resources that will assist the congregation in developing and sustaining a ministry of parish nursing practice. In reality the healthcare system needs to reach out to the community, actualizing their mission to the community, and relate to their constituency in their episodes of wellness as well as their episodes of illness. This involvement with the community is also one way of substantiating the non-for-profit status of the healthcare organization.

This partnership lives out the previously mentioned but often lacking "continuum of care." The congregant hopefully will reap the most benefit from such a partnership. If the congregant has a parish nurse somehow affiliated with a healthcare institution, a more fluid entrance and discharge from the hospital is possible. In addition the parish nurse may be invited to participate in patient care conferences during the congregant's hospitalization. The inclusion of a parish nurse in such a conference can bring new insights to the planning for the patient. The parish nurse knows the patient in times of wellness. In addition the parish nurse knows the congregant's housing and available family support. If outpatient care is required, perhaps the congregant will benefit from the knowledge and contacts that the parish nurse developed through affiliations with that hospital system or other agencies in the community.

There are different organizational frameworks for the ministry of parish nursing practice. Two of these organizing frameworks include a relationship with a sponsoring institution (See Appendix 21-B). The healthcare system affiliation and corresponding access to continuing education, theological reflection, evaluation, policy and procedure development, competency assessment, as well as nursing and physician consultation, may bring credibility to the ministry of parish nursing practice while relieving the congregation of concerns regarding the quality of the ministry of parish nursing practice.

The healthcare system that initiates a partnership of any sort with the congregation must accept that it bears a long-term responsibility to this relationship. Too often when the finances become tight or the intended results are not as quickly achieved, the healthcare institution will reduce or withdraw support from the ministry of parish nursing practice. At times healthcare institutions have terminated the relationship with the congregation leaving the congregation with no support to continue offering this ministry to their congregation. This is a very risky outcome for the healthcare institution as the congregation and community will learn the lesson that the healthcare institution cannot be trusted to live out commitments to the community. This can sometimes backfire when at a later date the healthcare system desires to connect with the community on another matter or program.

Although the development and integration of the ministry of parish nursing practice into the life of the congregation is considered a challenge, sustaining such a ministry over time is the true test. If there is a written partnership agreement between a healthcare institution and a congregation, either partner may be more thoughtful before discontinuing the ministry of parish nursing practice. Without outside sponsorship, the ministry is much more likely to disappear during a time of transition, such as the transfer, retirement, or leave of the clergy or the parish nurse.

Research in parish nursing reported that respondents whose ministry of parish nursing practice was anchored in a relationship with a healthcare institution were more likely to be in paid positions (Solari-Twadell, 2002). Remuneration for services offered through the ministry of parish nursing practice, however, is not necessarily always what parish nurses desire (Solari-Twadell, 2002). Parish nurses who are paid usually tend to work more hours and more fully develop the role of the parish nurse through more nursing interventions than those who are unpaid (Solari-Twadell, 2002). Clergy, lay ministers, and others supporting developing congregation-based parish nursing practices should consider the expected time, resulting presence, and responsibilities of the parish nurse. The parish nurse's services depend largely on her or his skills, the community's needs and resources, as well as the time that the parish nurse can commit to the ministry.

Capacities of the Parish Nurse Coordinator in Working Effectively with Clergy and Congregations

Just as the parish nurse needs to attend to the development of a particular skill set in working effectively in ministering to others, the parish nurse coordinator has or needs to develop specific capacities, skills, and abilities that will enhance working with clergy and congregations (see Chapter 19). Mentors are helpful to those who manage a parish nursing ministry, especially in the ways detailed in the following discussion (see Chapter 15).

Appreciation for the Power of Prayer

Pray always, not so much for what it is that you think is best but for the grace and blessing of God to be upon this work with others in developing the ministry of parish nursing practice. In Chapter 14, Langdon writes of the importance of listening for the will of God in your prayer. This is integral to the work of the PNC. As life-giving as this work may be, it is important to realize that it is not the work of one individual and that each person is a vessel used to accomplish the work of a God much more powerful and all-knowing than one person alone. So, pray always that this work may be servicing the greater work of God.

Listening Skills

Listening is an art. Lloyd and Ludwig-Beymer (1999) elaborated on the importance of listening at three key times: before service, at point of service, and after the service is completed. The clergy and congregation members need to feel that the PNC, who is their liaison to a large healthcare institution, hears their concerns, needs, and dreams. The healthcare system may already have the reputation of not listening or appreciating the position of the consumer. As the PNC, do not be surprised if a past occurrence with the healthcare institution left community members or congregations suspicious about the healthcare institution's interest in their congregation and its members.

Appreciation for Congregational History

Fite (1999) elaborates on the importance of taking the time to learn about the history of the congregation. Knowing the history may help the PNC to understand the present culture, decision making, celebrations, and ministries available to members of the congregation. This appreciation for history must be accompanied by a love of storytelling. Many members of the congregation will relate important information in the format of a story of something or somebody that had a significant impact on the development of the congregation.

Interest in and Understanding of the Culture of the Congregation

Entering a relationship with a congregation, one should understand and respect the culture of the congregation, the compatibility of the cultures of the healthcare institution and the congregation, and openness within each of these cultures to change (Fite, 1999). "Culture can eat change for breakfast" is a cute little description of a common phenomenon: culture can trump the parish nurse's ability to implement change. Understanding this description, one must see there is a deep appreciation for a culture's strength in managing information and change (Chaee-Ziolek, 2005). This is an especially important point because the ministry of parish nursing practice seeks to be a catalyst for change.

Appreciation of Politics

The congregation can be a political environment, yet congregants may not acknowledge this understanding. That seems quite contrary to what one might expect, given that "every congregation has a polity, a set of rules that governs its life" (Fite, 1999, p. 125). There are the formal leaders, documents, and rules, but as in any organization, there are the informal leaders, rules, and communication. The PNC must learn both. Understanding the nature of the politics within a congregation takes time, dedication, and appreciation for the power of informal leadership in influencing the success of programs and ministry.

The PNC must also be sensitive to the politics within the healthcare system. The success and longevity of the ministry of parish nursing practice may depend on knowing who the key supporters for the ongoing development of this ministry are throughout the organization. It is important that from the board level to staff level individuals are informed of the mission, purpose, and employees responsible for the development and ongoing supervision of the parish nursing initiative. Every opportunity should be taken to keep employees, from the president to the staff, knowledgeable about the difference the presence of the ministry of parish nursing is making for people in the community. The leaders of the healthcare institution will want to be clear on the benefits, given the investment being made in this effort.

Clarifying Expectations

Congregations historically are not well known for documentation. Whether it is job descriptions, policies and procedures, or history, there is often little written that undergirds or clarifies the organizational life of the congregation. This is understandable as the congregation is a voluntary organization. However, this is all the more reason for the PNC to be clear and explicit in spoken and written communication regarding expectations of the relationship between the healthcare institution, congregation, and parish nurse. As the ministry of parish nursing practice is integrated into the congregation, all parties absolutely must have congruent and consistent expectations. Clear communication and understanding will eliminate feelings of disrespect, taking unfair advantage of each other, or neglecting the integrity of each partner. Lack of clarity regarding the expectations of both partners can often be a fundamental cause for the demise of a parish nursing practice. Appendix C presents a planning tool that can assist in clarification of expectations.

Excellent Communication Skills

The role of the PNC is highly relational. The person in this position is in constant communication with either a parish nurse, pastor, administrator, lay minister, community member, community agency funder, or hospital staff member or leader. Some parish nurse managers and coordinators feel by the end of the day that they just want to go home and talk to no one! Because this administrative role interfaces with so many entities and people, ongoing enhancement of personal communication skills is necessary.

Good Organizing Abilities

The PNC, like the parish nurse, usually has multiple balls in the air at one time; therefore, multitasking is not an option. Slim budgets and limited precious time to accomplish all that needs to be done, as well as continual change, usually plague the PNC. All of these dynamics call for the PNC to foster good organization. Knowing where things are and understanding expected timelines for specific projects and who is expecting what from whom and when are important to managing the demands of this role and the complexity of the relationships. Appendix 21-D presents a process for developing a ministry of parish nursing practice in a congregation that PNCs may find helpful.

Ability to Follow Through in the Midst of Conflict

As much as stakeholders may want a ministry of parish nursing practice to succeed, a particular relationship with a congregation may not continue for a number of reasons. When all parties—the healthcare institution, congregation, clergy, and parish nurse—do not make this decision mutually, anger, resentment, and bitterness may result. This may be a very challenging time for the PNC. It is particulary important during this time that the PNC has a good support system, spiritual director and understanding supervisor who can assist in management of the associated feelings generated as a result of this change.

Development of a Ministry of Parish Nursing Practice

Advisory Board or Committee

Integration of the Ministry of Parish Nursing Practice is important in both the congregation and the healthcare institution. One way of integrating the ministry of parish nursing practice into the institution and creating ownership of the ministry is an advisory committee or board. This advisory board is separate and distinct from the Health Cabinet developed at the congregation. The advisory committee/board for the developing parish nursing program, services, or network functions under the auspices of a healthcare institution and provides counsel and consultation to the manager/coordinator of the ministry. This is accomplished through review and recommendations of ideas, policies and procedures, and future plans for growth and development as well as the strategic plan for the healthcare organization. The membership of the advisory board comprises approximately eight to 12 individuals from the healthcare organization, congregations, and community. The parish nurse manager chairs this advisory board/committee. Suggested participants of the board/committee include two parish nurses, two pastors from the community who have a ministry of parish nursing practice in their congregations, a hospital chaplain, a community outreach representative from the healthcare institution, the home-care administrator from the healthcare institution, and a representative from the foundation of the healthcare institution. A 2- to 3-year term on the advisory board/committee is recommended. All members of the committee should not leave their positions at the same time.

The advisory board/committee provides a sounding board for the parish nurse manager. The frequency of meetings can change. Initially the group might meet frequently (once a month), and when the operations of the ministry of parish nursing practice are established, they may move to a less frequent meeting schedule (two or three times a year). The chair of the board/committee plans the agenda for the meeting, with input from the membership of the board/committee.

The Health Cabinet

In *The Parish Nurse,* Westberg (1990) asserts that every congregation with a parish nurse should have a health cabinet or a wellness committee that can become a true support to the nurse and integrate the ministry of parish nursing practice into the life of the congregation. "The health cabinet is an umbrella group that promotes the healing ministry of the congregation" (McNamara, 2002, p. 8). The members have a comprehensive view of the congregation and already know individuals who are ready to help. Cabinet members are the eyes and ears of the congregation. They often know what programs are needed and can even identify health trends. Patterson (2003) describes a health cabinet as "composed of a small group of individuals drawn from health professionals and others who are interested in exploring issues of faith and health in a congregational setting" (p. 41). Besides support for the nurse, the health cabinet suggests health and wellness programs for the parish, educates the congregation about parish nursing, sets health ministry policy, develops promotional materials for the church bulletin, and evaluates ongoing success or needs of the health ministry program.

The health cabinet is a catalyst for change and encourages individuals to get involved, thus making them aware of how healing can come from each of them. The health cabinet's job is to make ministries of health possible (McNamara, 2002).

One parish nurse conducted a gifts assessment of the members of the congregation through the support of the health cabinet. The information gleaned from this endeavor identified people willing to take leadership roles for various services sponsored by the ministry of parish nursing practice. She had leaders who in turn identified volunteers for a greeting card ministry, drivers who would take congregants for physician visits, individuals who made meals for shut-ins, as well as those willing to do chore services and be companions to the elderly. Understanding the gifts and talents of each person facilitated the "multiplication of the ministers," offering congregational members the opportunity to use their gifts in service to others.

The Importance of Developing a Protocol for Working with Congregations

Advantages of a Protocol in Working with Clergy and Congregations

Introducing a parish nursing practice partnered with a healthcare institution involves offering various options for integrating the new entity into the congregation. This protocol has the following advantages.

- A consistent plan outlines institutional resources available to a congregation over time in integrating the ministry of parish nursing practice into the life of a congregation.
- A protocol clarifies the steps and expectations for all parties involved in developing the ministry of parish nursing practice.
- A protocol can constitute the groundwork for a plan and relationship upon which all parties can agree as they develop a ministry of parish nursing practice.
- A protocol identifies consistent learning that will be part of the development of the ministry of parish nursing practice.

- A protocol provides a common vision for the development of the ministry of parish nursing practice.
- A protocol encourages the development of a team approach to ministry.
- A protocol adequately informs all parties at the beginning of the work so they can be knowledgeable about the level of commitment required.
- A protocol provides an excellent opportunity for the PNC to get to know the pastor, congregation, and the culture of the congregation.

An example of a protocol for working with congregations in the development of a ministry of parish nursing practice is included in Appendix 21E.

Obstacles to the Use of a Protocol in the Development of the Ministry of Parish Nursing Practice

Early in the relationship, sensitivity to potential obstacles to the development and integration of the ministry is especially important. Some potential obstacles include the following:

1. The congregation does not see the need for a health cabinet or committee to support the work of the parish nurse. Maybe a group already exists in the congregation and is a good match for the ministry of parish nursing practice. For example, in some congregations a group such as "social concerns" may support the parish nurse. However, if no group exists and no interest in providing a task force or group of members in the church to take up the leadership can be found, concern regarding the future integration of the ministry of parish nursing practice into the life of the congregation is warranted.

2. The pastor or lead clergy is not able to participate in the development of the mission and vision of the ministry of parish nursing practice in the congregation. Very few seminaries prepare pastors for the important intersection of health and faith (Carson & Koenig, 2002). The pastors may see their role as tending to the sacramental life of the church and worship liturgy. They may not understand their role in health promotion or see the congregation as a health place in the community. In addition, they may not understand the language of health and healthcare, which may limit communication with clergy (Story, 2003).

3. Unspoken agendas can also interfere with the development and integration of the ministry of parish nursing practice. For example, one member of a task force for the development of the ministry of parish nursing practice in a congregation was a physician, practicing in a hospital that was in competition with the potential parish nurse sponsor hospital. Throughout the early work of the task force this physician was consistently raising questions that began to create tension in the group. Finally, the physician questioned the alignment with the partnering healthcare institution rather than the one in which he was employed. The work of the group could not continue until the task force resolved this issue. The PNC absented herself from the next meeting of the task force so that the agenda of the physician task force member could be discussed openly without the presence of the PNC.

4. Lack of understanding of the ministry of parish nursing practice can interfere with the development and integration of the ministry of parish nursing. For example, pastors may be afraid of liability issues, even when told the nurse is covered as an employee of the hospital. In other cases, pastors may not understand health or disease prevention. They have a basic knowledge of the scriptural commands regarding health, healing, and wholeness, but they have not had the opportunity to explore what this can mean for their ministries and the ministries in their congregation (Carson & Koenig, 2002). Taking time to bring key members of the congregation to a similar level of understanding regarding the ministry of parish nursing practice is important. The work of the task force cannot proceed beyond the person on the task force that has the least understanding of the ministry of parish nursing practice.

5. Competing interests may also create problems for the task force to move ahead with developing and integrating the ministry of parish nursing practice. A nurse member of the

task force may desire to become the parish nurse. If the group decides that the selection of the parish nurse should be done through advertising for the position to ensure that the best person for the position is chosen, the nurse task force member may have a conflict of interest. Unknowingly she or he may want to curb this decision due to the personal interest in the parish nurse position. Each member of the committee must have an opportunity to tell the group why he or she is part of the committee/task force/health cabinet so that all understand the purpose of participation for each member of the group.

6. Adding new members at different points can be very disruptive to the work group. When this occurs, time to restart the group and ensure that each member has a similar understanding of the work of the group, the ministry of parish nursing practice, and the function of the partnership with the healthcare organization must be a priority.

7. Lack of communication is always a problem for any work group. Time frames, clarity of the work, and level of commitment needed from the group members must be clearly communicated. In one congregation the pastor recruited the members of the task force. As the work proceeded the PNC could sense that the members of the group were becoming irritated. Finally at one of the meetings the PNC raised her concern regarding the temperament of the group. They were open with the PNC, explaining that the pastor had not communicated clearly to the members all that would be entailed in their participation on the task force. Even though the PNC had explained to the pastor the details of working together with the task force, those expectations were not communicated to the task force members.

Recommendations for Relationship Development

In a 1995 issue of *Preventive Care* an article "Eleven Tips for Partnering with Local Churches" identified the following suggestions for wellness professionals in working with congregations: 1) start with the basic question of how the church sees itself; 2) probe the mindset of the clergy; 3) look beyond traditional religious ties and seek different religious denominational partners; 4) contact your clergy friends; 5) meet church leaders in their environment; 6) contact the regional ecumenical pastors organization; 7) discuss access to healthcare and appropriate use of healthcare resources; 8) focus on the term *health*; 9) be clear about the resources that the healthcare organization can commit; 10) offer to begin the partnership slowly; and 11) dedicate a liaison to the congregation and ensure the congregation knows who that person is.

These friendly tips are easy to list but are often complex and time-consuming to actualize. It is important when engaging in working with congregations, that there is the realization that what is vital are the forming and sustaining of relationships. Problems will be much easier to weather with solid relationships at the foundation. Relational work is time-consuming and energy-absorbing, and it takes dedication. Members of the healthcare institution must understand their investment with the money they are dedicating to the ministry of parish nursing practice. The investment is in the successful integration of the ministry of parish nursing practice into both the strategic plan of the healthcare institution and the life of the congregation. This will result in a valuing at both the healthcare institution and the congregation of the developed network of relationships that creates an environment of health that otherwise would not be present throughout the community. However, if it does not understand this significant work, the healthcare institution may not meet the professed expectations of the relationship, thus destroying it and engendering distrust and disrespect. For this reason, institutions and congregations must develop and integrate the ministry of parish nursing practice diligently, faithfully, and deliberately. The well-being of many is at stake. The PNC is the connector. The successful negotiation of the relationships involved can often depend on the spiritual leadership of the PNC. The purposefulness of her or his leadership in representing each partner, in addition to acknowledging the grace of God, sustains the belief of the difference that can be made through the efforts of all involved

REFERENCES

Carson, V., & Koenig, H. (2002). *Parish nursing: stories of service and care*, Philadelphia, PA: Templeton Foundation Press.

Chase-Ziolek, M. (2005). *Health, healing, and wholeness: Engaging congregations in ministries of health*. Berea, Ohio: Pilgrim Press.

Djupe, A., Olson, H., Ryan, J., & Lantz, J. (1994). *Reaching out: parish nursing services*. National Parish Nurse Resource Center. Park Ridge, IL: Lutheran General HealthSystem.

Eleven tips for partnering with local churches. (1995). *Preventive Care*, (1)7: 26–28.

Fite, R.C. (1999). The congregation as a workplace. In P.A. Solari-Twadell & M.A. McDermott (Eds). *Parish nursing: promoting whole-person health within faith communities*. Thousand Oaks, CA: Sage.

Lloyd, R. & Ludwig-Beymer, P. (1999). Listening to faith communities: collaboration with those served. In P.A. Solari-Twadell & M.A. McDermott (Eds). *Parish nursing: promoting whole-person health within faith communities*, pp. 107–121. Thousand Oaks, CA: Sage.

McNamara, J.W. (2002). *The health cabinet*. St. Louis: International Parish Nurse Resource Center.

Pape, L. (2002). The role of the healthcare institution in pastor and parish nurse team building. In L. Vandecreek & S. Mooney (Eds). *Parish nurses, health care, chaplains and community clergy: navigating the maze of professional relationships*. New York: Hayworth.

Parish nursing's pioneer: a JCN interview. (1989, Winter). *Journal of Christian Nursing*.

Patterson, D. (2003). *The essential parish nurse: ABCs of congregational health ministry*. Cleveland: The Pilgrim Press.

Solari-Twadell, P.A. & McDermott, M.A. (Eds). (1999). *Parish nursing: promoting whole-person health within faith communities*. Thousand Oaks, CA: Sage.

Solari-Twadell, P.A. (2002). The differentiation of the ministry of parish nursing practice within congregations. *Dissertation Abstracts International*, 63(06). 569A. UMI No. 3056442.

Story, C. (2003). Barriers, difficulties, and challenges. In S. Smith (Ed). *Parish nursing: a handbook for the new millennium*. New York: Hayworth.

Westberg, G. (1990). *The parish nurse*. Minneapolis: Augsburg Press.

APPENDIX 21A

Properties of a Congregation and Healthcare Institution

Congregation

1. Congregations are voluntary organizations. Most services offered by a congregation are provided through people who volunteer.
2. Congregations usually have a change in the designated leadership (clergy) on a rotating basis every several years.
3. Congregations are not accustomed to administrative practices such as policies and procedures, regular personnel evaluations and contracts.
4. Congregations do not have external licensing bodies that periodically review their practices.
5. Congregations usually have relatively small organizational budgets that a few individuals oversee.
6. Congregations most often are part of a larger denominational body that professes the same beliefs.
7. Congregations are less comfortable with physical health and disease and more comfortable with health promotion and disease prevention.

Healthcare Institution

1. Healthcare institutions are operated through employees who are paid to work for providing specific services to others.
2. Healthcare institutions have a designated leadership that usually remains consistent over a number of years.
3. Healthcare institutions function on administrative practices that are well documented and implemented.
4. Healthcare institutions have different regulatory bodies and licensing organizations that systematically come to review the function of the operation.
5. Healthcare institutions usually have very large operating budgets that are managed by specific individuals within the organization and overseen by a board of directors.
6. Healthcare institutions may belong to a larger system, but some are entities that function without any larger organizational affiliation.
7. Healthcare institutions are more comfortable with physical health and disease and spend fewer resources on health promotion and disease prevention.

Four Models of Institutional Frameworks for the Ministry of Parish Nursing Practice

The institution can be defined as a hospital, healthcare system, home care agency, community coalition, public health department, hospice, long-term care facility, health maintenance organization, school of nursing, or community agency (Solari-Twadell & Mc Dermott, 1999, p. 5).

MODEL 1: DISTINGUISHING FEATURES OF A PAID INSTITUTIONAL ORGANIZATIONAL FRAMEWORK

1. Consultation and continuing education are available from the sponsoring institution for pastors and lay leaders on the development of a parish nurse program.
2. The parish nurse receives financial compensation for providing parish nursing services. This payment can be salaried, hourly or a stipend.
3. Selection of the parish nurse including advertising and interviewing is done in partnership with both the institution and congregation participating.
4. There is an installation (commissioning) of the parish nurse held at the congregation with involvement of representatives from the sponsoring organization emphasizing the integration of the parish nurse into the ministerial team of the congregation.
5. Access to basic preparation in parish nursing and an orientation to the sponsoring institution and the congregation (if necessary) are facilitated for the parish nurse.
6. The parish nurse receives ongoing continuing education through the congregation's relationship with the sponsoring institution.
7. The parish nurse networks with other parish nurses through the relationship with the sponsoring institutional organization.
8. The parish nurse receives assistance in identification of referral resources from the sponsoring institutional partner.
9. The parish nurse receives ongoing continuing education and spiritual development opportunities through the relationship with the sponsoring organization.
10. The parish nurse may receive benefits and reimbursement for travel through either the sponsoring organization or congregation.
11. The parish nurse uses a documentation system that results in regular reports for both the congregation and sponsoring institution.
12. The parish nurse and/or the congregation may receive liability insurance through the relationship with the sponsoring institution.
13. The position description for the parish nurse is endorsed by both the congregation and the sponsoring institution.
14. Suggested policies and procedures related to the ministry of parish nursing practice are available from the sponsoring institution.
15. Physician resources and consultation are available through the relationship with the sponsoring institution.
16. A process for evaluation of the parish nurse is suggested by the sponsoring institution.
17. External funding for the congregation, such as that from grants, is pursued in partnership with the sponsoring institution.
18. There is a written contract or covenant which stipulated the conditions of the partnership to support the ministry of parish nursing practice.

MODEL 2: DISTINGUISHING FEATURES OF AN UNPAID INSTITUTIONAL ORGANIZATIONAL FRAMEWORK

1. The parish nurse receives no financial compensation for providing parish nursing services, or the parish nurse may create an understanding with the congregation that the service provided to the congregation through the ministry of parish nursing practice as her or his personal stewardship offering to the congregation.

MODEL 2: DISTINGUISHING FEATURES OF AN UNPAID INSTITUTIONAL ORGANIZATIONAL FRAMEWORK—cont'd

2. The Parish Nurse Coordinator that represents the sponsoring organization is paid by the sponsoring institution for the work she or he is doing with congregations in developing the ministry of parish nursing practice.
3. Consultation and continuing education may be available from the sponsoring institution for pastors and lay leaders on the development of a parish nurse program.
4. Assistance in the selection of the parish nurse including advertising and interviewing may be provided by the sponsoring institution, with the final decision being made by the pastor and congregation.
5. There is an installation (commissioning) of the parish nurse held at the congregation with involvement of representatives from the sponsoring organization emphasizing the integration of the parish nurse into the ministerial team of the congregation.
6. Access to basic preparation in parish nursing and an orientation to the sponsoring institution and the congregation (if necessary) may be facilitated for the parish nurse.
7. The parish nurse receives ongoing continuing education through the congregation's relationship with the sponsoring institution.
8. The parish nurse networks with other parish nurses through the relationship with the sponsoring institutional organization.
9. The parish nurse receives assistance in identification of referral resources from the sponsoring institutional partner.
10. The parish nurse receives ongoing continuing education and spiritual development opportunities through the relationship with the sponsoring organization.
11. The parish nurse may use a documentation system that results in regular reports for both the congregation and sponsoring institution.
12. The parish nurse and/or the congregation in most arrangements needs to secure liability insurance independent of the sponsoring institution.
13. The position description for the parish nurse is endorsed by both the congregation and the sponsoring institution.
14. Suggested policies and procedures related to the ministry of parish nursing practice may be available from the sponsoring institution.
15. Physician resources and consultation may be available through the relationship with the sponsoring institution.
16. A process for evaluation of the parish nurse is suggested by the sponsoring institution.
17. External funding for the congregation, such as that from grants, may be pursued in partnership with the sponsoring institution.
18. There may be a written contract or covenant which stipulated the conditions of the partnership to support the ministry of parish nursing practice.

MODEL 3: DISTINGUISHING FEATURES OF A CONGREGATIONAL PAID ORGANIZATIONAL FRAMEWORK

1. There is no contract or covenant with any sponsoring institution.
2. The parish nurse receives financial compensation for providing parish nursing services. This payment can be salaried, hourly or a stipend.
3. There may or may not be a selection process for the parish nurse including advertising and interviewing. If there is a selection process, that is usually managed by an established task force of the congregation.
4. There may or may not be an installation (commissioning) of the parish nurse held at the congregation emphasizing the integration of the parish nurse into the ministerial team of the congregation.
5. Access to basic preparation in parish nursing and an orientation to the congregation will need to be negotiated by the parish nurse in accepting the parish nurse position.
6. The parish nurse seeks a network of other parish nurses in the geographic area.
7. The parish nurse identifies referral resources in the community.

Continued

Four Models of Institutional Frameworks for the Ministry of Parish Nursing Practice—cont'd

MODEL 3: DISTINGUISHING FEATURES OF A CONGREGATIONAL PAID ORGANIZATIONAL FRAMEWORK—cont'd

8. The parish nurse identifies opportunities for ongoing continuing education and spiritual development.
9. The parish nurse negotiates reimbursement for travel through the congregation.
10. Documentation processes are established by the parish nurse in conjunction with the pastor, health cabinet, or lay leadership of the congregation, taking into considerations the requirements of the nurse practice act of the state and the professional accountability of the parish nurse.
11. The parish nurse and congregation seek out and purchase liability insurance.
12. The position description for the parish nurse is developed and endorsed by both the pastor and congregation.
13. Policies and procedures related to the ministry of parish nursing practice are developed by the parish nurse and endorsed by the congregation.
14. Physician resources and consultation are sought by the parish nurse.
15. A process for evaluation of the parish nurse is determined by the pastor or lay leadership of the congregation in conjunction with the parish nurse.
16. The parish nurse may seek external grants to fund her or his work in the congregation.

MODEL 4: DISTINGUISHING FEATURES OF A CONGREGATIONAL UNPAID ORGANIZATIONAL FRAMEWORK

1. There is no contract or covenant with any sponsoring institution.
2. The parish nurse receives no financial compensation for providing parish nursing services.
3. There may or may not be a selection process for the parish nurse including advertising and interviewing. If there is a selection process, that is usually managed by the pastor.
4. There may or may not be an installation (commissioning) of the parish nurse held at the congregation emphasizing the integration of the parish nurse into the ministerial team of the congregation.
5. Access to basic preparation in parish nursing and an orientation to the congregation will need to be negotiated by the parish nurse in accepting the parish nurse position.
6. The parish nurse seeks a network of other parish nurses in the geographic area.
7. The parish nurse identifies referral resources in the community.
8. The parish nurse identifies opportunities for ongoing continuing education and spiritual development.
9. The parish nurse negotiates reimbursement for travel through the congregation.
10. Documentation processes are established by the parish nurse in conjunction with the pastor, health cabinet or lay leadership of the congregation, taking into considerations the requirements of the nurse practice act of the state and the professional accountability of the parish nurse.
11. The parish nurse and congregation seek out and purchase liability insurance.
12. The position description for the parish nurse is developed and endorsed by both the pastor and congregation.
13. Policies and procedures related to the ministry of parish nursing practice are developed by the parish nurse and endorsed by the congregation.
14. Physician resources and consultation are sought by the parish nurse.
15. A process for evaluation of the parish nurse is determined by the pastor or lay leadership of the congregation in conjunction with the parish nurse.
16. The parish nurse may seek external grants to fund her or his work in the congregation.
17. There may be a team of parish nurses that work together to fulfill the functions of the parish nurse with one nurse taking the lead in coordinating the ministry of parish nursing practice for the congregation.

APPENDIX 21C

Planning Tool for Use in Developing Parish Nurse Programs

Organizational Framework	Institutional Paid	Institutional Unpaid	Congregational Paid	Congregational Unpaid
Factors for consideration in planning				
Education and consultation development				
Parish nurse paid or unpaid				
Advertising, interviewing selection				
Basic preparation for the parish nurse				
Ongoing continuing education for the parish nurse				
Networking for the parish nurse				
Development of referral sources for the parish nurse				
Liability insurance for the congregation and parish nurse				
Nursing and pastoral				
Supervision for the parish nurse				
Evaluation of the parish nurse				
Benefits for the parish nurse				
Documentation system				
Position description				
Physician consultation				
Budget				
Policies and procedures				

APPENDIX 21D

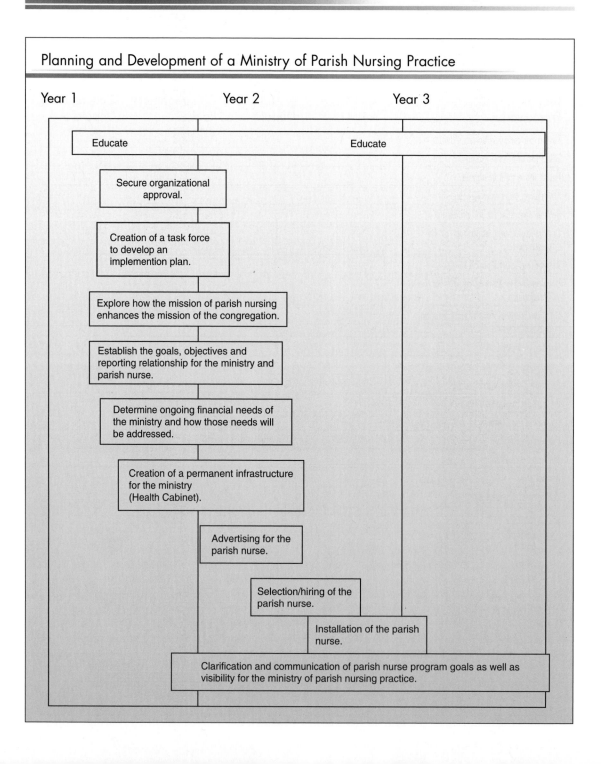

Planning and Development of a Ministry of Parish Nursing Practice

Year 1   Year 2   Year 3

Educate   Educate

Secure organizational approval.

Creation of a task force to develop an implemention plan.

Explore how the mission of parish nursing enhances the mission of the congregation.

Establish the goals, objectives and reporting relationship for the ministry and parish nurse.

Determine ongoing financial needs of the ministry and how those needs will be addressed.

Creation of a permanent infrastructure for the ministry (Health Cabinet).

Advertising for the parish nurse.

Selection/hiring of the parish nurse.

Installation of the parish nurse.

Clarification and communication of parish nurse program goals as well as visibility for the ministry of parish nursing practice.

APPENDIX 21E

Suggested Protocol for Working with Congregations to Develop a Ministry of Parish Nursing Practice

STEP 1: INVITATION TO DIALOGUE

This is the initial meeting with the pastor and others from the congregation invited to explore the development of a formalized health ministry in their congregation. It is best if this meeting is held at the congregation. Specific information regarding the ministry of parish nursing practice—including the requirements of the relationship such as the requirements for documentation and evaluation—is shared. Materials that enhance the understanding of the ministry of parish nursing practice include the following:

- Information about the healthcare institution, including the institution's mission and the mission of the parish nursing office of the healthcare institution
- A basic information packet that includes articles on the ministry of parish nursing practice. *The Parish Nurse* by Reverend Granger Westberg (1990) and *The Health Cabinet* by Jill Westberg McNamara (2002)
- Specific information regarding the infrastructure that supports the parish nursing office within the healthcare institution. For example, the manager for the ministry of parish nursing practice reports directly to the vice president of mission and advisory committee members are identified.
- Information on the institutional model and the advantages it provides to the congregation. Examples of the advantages are the following: (1) ongoing continuing education for the nurse; (2) opportunities for theological reflection for the parish nurse; (3) regular meetings with other clergy and congregations that have a ministry of parish nursing practice; (4) assistance in the formation of a task force or health cabinet in the congregation; (5) assistance in the selection of a parish nurse.
- Suggested timeline for the development of the ministry of parish nursing practice within a congregation.

By the end of this meeting there should be some clarity as to the interest in proceeding with the proposed work of initiating a ministry of parish nursing practice.

STEP 2: FORMATION OF A PARISH NURSE TASK FORCE/EXPLORATORY COMMITTEE

Purpose of the task force: investigate the extent of health ministry already present in the congregation and the feasibility of further developing this mission by creating a ministry of parish nursing practice.

Work of the task force: (a) identify all that are currently providing ministries of health to members of the congregation; (b) develop a mission statement for ministries of health within the congregation; (c) create overarching goals for the ministry of parish nursing practice in the congregation because the parish nurse must understand the congregation's priorities for ministry (Djupe et al, 1994); (d) list the qualifications for a parish nurse; (e) document the process for selecting and hiring of the parish nurse; (f) lay the foundation for a health cabinet.

Length of time for the task force to accomplish the work: 6 months to a year.

Agenda for the meetings between the task force and the parish nurse manager/coordinator and the task force.

Meeting 1 Agenda

Prayer
Introduction of members
Clarification of purpose (task force versus health cabinet)
Establish role of members (i.e., chair, record keeper)
Review purpose of group
Discussion for the purpose of clarifying the level of understanding of parish nursing
Create mutual definitions of *health, wellness, congregation,* and *nurse*
Identification of health ministry presently available in the congregation

Continued

Suggested Protocol for Working with Congregations to Develop a Ministry of Parish Nursing Practice—cont'd

STEP 2: FORMATION OF A PARISH NURSE TASK FORCE/EXPLORATORY COMMITTEE—cont'd

Preparation for next meeting—development of the mission
Statement for health ministry for the congregation
Confirmation of next meeting
Closing prayer
    Materials for the meeting: Mission statement of the congregation
       Listing of current ministries in the congregation
       Demographics of the congregation
       Results of any needs assessments that have been done in the congregation

Meeting 2 Agenda

Prayer
Discussion review of demographics of the congregation
Review of the mission statement of the congregation
Development of the mission statement for health ministry
    Identification of communication strategies to inform and/or solicit input from congregation on work of the task force
    Considerations regarding a parish nurse candidate (i.e., congregation member or not a congregation member, denomination of the candidate,
and advertising for candidates for the parish nurse position)
Preparation for the interview process—format, process, questions, timeline
Next meeting date
Closing prayer

Meeting 3 Agenda—Follows the interviewing of the candidates

Prayer
Candidate considerations
Review of interview with different candidates
Recommendation for parish nurse to pastor
Basic preparation of the parish nurse
Orientation for the parish nurse—parish, institution,
Installation of the parish nurse
Transition from a task force to a health cabinet
Ongoing relationship with the institution
Closing prayer

STEP 3: ESTABLISH AN ONGOING WORK PATTERN WITH THE PASTOR, HEALTH CABINET, AND PARISH NURSE

Frequency of meetings
Documentation/implementation
Installation of the parish nurse
Commissioning the members of the health cabinet
Orientation of the parish nurse
Establish an evaluation process—parish nurse, program, and partnership

Policies and Procedures for the Ministry of Parish Nursing Practice

22

Deborah Ziebarth

The parish nurse practice standards are stated in the document *Scope and Standards of Parish Nursing Practice* (ANA, 1998). This document represents the combined efforts of the American Nurses Association and the Health Ministries Association in describing the parish nurse practice standards that, for the most part, create the accountabilities for the unique ministry of parish nursing practice. The accountabilities of the ministry of parish nurse practice continue to be defined by state professional nursing regulations and by parish nurse community standards. State boards of nursing and the Public Heath Department promulgate state requirements for all registered nurses and healthcare institutions. Community standards refer to regional standards of practice established by the other parish nurse programs operating from within an area. With national, state, and community professional standards in place, the accountabilities become operational with essential support from policies and procedures. Policies and procedures provide the support, direction, or undergirding that clarify the accountabilities for the practice.

Policies and procedures support the ministry of parish nursing practice with specificity that describes the operation of the practice. Policies and procedures can conceptualize the parish nurse practice in a particular work environment, laying the foundation for a quality program, while reflecting the philosophy of the supporting organization. Policies and procedures that are very specific to environmental and organizational expectations help to further define the requirements of practice and allow the parish nurse to develop performance standards. Parish nurse policies and procedures describe the practice and state practice competencies and program outcomes to be satisfied. During the annual performance review, evaluation of practice competencies can be measured for the individual parish nurse. Ultimately, the parish nurse gains confidence and skills in performing practice competencies: moving from meeting standards to exceeding standards.

Program outcomes can be identified and assessed through directives provided by policies and procedures. The program outcomes serve as a basis for ongoing development of a visionary statement with mission-driven objectives for the parish nurse program. The supporting organization or congregation establishes program outcome expectations. These outcome expectations may be the collection of statistical information or be measured by other identifiable quality indicators. Refer to policy *Quality Improvement and Outcome Collection/ Projects* (see Appendix 22A and Chapter 20).

Policies and procedures become an essential part of the new parish nurse orientation and preceptorship. As the new parish nurse becomes familiar with the policies and procedures, the job expectations become clearer. Policies and procedures describe the congregant population that is receiving care; the complexity and range of their needs; how the needs are assessed; and how the interventions are planned and evaluated. This knowledge gives the parish nurse professional boundaries of the practice with clear role expectations and accountabilities.

The initial effort of policy and procedure development will help to do the following:

- Identify the ministry of parish nurse practice accountabilities.
- Standardize best practices.
- Establish performance and outcome accountabilities.
- Reduce the amount of time and effort spent on problem solving and decision making.
- Provide direction to those that succeed the current parish nurse or parish nurse coordinator/manager.
- Educate those not familiar with the ministry of the parish nurse practice.
- Be a reference point for future alterations or changes in the ministry of parish nursing practice.

Definitions

Understanding the definitions of policies, procedures, and guidelines is an important preliminary step.

Policy

A policy is a statement that sets forth an expectation and establishes a program's position on a particular issue. Policies are the guides to thinking and action; they spell out the required, prohibited, or suggested courses of intervention. A policy sets boundaries in which to act when performing activities and making decisions.

Six general areas in parish nursing will require policy formation. They are the following:

- Areas in which confusion about the nurse's responsibilities might result in neglect. These are necessary to a client's welfare. (*Blood Pressure Screening, Transportation, Abuse and Neglect, Medical Emergencies,* etc.)
- Areas pertaining to protection of the client rights. (*Client's Rights and Responsibilities, HIPAA, Referrals to, Referrals from, Documentation Records,* etc.)
- Areas defining relationships. (*Relationships Between Clergy, Parish Nurse, and Organization; Collegiality,* etc.)

- Areas involving personnel management. (*Annual Evaluation, Mileage, Family Leave, Supervision, Selection of the Parish Nurse, Termination,* etc.)
- Areas involving the work environment and safety. (*Visitation in a Home, Visitation at Various Healthcare Institutions, Personal Safety,* etc.)
- Areas pertaining to professional and administrative expectations. (*Competencies, Orientation Manual, Orientation and Preceptorship Program, Continuing Education, Quality Improvement and Outcomes, Documentation,* etc.)

The supporting organization or congregational site of a parish nurse program may have policies and procedures that are related to personnel management, work environment, and safety. The nurse should be familiar with all policies and procedures that may affect the ministry of parish nursing practice. Appendix 22A presents policy examples.

Procedure

A procedure defines a series of steps in an intervention. Procedures describe how a policy is to be executed. Procedures show the protocol to be taken to complete an intervention or task. These are mostly very specific to the department or program. Procedures establish a consistent method of accomplishing an intervention and help ensure that all staff use a standardized approach. Paige (2003) explains, "A procedure may have some variation in steps as long as the same outcome is obtained. The steps in the procedure should be written general enough to allow for this variation. The use of command words (for example, *must, shall*) should only be used when directing nondiscretionary interventions" (p. 47). Nondiscretionary interventions are those that are considered to be of highest importance. An example of a nondiscretionary intervention is that the parish nurse *must* have a current, registered nurse license to practice in a parish nurse role.

Because they provide direction, procedures become essential for providing nursing interventions and achieving program outcomes for parish nurses. To that extent, procedures should not detail nursing interventions that are not performed and should not establish unrealistic expectations of the parish nurse.

Guidelines

Some policies and procedures are really just process guidelines. Paige (2003) explains, "Guidelines become policies and procedures by default because it's easier for staff to keep track of all necessary information in one location—the policy manual" (p. 46). Guidelines can be operational related to aid in decision making or can provide the parish nurse evidenced-based research to support a policy. Administrative guidelines provide the nurse with instructions of how to fill out a form or how to sign out equipment. A guideline can be attached to a policy or can stand alone. It may be based on published standards.

The following are the three types of guidelines for parish nursing:

- Operational guidelines are suggested to aid in operational decision-making (e.g., how to set up a community-based blood pressure screening).
- Practice guidelines are clinical practice statements based on research to assist the parish nurse and client with decisions about appropriate healthcare decisions (e.g., blood pressure standards).
- Administrative guidelines help organization-supported programs that have several parish nurses operate more effectively (e.g., guidelines for signing out education equipment).

Policy and Procedure Format

A policy and a procedure often appear together on one document with the policy statement first and the procedure protocol following. Many formats exist for policy and procedure development, but the final product should include the following:
Policy statement with a clear definition and purpose (*what, when, who, why,* and *where* may be included)

- Procedure statement that offers protocol for the policy
- Responsibility for implementing the procedure
- Target audience to receive or to be impacted by the procedure
- Steps necessary to carry out the procedure
- Expected outcomes from the procedure
- Method of documenting and communicating the results of the procedure

- Supporting documentation and regulations can be included for reference to the user. Current references are suggested (e.g., books, journal or magazine articles, product literature, *Scope and Standards of Parish Nursing Practice,* symposium material, documentation tools, or guidelines).

Development and Revision

The policy and procedure manual is a collection of legally binding documents and must be kept current in its content. Additions and/or modifications become necessary for a variety of reasons. These may include the following:

- Renewal date expiration
- Changes in supporting organizational or congregation-site practices (e.g., mandatory CPR Instructor Training for all parish nurses)
- Changes in parish nurse role expectations (e.g., decreased hours for parish nurse practice *or* organizational program using parish nurses in discharge referral program)
- Implementation of a new program of service (e.g., congregation adds senior daycare program with new parish nurse expectations *or* organizational supported parish nurse program with a new targeted population, thus requiring documentation of new or additional stats)
- New health-related regulation (e.g., HIPAA or State Patient Privacy Regulations, changes in acceptable abbreviations)
- Application of research or best practice models, quality improvement (e.g., blood pressure standards)
- The addition of technology (e.g., moving from manual documentation to a computerized health information system)

Because any one of these conditions may affect the parish nurse role or scope of practice expectations from the supporting organization or congregation, regular changes to the policy and procedure manual become necessary.

Compliance

The extent to which a policy will be binding depends on the difficulty of its implementation. If a parish nurse policy fails to take into account the constraints within a congregational setting, one should not expect its implementation or use. Developing policies feasible in the actual setting will minimize deviation or exceptions.

The degree to which a parish nurse is led to believe that departmental policies constitute mandatory matters will also affect compliance. Setting the expectation that a policy must be followed and holding to that expectation is essential for the effective use of policies. If a policy appears "not to matter, one could question the need for its development" (Rowland & Rowland, 1997, p. 168).

Compliance with policies in a parish nurse program can vary greatly based on parish nurse program models. In an unpaid parish nurse program, policies may become burdensome to develop and even more difficult to follow. The parish nurse may work very limited hours, thus making development and compliance of policies and procedures low on the priority list and client care ranked high. In any congregation-supported parish nurse program, the congregational personnel committee and leadership may have limited knowledge of parish nurse practice standards that are considered an essential part of a quality parish nurse program. The congregation cannot be expected to enforce what they do not know. Having basic quality indicators for congregational paid or unpaid parish nurse program models are helpful for a congregational personnel committee or leadership in evaluating their parish nurse program. Included is a *Building Blocks for a Parish Nurse Program* tool (Table 22-1)

TABLE 22-1   Building Blocks for a Parish Nurse Program

The following should be present in any parish nurse program

	Yes	No	In Process	Other
1. The Parish Nurse (PN) has a current, valid license as a registered nurse in the state of practice.				
2. PN has completed a Basic PN Preparation Course.				
a. Course uses curriculum of International Parish Nurse Resource Center.				
b. Course not less than 35 contact hours.				
3. PN has copy of *Scope and Standards of Parish Nursing* (ANA).				
4. PN has copy of state's nurse practice act.				
5. Parish nurse is a member of pastoral staff.				
a. PN has a written job description.				
b. PN attends staff meetings.				
c. PN has the support of a dedicated committee.				
d. Committee reports/relates to governing body of the church.				
6. PN has an office space for confidential interactions.				
7. PN collects and records health data.				
a. Health data are recorded in a standardized, systematic, concise, retrievable form.				
b. Health data are kept locked and confidential.				
8. PN evaluates program yearly.				
9. PN/congregation engages in a yearly performance appraisal.				
10. PN maintains current knowledge in nursing practices.				
11. PN aware of legal/ethical activities of practice.				
12. Written polices and procedures are available to describe PN practice.				

Source: Wisconsin Parish Nurse Coordinator's Group, 2003.

that was created by the Wisconsin State Coordinator's Group. The checklist has proven a useful tool for congregational supported parish nurse programs (Wisconsin State Coordinator's Group, 2003).

Looking closely at our unique professional practice standards in the *Scope and Standards of Parish Nursing Practice,* one finds close proximity to the *American Nurses Association Standards of Clinical Nursing Practice.* Now compare these standards to your state's *Nursing Regulatory Standards*; again they are very similar. *Relevant Legal, Professional Standards and Guidelines for Parish Nursing in Wisconsin* takes a comparative look at essential standards for every parish nurse (Ziebarth, 2002).

Relevant Legal, Professional Standards and Guidelines for Parish Nursing in Wisconsin

Essential standards include: current nursing license, perform and document assessment, perform and document (nursing) diagnosis, perform and document planning, perform and document implementation/interventions, perform and document outcomes, perform and document evaluation, quality-of-care nursing practice, ethically based practice, research-based practice, research utilization, collaboration, collegiality, continuing education, and performance appraisal of the nurse. The parish nurse practice framework is solid. Policies and procedures operationalize these standards in a particular congregational site or parish nurse model (Table 22-2). Ask yourself the five "W's", (*what, where, who, when, why*), and ask "how" for each standard. These questions will define your job expectations and begin your parish nurse program policy and procedure development process.

In most organization-supported parish nurse programs some familiarity with policy and procedure standardized formatting exists. The employer considers development and compliance to organization and department policies and procedures a job expectation. The problem may arise when an organization-supported parish nurse program uses only organizational policies and procedures. Organizational (healthcare institutions) policies neglect the third party, the congregation. In organization-supported parish

nurse policy development, one must pay close attention to these three details:

1. The professional practice boundaries
2. The specific congregational site environment
3. The congregational site leadership.

Keeping these details in mind, policymakers can write realistic and appropriate policies.

Criteria for Evaluating Appropriateness of Policies

The general process of applying policy evaluation criteria as stated in the fourth edition of the *Nursing Administration Handbook* (Rowland & Rowland, 1997) to parish nursing policy development remains very similar. The criteria by which one can judge the effectiveness of policies relates to the degree to which they facilitate the achievement of the parish nurse program objectives.

Policies that do this will most likely contain these three characteristics:

- The purpose can be stated in the terms of outcomes to be achieved as a result of implementation.
- The expected outcomes can be shown to be instrumental in achieving the program's vision and objectives.
- The policy and procedure content is directly related to their stated purposes and reflects relevance to the parish nurse program.

Language and Flexibility

Liebler, Levine, Rothman (1992), note that policies permit and require interpretation. Use of language such as "whenever possible" or "as circumstances permit" give the needed flexibility. It is important in developing policies that they are somewhat futuristic. This is important in that they should be in force, with little change, for long periods of time. Broader language helps anticipate change.

Language that causes contradictions within and between policies and their related procedures should be avoided; such language could confuse any nurse. A procedure should have the same title when it is mentioned in other policies. A careful development compares the procedures to other documents, an essential step in decreasing confusion.

A few suggestions from the *American Hospital Association* (1962) to keep in mind when writing

---

TABLE 22-2   Relevant Legal, Professional Standards and Guidelines for Parish Nursing in Wisconsin*

Parish Nurse Activities	WI Board of Nursing Chapter 5	WI Board of Nursing Chapter 6	American Nurses Association Standards of Clinical Nursing Practice
Current License	X	X	X
Perform/Document Assessment		X	X
Perform/Document Diagnosis			
Perform/Document Planning		X	X
Perform/Document Implementation/Interventions		X	X
Perform/Document Outcome		X	X
Perform/Document Evaluation		X	X
Quality of Care of Nursing Practice			X
Ethically Based Practice			X
Research-Based Practice			X
Research Utilization			X
Collaboration			X
Collegiality			X
Continuing Education			X
XPerformance Appraisal of Nurse			X

*Note: This tool *does not* include all standards and guidelines for the registered nurse.
Please also refer to the following:
Wisconsin Nurses Association (WNA) Board Of Nursing, Chapter 7, for Rules of Conduct
American Nurses Association (ANA) Code of Ethics.
Source: D. Ziebarth, Manager of Community Benefit Outreach (Parish Nursing & Community Outreach Nursing), Waukesha Memorial Hospital, Waukesha, WI.

---

policies/procedures and organizing them into a manual follow.

- Use concise, simple language; keep it easy to understand and next to impossible to misunderstand.
- Remember that the policies are guides for making decisions about what to do, so keep them realistic and be sure they truly reflect the objectives of the department.
- Organize the manual as simply as possible so that it will be easy to use.
- Give thought to indexing, to dating entries, and to the need for keeping it updated. Provide for incorporating policy changes into the manual.
- Plan for periodic review of policies and set up a timetable for such review.

- In reviewing, evaluate effectiveness and workability; review experiences of staff in carrying out the policies; and verify that policies are being followed.
- Be objective about changes; do not let policies become sacred.
- When changes are made, provide for informing all personnel.

A Policy Team/Committee Approach

Although ensuring the accuracy and relevancy of the policy and procedure manual is ultimately the responsibility of the parish nurse and parish nurse administrator, the task can be shared with others. When an organization-supported parish nurse model employs multiple parish nurses, a policy team or policy committee can be a most effective use of skills and time.

In a Shared Governance Structure Model, parish nurses are decentralized into committees. This approach allows nurses to retain influence about decisions that affect their practice, work environment, professional development, and personal fulfillment. "It enhances the nurse's ability to take more responsibility and accountability for themselves and their peers" (Rowland & Rowland, 1997, p. 120).

Parish nurses are initially assigned to a committee that aligns with their skills and interest. One parish nurse shared governance structure model has four working committees: 1) Public Relations; 2) Practice and Standards; 3) Documentation and Education; and 4) Social Events. Refer to the policy titled *Shared Governance Committee Participation* on p. 275. In a congregation-supported parish nurse model, a committee that expands the parish nurse practice, along with congregational leadership, can be encouraged to participate in policy and procedure development.

Continuum Folder

Creating a continuum "folder of items to be considered for inclusion or documentation related to policy or procedures that might require modification" can facilitate the process of policy and procedure revision (Amann, 2001, p. 71). Anyone is encouraged to add to the folder at any time. Then, on a quarterly basis, the policy committee/team can review the contents. A more frequent review of the folder contents and of the policy and procedure manual ensures changes are made on a timely basis and significant modifications are not delayed.

"Policy team members should be assigned policies based on their skills, familiarity in a particular area, and specific interest. Capitalize on team member's writing ability and previous work on policy development" (Amann, 2001, p. 69).

The following steps may be taken to ensure that the parish nurse team/committee reaches its desired outcome:

- The development of format guidelines for policies and procedures. The guidelines should include how to write a policy statement, how to write a procedure, how to cite references, how to submit a format draft and finally, publication and distribution.
- Schedule and hold a meeting to review the "folder" contents.
- Develop a list of new policy and procedures to be added to the manual, and flag old items that require revisions.
- Assign the new policy and procedure on the list and flagged items for revisions to team/committee members and ask them to procure the documentation and reference materials necessary to develop the policy or/and procedure (e.g., documentation or reference materials may include policies from other parish nurse programs, related policies from the supportive organizational and congregational sites, and research resources from literature searches).
- Development of a timeline is important, as it will define the project in terms of resources and expectations.
- Following a format for either new policy/procedure development and revisions, request that the team/committee member develop the first draft. Come together as a team to consider the drafts and make content recommendations.
- The assigned team/committee member will make all necessary changes to the draft and will present the policy/procedure in a completed form, ready for publication.
- Each policy or procedure must be dated on any inclusion or revision and signed by the author and other appropriate leadership.
- The policy manual's table of contents will need to be updated, along with distribution, when new documents replace old.

In large, organization-based parish nurse programs with multiple community-based sites, each parish nurse will need to have a personal copy of the policy and procedure manual.

Distribution of Policies

The team/committee may want to include these two additional tools during the time of policy and procedure distribution:

- An instruction sheet for updating the orientation manual or the individual manual. This instruction sheet list items to delete, add, or replace.

- A signature sheet to collect the nurse's signature indicating that she or he has read the new policy and procedure and is accountable for the content. This facilitates tracking compliance and can be kept in the nurse's file and considered at annual evaluation time.

Joint Commission on Accreditation of Healthcare Organizations

The Joint Commission on Accreditation of Healthcare Organizations (JCAHO) establishes standards, evaluates care, and grants accreditation for healthcare institutions that meet standards. In an organization-supported (healthcare institution) parish nurse program, attention to JCAHO standards is important. Although JCAHO standards were not written with a parish nurse program in mind, they are adaptable. The effort to adapt JCAHO standards can raise practice standards. It will also help align the parish nurse program's practice objectives with other nursing departments within the institution.

Examples of Joint Commission standards that can guide policy and procedure development for an organizational supported (healthcare institution) parish nurse program are:

- NR .3   Nursing policies and procedures, nursing standards of patient care, and standards of nursing practice are the following:
- NR .3.2   Policies are defined in writing.
- NR .3.3   Policies are approved by the nurse executive or a designee(s).
- Leadership .2.3   Directors develop and implement policies and procedures that guide and support the provision of services.
- Leadership .2.8   Directors provide for orientation, in-service training, and continuing education of all persons in the department.
- Human Resources .1   The hospital's leaders define the qualifications and performance expectations for all staff positions.
- Human Resources .4   An orientation process provides initial job training and information and assesses the staff's ability to fulfill specified responsibilities.
- Human Resources .4.2   Ongoing in-service and other education and training maintain and improve staff competence.
- Human Resources .5   The hospital assesses each staff member's ability to meet the performance expectations stated in his or her job description.
(Joint Commission on Accreditation of Healthcare Organizations [JCAHO] 2000, p. 12.)

A Multidisciplinary Approach to Intradepartmental Policy and Procedure Development for an Organization-Supported Parish Nurse Department

Although parish nursing is a distinct community-based nursing department in which nurses perform all duties in the community, it can benefit from working with other organization-based departments in policy and procedure development. Various departments—nursing and non- nursing—perform similar tasks that require a department-specific policy related to the process. When one compares similar organizational policies that are varied in content, confusion and misinterpretation result. Through a multidisciplinary approach, intradepartmental policies can benefit an organization.

The Joint Commission on Accreditation of Healthcare Organizations (JCAHO) supports a multidisciplinary focus that specifically addresses policy and procedure development and has changed its criteria pertinent to the nursing process. "The objective of these changes is to stimulate a cross-functional approach to performance and performance improvement. The emphasis is on constructing a collaborative approach to delivering patient care services" (Rowland & Rowland, 1997, p 166). They have issued a standard to require all departments to devise policies in collaboration with associated departments. JCAHO does not base practice standards on distinct departments or disciplines. Instead, they emphasize "overriding professional boundaries and constructing a collaborative approach to delivering patient care. The intent is to standardize the practice for all staff and describe accepted methods for carrying out care activities. Collaboration with a multidisciplinary team for policy and procedure development, which may impact more than one department, decreases errors and creates opportunities to determine best practices" (*Solve the Policy and Procedure Puzzle*, 2003, p. 46). The combined effort to create policy and procedures through a multidisciplinary approach will also decrease effort and time.

Associated departments should be encouraged to participate in a policy team/committee to address inseparable boundaries. These departments could include representation from human resources, community education, pastoral care, visiting nurses, social work, care coordinators (or discharge planners), heart care center, and of course, parish and community nursing.

The team/committee's assignment is the following:

- Review the policy manual's table of contents for associated departments for same or similar topics.
- Combine policies and procedures into an intradisciplinary revised policy and procedure, whenever possible.
- Use broader language, if necessary, to be inclusive of community (e.g., use *site* as an alternative to *unit*. Use *site leadership* as an alternative to *unit management* or *pastor*.)

Organizational, Departmental, and Site (Congregational) Policies

Some organizational policies (e.g., termination of employment, annual performance, and family/medical leave) that are written with all employees in mind can be adapted to umbrella a parish nurse program when language that includes the third party, the congregation, is added.

Other organizational policies (e.g., domestic abuse, child abuse and neglect, elder abuse, confidentiality, infection control and collegiality) that are written with all employees in mind may already be general enough in language to include an employee at a community site. In that case, an additional departmental or site (congregational) policy is unnecessary.

The following four options can be adapted or incorporated into an organizational policy into parish nurse department policy development:

- With a multidisciplinary approach, an organizational policy can be adapted to include community-based employees, such as a parish nurse.
- A parish nurse department policy can reference an organizational policy.
- A site (congregational) policy can either reference an organizational policy or another site (congregational) policy.
- A site (congregational) policy can also adapt the core content from an organizational policy.

Appendix 22B presents several variations of an organizational policy related to termination of employment.

Policy and Procedure Manual

The policy and procedure manual is an important tool that needs to be kept visible to facilitate frequent use. It optimally serves as a reference for administrative, operational, and clinical questions. It can also explain the unique services of the ministry of parish nurse practice. Some parish nurse programs have opted to keep the policy and procedure contents in the orientation manual, along with documentation tools and guidelines. Others have found it most helpful to keep their policies and procedures separate and simply compiled in a three-ring binder. If more than one parish nurse is employed, more than one manual must be available. All parish nurses should have their own policy and procedure manual at the congregational site.

Policy and Procedure Manual Content

The content of the policy and procedure manual varies greatly between parish nurse programs, services, and networks. The variations of content are based on the specific setting and the model in which one practices. Including current documentation tools, reports, and other instruments mentioned as attachments or referenced on policies further ensures the policy's consistency and compliance. Because the manual is intended to be useful, it may also contain sections devoted to guidelines and the professional practice of parish nursing can also be added (e.g., the state's nurse practice act and the parish nurse scope of practice). In addition, developing a content outline often helps team members visualize the contents and easily locate desired documents.

BOX 22-1   Essential Policies for a Parish Nurse Program Model

Key points to consider are noted in parentheses.
- Abuse—Child, Adult, and Elder (know state regulations surrounding professional expectations, referrals, nearest shelter, etc.)
- Annual Parish Nurse Evaluation (RN license renewal, client evaluations, site leadership evaluation, professional and program goals, etc.)
- Blood Pressure Screening (use of nurses and nonnurses as screening volunteers, AHA guidelines, documentation, equipment standards, etc.)
- Confidentiality of Client Personal Health Information (defined, private health information shared, etc.)
- Death in the Home and other Medical Emergencies (CPR, 911, DNR bracelet, documentation, family notification, etc.)
- Documentation and Maintenance of Client Records (who is owner, transportation of records, storage, how long kept, how destroyed, how to receive client copies, etc.)
- Family/Medical Leave and Leave of Absence (establish guidelines, with whom and when contacts are made, etc.)
- Home and Hospital Visits (role expectation, how often, communication, etc.)
- Infection Control (hand washing, wound care, etc.)
- Personal Safety (sexual harassment, firearms, dogs, environment, etc.)
- Professional Development (CEUs, conferences, etc.)
- Referrals to Agencies (documentation, networking, follow-through, etc.)
- Relationship between the Congregation and the Parish Nurse (contract, professional liability insurance, role expectations, job description, office hours, meetings, etc.)
- Safety, Home Visits (home safety checklist, etc.)
- Termination of Employment (resignation vs. discharge)
- Transportation of Clients (role expectation, car insurance, documentation, etc.)
- Volunteers, use of (training, liability, management, etc.)

Table of Contents

The organization of a policy and procedure manual's table of contents may have policies simply listed, numbered, or alphabetized. The manual may be organized to begin with policies or highest-level documents and proceed to procedures, which serve to operationalize the policies. Policies can also be divided into categories.

Four examples of category content division of a parish nurse policy manual are the following:
- Nursing value, client relationship, professional relationship, and other values
- Administrative operations—external, administrative operations—internal, professional development, and community screening
- Administration of the parish nurse program, marketing, the parish nurse practice, parish nursing services, safety issues, and personnel issues
- Administration, committees, parish nurse ministry services, scope of practice, safety and infectious disease, and personnel

Appendix 22C presents several examples of a policy and procedure manual's table of contents. They represent a variety of parish nurse program models. Box 22-1 presents policies essential for any parish nurse program model. Box 22-2 lists

---

BOX 22-2   Additional Policies and Procedures that Hospital-Supported Parish Nurse Programs May Use

- Client Rights and Responsibilities
- Collegiality
- Competencies and Mandatory Education
- Community Educational Events
- Health Insurance Portability and Accountability Act (HIPAA)
- Orientation and Mentoring
- Orientation Manual, Use of
- Outcome Projects, QI
- Referrals from Hospital Staff
- Selection of a Parish Nurse
- Shared Governances Structure for Parish Nurse Department
- Supervision of Parish Nurse Job Performance

additional policies and procedures that hospital-supported parish nurse programs may use.

Conclusion

The development and regular review of policies and procedures for the ministry of parish nursing practice creates a road map for those that are new to the ministry and provides ongoing points of clarification for parish nurses. The development for policies and procedures can be time-consuming and educational for all parties involved in the process. Having the policies in place before any problems arise prevents rash decisions made with little prior thinking or review of necessary documents and individuals. The ministry of parish nursing practice is often called a pioneering effort. Pioneers often document where they err and what they learn so that those coming after them can avoid the same dilemmas. Creation of the necessary policies and procedures promotes development of relationships, clarification in thinking, and opportunities for problem identification and resolution before the problem occurs. Policy and procedure development is good stewardship of all God's gifts that have been given through the ministry of parish nursing practice.

REFERENCES

Amann, C. (2001). The policy and procedure manual: keeping it current. *Management File,* 49(2): 69-71.

American Hospital Association, Division of Nursing Services. (1962). Setting up a policy manual. *Practical approaches to nursing services.* 1(1).

American Nursing Association & Health Ministries Association (1998). *Scope and standards of parish nursing practice.* American Nursing Publishing Company. Washington, DC.

Joint Commission on Accreditation of Healthcare Organizations (JCAHO). (2000). *Comprehensive accreditation manual for hospitals: the official handbook.* Oakbrook Terrace, IL.

Liebler, J.G., Levine, R.E. & Rothman, J. (1992) *Management principles for health professionals,* (ed. 2). Gaithersburg, MD: Aspen.

Paige, B. (2003). Solve the policy and procedure puzzle. *Nursing Management,* 34(3): 46-47.

Rowland, H.S & Rowland, B.L. (1997). *Nursing Administration Handbook,* (ed 4). Gaithersburg MD: Aspen.

Waukesha Memorial Hospital. (2004). *Human resource policy: termination of employment.* Waukesha, WI: Author.

Waukesha Memorial Hospital. (2004). *Parish nurse policy: community benefit outreach.* Waukesha, WI: Author.

Waukesha Memorial Hospital. (2004). *Parish nurse policy: client rights and responsibilities.* Waukesha, WI: Author.

Waukesha Memorial Hospital. (2004). *Parish nurse policy: collegiality.* Waukesha, WI: Author.

Waukesha Memorial Hospital. (2004). *Parish nurse policy: competencies and mandatory education.* Waukesha, WI: Author.

Waukesha Memorial Hospital. (2004). *Parish nurse policy: community education events.* Waukesha, WI: Author.

Waukesha Memorial Hospital. (2004). *Parish nurse policy: HIPAA.* Waukesha, WI: Author.

Waukesha Memorial Hospital. (2004). *Parish nurse policy: orientation and preceptor program.* Waukesha, WI: Author.

Waukesha Memorial Hospital. (2004). *Parish nurse policy: referrals from hospital staff.* Waukesha, WI: Author.

Waukesha Memorial Hospital. (2004). *Parish nurse policy: selection of a parish nurse.* Waukesha, WI: Author.

Waukesha Memorial Hospital. (2004). *Parish nurse policy: shared governance structure in parish nursing.* Waukesha, WI: Author.

Waukesha Memorial Hospital. (2004). *Parish nurse policy: supervision of the parish nurse job performance.* Waukesha, WI: Author.

Waukesha Memorial Hospital. (2004). *Parish nurse policy: quality improvement and outcome collection & projects.* Waukesha, WI: Author.

Wisconsin State Coordinator's Group. (2003). *Building blocks for a parish nurse program.* Unpublished.

Ziebarth, D. (2002). *Relevant legal, professional standards and guidelines for parish nursing in Wisconsin.* Unpublished document.

Policy Examples

Title: Client's Rights and Responsibilities

PURPOSE:

To provide guidelines for informing clients of their rights and responsibilities within the parish nurse program.

POLICY:

The parish nurse is responsible for informing clients of their rights and responsibilities. The following rights and responsibilities are to be acknowledged in delivering parish nursing services.

PROCEDURE:

The parish nurse will review the department brochure, *Parish Nursing Programs* with new *Case-Managed Clients.*
Special attention will be noted of client rights.
Expect appropriate and respectful care that considers your values and beliefs.
Be treated with dignity.

Participate to the fullest extent possible in planning your care.
Be informed in terms you can understand.
Have an assessment of any pain you might experience.
Complete a living will or healthcare durable power of attorney document.
Expect your medical information to be kept confidential and private.
Know that there is a hospital policy and procedure for responding to client complaints.
Attention will also be noted of client responsibilities.
Cooperating in your own health care.
Providing accurate information.
Information about expressing concerns or complaints is also provided on the department brochure.

REFERENCE:

Parish Nursing Programs Brochure

Source: Waukesha Memorial Hospital, Community Benefit Outreach, Parish Nursing, Waukesha, Wisconsin.

Title: Collegiality

PURPOSE:

To guide the parish nurse in promoting the professional role of the parish nurse through appropriate informal and formal teaching and collaboration with colleagues.

POLICY:

The parish nurse contributes to the professional development of other healthcare professionals, colleagues, and students.

PROCEDURE:

All student mentorship programs will abide by the school agreement policy.
The parish nurse participates in developing and evaluating educational objectives for the healthcare professional or student.

The parish nurse creates an environment conducive to learning with educational objectives of the healthcare professional or student in mind.
The parish nurse promotes an informal mentoring relation with other departmental colleagues.
The parish nurse may provide appropriate speaker services—at the request of colleges, high schools, and community sites—on the role of the parish nurse.

REFERENCE:

Source: Waukesha Memorial Hospital, Community Benefit Outreach, Parish Nursing, Waukesha, Wisconsin.

Title: Competencies and Mandatory Education, Parish Nurse Department

PURPOSE:

To ensure that the nurses are knowledgeable of current general health information and possess the necessary skills to fulfill their roles, as described in the parish nurse job description.

POLICY:

All parish nurses will complete measurable departmental competencies and selected mandatory education requirements on an annual basis.

PROCEDURE:

Each nurse will be able to show proof (record of attendance) of completed competencies and attendance at mandatory educational events at the annual evaluation.

Competencies include CPR instructor training, community education, Windows 2000, home safety assessment, HIPAA, outcome

documentation, age-specific critical behavior, and integration of health and faith.

Mandatory education includes adult and child assessment, pain assessment, age specific, organ donation, blood pressure/heart health, and organization's all-staff education.

The Competency Verification Form of required departmental competencies and mandatory education will be kept in each nurse's educational file in the (organization's) parish nurse office.

The Competency Verification Form will be completed at the time of the nurse's annual evaluation and will be reviewed by the coordinator/manager at that time.

REFERENCE:

Source: Waukesha Memorial Hospital, Community Benefit Outreach, Parish Nursing, Waukesha, Wisconsin.

Title: Community Educational Events

PURPOSE:

To provide guidelines in planning and evaluating community-based educational events.

POLICY:

Parish nurses shall provide quality health educational programming for their congregational sites.

PROCEDURE:

The nurse will use the teaching plan*, which contains:
  Topic/subject
  Target audience (teen, seniors, women, etc.)
  Format/time span (lecture, interactive, presentation, etc.)
  Resources used
  Materials or equipment needed (overhead projector, posters, handouts, CD player, etc.)

  Objectives
  Evaluation
Use the Educational Program Evaluation Tool (orientation manual).
Submit a completed Activity Tracker Form (orientation manual) with an attached Teaching
Plan (orientation manual) with monthly reports to department coordinator/manager.

REFERENCE:

Source: Waukesha Memorial Hospital, Community Benefit Outreach, Parish Nursing, Waukesha, Wisconsin.
*Teaching plans will be shared with other parish nurses.

Title: Health Insurance Portability and Accountability Act (HIPAA) Standards for the Parish Nurse Department

The following policy may apply to an organizational healthcare institution–supported parish nurse program.

PURPOSE:

To instruct in the effective use of adapted federal HIPAA standards.

POLICY:

The parish nurse is a healthcare provider that is employed by a HIPAA-covered organization. This department has adapted federal HIPAA standards and has effectively incorporated these into practice.

PROCEDURE:

Nurses will perform within these HIPAA standards when performing their roles.

Notice of Privacy Practices (NPP)/Acknowledgment:

Available in English, Spanish, large print and audiotape.

When the nurse is making initial contact with the patient/client, the NPP should be given and the Acknowledgment form signed by the client.

The signature on the *Acknowledgment* form states that he or she has received the NPP.

The client may use the *NPP* Explanation form information in obtaining signature.

The patient should have the right to decline nursing interventions.

The interventions are to be documented on the appropriate documentation forms.

If you have made a good effort to deliver the NPP and obtain the client's signature and the client has chosen to receive the nursing interventions but not to sign the Acknowledgment form, the nurse may indicate on the Acknowledgment form that the client refused to sign and have two signatures as witnesses.

The NPP Acknowledgment form only needs to be signed once.

The signed Acknowledgment form will be kept with the client records for 6 years.

Community Cards:

Community clients may complete a *Community NPP Card.*

Their signature indicates that they have already signed an NPP Acknowledgment form and do not need to sign another NPP Acknowledgment form in the future at any entity.

Resources and Referrals Given to the Client:

Resources and referrals may be given to a client without an NPP/Acknowledgment form.

Client contact documentation on the Daily form, when a resource or referral solely is provided, should not include names.

Referrals from Pastor and Pastoral Associate:

The client is always encouraged to come to the nurse first.

When a referral comes from another source, encourage privacy of protected health information (PHI).

Marketing:

You may market a community service by condition.

Example: Send a flyer about flu shots to all patients with diabetes.

The patient has the immediate opportunity to opt-out through one of the following:

Throwing the flyer in the trash.

By not showing up for the community outreach service.

By completing the opt-out form or following the instructions that are in the flyer regarding opting out. This should be returned to the nurse to ensure that there are no future mail-outs to the individual.

Education:

You can host community educational events at community sites without an NPP/Acknowledgment, if the events have been publicized and if the information provided at the event is given directly to the individual.

Screening:

All blood pressure screening clients need to have an *NPP/Acknowledgment* form completed.

The signed Acknowledgment form must be kept for 6 years with client records.

Hospital and Other Visits:

If site leadership wants to have the nurse visit a client, then he/she needs to ask for the client's permission first; or

Title: Health Insurance Portability and Accountability Act (HIPAA) Standards for the Parish Nurse Department—cont'd

The nurse needs to call the client and ask if the client would like to have a visit; *or*

The nurse first stops at the entrance to the client's hospital room and asks if the client would like to have a visit from the parish nurse.

The nurse may then visit by first introducing self and describing role; *or*

The nurse sends out a notice to all community site population that members may receive a visit from the nurse if hospitalized. The notice should read, "If you do not want to receive this service, please contact the site office with the request not to be visited."

Confidentiality:

All community sites need to sign the Confidentiality Business Agreement.

The PHI of a client cannot be shared without the client's permission.

This permission is received when a client signs the Authorization to Release Medical Information form or verbally when the nurse asks the client (e.g., "May I share this information with the site leader?").

If permission is given, document the verbalized permission on the client's chart that only "need to know" information is to be shared.

If the client requests that their PHI is not to be shared, then the nurse cannot share any PHI.

It is important that the nurse documents that the client either gave permission or did not give permission to share PHI.

In rare occasions when the client cannot be asked (such as an emergency) or when the nurse determines that limited PHI needs to be shared with an agency, such as public health, a *Disclosure Log form* must be completed and e-mailed directly to the privacy officer.

Care Management* Clients/Documentation:

All Care Managed Clients will be asked to sign an Acknowledgment form upon receipt of the NPP.

A NPP Community Card will also be provided.

Retention and Transportation of Documentation:

All client hard copy documentation will be kept at the community site in locked files/cabinets unless the documents are in transport, in which case these documents will be in a closed file box or in a zippered case. The doors of the vehicle will be kept locked at all times.

If the nurse has terminated his or her position at the community site, all documents will be transported to the hospital and kept in the parish nurse office.

Client documentation will be kept at the community site for 7 years after which it is to be transported to the hospital and shred in the parish nurse office.

Computers:

PHI cannot be maintained on home computers or at the community sites.

PHI should be maintained on organization computer equipment that ensures secured information.

Volunteers:

For the volunteers to *not* be a part of our workforce, they need to be the community site's responsibility; the community site needs to distribute a job description under their authority.

Children in Community Sites:

When the school is located in a church or when the nurses are treating children in all other community sites, the parents will be contacted before treatment and asked if they want the nurse to perform any nursing interventions with the child.

This permission will need to be documented on the client's record and an *NPP Acknowledgment* form will be sent or hand delivered to the parent.

In the case of an emergency, age-appropriate care will be provided by the nurse.

REFERENCE:

Source: Waukesha Memorial Hospital, Community Benefit Outreach, Parish Nursing, Waukesha, Wisconsin.
*Care Management currently is defined as a process of care initiated when an individual or family experiences a precipitating event, which incorporates or begins with a major physical component. Care management leads the individual or group in the direction of health/wellness or quality of life as defined or experienced by the professional or client(s). To be counted as an individual or group that is "care-managed," one should anticipate a minimum of three follow-up contacts within 6 months.

Title: Orientation and Preceptor Program, Parish Nurse Department

PURPOSE:

To provide a procedure for the orientation and preceptorship of a new parish nurse.

POLICY:

All new nurses benefit from a quality orientation process. The parish nurse has a unique practice in that the environment is community-based. It requires the parish nurse to work in an independent practice model with professional boundaries practiced. Experienced (expert) parish nurses will precept inexperienced (amateur) parish nurses. Every parish nurse will foster an informal mentoring relationship with other parish nurse colleagues in the department.

A parish nurse preceptor needs to meet these qualifications:

Employed by the organization in the parish nurse role for no less than 3 years.
Completed the organization's preceptor training.
Completed the parish nurse preceptor competency verification form.
Met standards as specified in the parish nurse preceptor job description.

PROCEDURE:

It is assumed that the new parish nurse will have already attended a basic parish nurse preparation course or plan to attend one within the first 3 months of hire.

New parish nurse will do the following:

Attend the first 2 days of the organization's orientation.
Meet with parish nurse coordinator/manager (mailbox room key, laptop, computer access request, voicemail, pager, business cards, parish office door code).
Complete the Parish Nurse Organization and Community Resource Contact Checklist. (This checklist takes approximately 2 weeks to complete.)
Contact the assigned parish nurse preceptor and follow her at her site for 2 weeks. (During these two weeks complete the Parish Nurse Orientation Checklist.)
Read the parish nurse orientation manual.
Meet with the congregational health ministry committee accompanied with the parish nurse coordinator/manager. The parish nurse coordinator/manager will discuss committee expectations and parish nurse expectations at this meeting.
Contact two other parish nurses for site visits (1 week).
Document all hours in steps 1 through 6 as orientation times on timecard.
Site placement.
Preceptor program continues for 5 months. Contact assigned preceptor once a week for 8 weeks and then once a month for 3 months.
Schedule to meet with preceptor and parish nurse coordinator/manager for a 3-month evaluation.

REFERENCES:

Parish Nurse Preceptor Competency Verification Form
Parish Nurse Preceptor Job Description
Parish Nurse Organization and Community Contact Resources Checklist
Parish Nurse Orientation Checklist
The Parish Nurse Orientation Manual
The Role of the Health Ministry Committee

Source: Waukesha Memorial Hospital, Community Benefit Outreach, Parish Nursing, Waukesha, Wisconsin.

Title: Orientation Manual, Use of

PURPOSE:

To enable parish nurses to keep current information in their Orientation Manuals.

POLICY:

The orientation Manual provides needed resources for the Parish Nurse practice. It is the responsibility of each nurse to keep his or her orientation manual current.

PROCEDURE:

Every new parish nurse will receive a copy of the parish nurse department orientation manual on hire.

When new contents are added or when revisions occur, copies will be distributed to every nurse via mailboxes or at monthly meetings, with instructions to add to or change current forms in their manual.

The office and documentation committee and/or coordinator/manager will review and/or update the manual annually or as needed.

All changes must be reviewed and approved by coordinator/manager and committee.

REFERENCE:

Parish Nurse Department Orientation Table of Contents and Manual

_____

Source: Waukesha Memorial Hospital, Community Benefit Outreach, Parish Nursing, Waukesha, Wisconsin.

Title: Referrals from Organization's Staff

PURPOSE:

To provide guidelines for referring patients to the parish nurse program.

POLICY:

Referrals from organization's staff will be routed to the parish nurse office to ensure continuity of care in the delivery of service to patients. Parish nurses are available to provide supplemental education, emotional support, advocacy or spiritual care for the organization's patients after hospitalization when such care is not available through existing community support systems.

PROCEDURE:

Staff will determine the appropriateness of completing a referral for parish nurse services during the inpatient stay in the following circumstances:

When patient already has a relationship/connection with a current parish nurse site (refer to parish nurse directory page for assistance).

The client needs spiritual or emotional support and has no current resources.

The client's caregiver needs spiritual or emotional support.

The client needs reinforcement of health teaching.

Patients should not be considered for referral if their needs include any of the following:

The client needs homecare services, including procedures, medication administration, and/or supervision.

The client needs transportation services.

The client or family needs household support (meals, yard work, etc.).

The client needs immediate home healthcare support.

Title: Referrals from Organization's Staff—cont'd

Staff will complete the Parish Nurse Referral for Services Form and route it to the parish nurse department.

Staff will contact the coordinator/manager by phone to convey information and set up a contact with the parish nurse.

The coordinator/manager of parish nursing will confirm the referral and assign the case to the appropriate parish nurse.

The nurse will contact the patient and/or family in a timely manner to assess and provide care as appropriate.

The nurse will document care as appropriate and will also provide feedback to the coordinator/manager regarding the care required and delivered.

REFERENCES:

Parish Nurse Directory
Parish Nurse Referral for Services Form
Guidelines for Referral to Parish Nurses Guidelines

Source: Waukesha Memorial Hospital, Community Benefit Outreach, Parish Nursing, Waukesha, Wisconsin.

Title: Selection of the Parish Nurse

PURPOSE:

The purpose of this policy is to establish a protocol for the selection of the parish nurse.

POLICY:

The parish nurse who serves a designated congregation will be selected through a process that includes both the healthcare institution and the congregation to be served.

PROCEDURE:

The positions are advertised by the organizations, through traditional methods, and in the congregation.

The prospective candidates will complete an online application and submit resumés with required spiritual assessment.

The first preliminary interview is completed by human resources.

The second interview is completed by the parish nurse coordinator/manager and/or designated parish nurses.

The third interview is completed by the congregation.

The organization may have representation at the community site interview.

The final decision as to the parish nurse selection is made by all the individual interviewers.

REFERENCES:

Parish Nurse Interview Guide
Organization's Hiring Policy

Source: Waukesha Memorial Hospital, Community Benefit Outreach, Parish Nursing, Waukesha, Wisconsin.

Title: Shared Governance Committee Participation

PURPOSE:

To establish guidelines for participation in the department's shared governance structure, which empowers nurses to contribute to decisions that directly affect community-based practice and standards of client care.

POLICY:

Each nurse participates in one of four shared governance committees. They are the following:
- Documentation and Office Management Committee
- Public Relations/Networking Committee
- Social Events Committee
- Standards Committee

PROCEDURE:

During orientation, nurses will be assigned a shared governance committee based on skills, familiarity in a particular area, and specific interest.

Committees will meet in whole or in part on a monthly basis, as appropriate to complete an assignment. Meeting time will be provided during the regular monthly staff meetings, whenever possible.

Individual duties of committee members will be decided by the committee and will be based on skills, familiarity in a particular area, and specific interest.

It is desired that all committee members will participate equally and will network with the manager and other peers.

If a member cannot attend the committee meeting, he or she will be expected to contact another member of the committee and have ready any work assignment due to share in his or her absence.

Decision making that affects the whole department will be presented to the staff during the committee report time to assess feedback, whenever possible.

Rotation or reassignment of a committee member to another committee will be decided between that individual member and the manager.

Committee assignments include but are not limited to the following:

Documentation and Office Management Committee:
- Creates and revises documentation tools.
- Assists with statistical collection.
- Assists with selection and scheduling continuing education and resource speakers. Responsibilities will include scheduling room and caterer for educational events held outside regular monthly staff meetings and follow-up with speakers.
- Assists with ordering and management of department educational resources.
- Assists with ordering and management of department office supplies and equipment.
- Manages department orientation manual.
- Assists with the department orientation and preceptorship of new hires.
- Schedules monthly meeting chairs/minutes.
- Updates bulletin boards in office.

Public Relations/Networking Committee:
- Christmas letter development and distribution.
- Hospital directory updates.
- Parish nurse brochure development and distribution.
- Program awareness.
- Client surveys.
- Service Projects (e.g., CCWC clothes drive, Easter baskets distribution, etc.).

Social Events Committee:
- Pastor/parish nurse meetings.
- Annual day retreat.
- Annual Christmas party.
- Annual cafeteria Christmas event.
- Schedules rooms and coffee for monthly staff meetings.
- Assists with staff cards/gifts.
- Bowling bash participation promotion and sign-up.
- Assists with parish nurse symposium and Wisconsin Nurse Association Parish Nurse preconference registration, reservation, and transportation planning.

Standards Committee:
- Assists with policy/procedure development and revisions.
- Assists with annual scope of practice tool completion and 6-month evaluation.
- Interview participation.
- Assists with job description revisions.
- Assists with evaluation tools and interview guide tool development and revision.
- Assists with the development and maintenance of competencies and mandatory education (e.g., assists with scheduling competency and mandatory education and the development and maintenance of take-home education kits).

REFERENCE:

Source: Waukesha Memorial Hospital, Community Benefit Outreach, Parish Nursing, Waukesha, Wisconsin.

Title: Supervision of Parish Nurse Job Performance Problems

PURPOSE:

To provide a protocol for the parish nurse coordinator/manager when a parish nurse has job performance issues.

POLICY:

Parish nurses that are demonstrating performance problems will be monitored on a regular basis by parish nurse coordinator/manager according to the mutual development of performance behaviors and goals.

PROCEDURE:

Parish nurses demonstrating performance problems will meet with the parish nurse coordinator/manager to discuss the specific parish nurse performance issue.

The parish nurse coordinator/manager will put in writing the content of the coaching session.

The parish nurse coordinator/manager and parish nurse will develop a plan. This plan will include specific recommendations for improvement and time parameters for evaluating the parish nurse performance.

The parish nurse coordinator/manager will then contact the pastor of the congregation served to discuss the identified performance problems and the plan, which has been developed to address the performance problem. Time parameters will also be established.

Improvement over performance problems will be noted on the parish nurse annual performance evaluation.

If the performance problem persists, the disciplinary policy and performance improvement action process will need to be reviewed with the pastor of the congregation and the parish nurse. The performance improvement policy will be adhered to in continuing to address the performance problems.

REFERENCE:

Organization's Performance Improvement Policy

Source: Waukesha Memorial Hospital, Community Benefit Outreach, Parish Nursing, Waukesha, Wisconsin.

Title: Quality Improvement and Outcome Projects

PURPOSE:

To provide protocol for the nurse regarding the participation in organizational and departmental quality improvement (QI) and outcome projects.

POLICY:

Parish nurses, in most cases, have a longitudinal relationship with clients.

All parish and community health outreach nurses participate in departmental QI and outcome collection/projects. Evaluating current practices, collecting outcome data, and applying research-based best practices are ongoing and essential.

QI projects are designed to improve services. Applying research-based information or best practice models may be one way to achieve improvement in the parish nurse service.

Outcome collection/projects are designed to show program and clinical value. They may include collection of specific data and/or participation in disease-specific client care.

PROCEDURE:

Outcome data collection includes the following:

Specific monthly statistical data of targeted populations, referrals, educational events, and care-managed clients (ongoing).

Client surveys (ongoing).

Quality indicators such as the following:
   Enhanced independent living.
   Medical devices obtained/medication assistance obtained.
   Injury prevention.
   Hospital admission or emergency room visit avoidance.
   Enhanced quality of life.

Outcome projects may require specific data collection. This data may be clinical (e.g., such as test results) or demographical. All personal health information is protected.

Participation in disease-specific client care.

Collaborative community screenings or testing.

Collaborative community educational or promotional events.

One-on-one health counseling.

REFERENCES:

Daily, Monthly, and Activity Tracker Documentation Forms
Client Survey Form
Client Outcome Guidelines (Quality Indicators)
Outcome Projects

Source: Waukesha Memorial Hospital, Community Benefit Outreach, Parish Nursing, Waukesha, Wisconsin.

APPENDIX 22B

Examples of Organizational Policies on Termination

Title: Termination of Employment (Organizational Policy)

POLICY/PURPOSE STATEMENT:

To provide guidelines to facilitate termination of employment.

PROCEDURE:

Communication of accurate information relating to the resignation or termination of employment shall be submitted to the human resources department in a timely manner to provide appropriate terminal benefits, update of employee records, and deletion of access codes to the various information systems.

Return of keys, ID badges, and other company property is the responsibility of the respective department manager.

RESIGNATION:

When an employee chooses to resign, the department manager should advise the employee of the appropriate minimum notice required and ask the employee to submit the resignation in writing specifying the last day of work and the reason for leaving.

Appropriate notice for an hourly employee is 2 weeks before separation.

Appropriate notice for an exempt employee is 4 weeks before separation.

The department manager will submit the letter of resignation and completed employee termination paperwork to the respective human resources department to process records and benefits in a timely basis.

If the resignation is for retirement, the employee should be referred as early as possible to the human resources department for pension and other related counseling.

DISCHARGE:

A department manager may discharge an employee without notice anytime during the introductory period.

A department manager may discharge an employee without notice for misconduct as outlined in the performance action policy.

The department manager will submit the employee's completed paperwork and any related documentation to human resources in order to process records and benefits on a timely basis.

Source: Waukesha Memorial Hospital, Waukesha, Wisconsin.

Title: Termination of Employment (Organizational Policy, Adapted for Parish Nursing Program)

The following is the same organizational policy adapted through a multidisciplinary approach to include a parish nursing program.

POLICY/PURPOSE STATEMENT:

To provide guidelines to facilitate termination of employment.

PROCEDURE:

Communication of accurate information relating to the resignation or termination of employment shall be submitted to the human resources department in a timely manner to provide appropriate terminal benefits, update of employee records, and deletion of access codes to the various information systems.

Return of keys, ID badges, and other company or community site property is the responsibility of the employee and the respective department coordinator/manager.

RESIGNATION:

When an employee chooses to resign, the department coordinator/manager should advise the employee of the appropriate minimum notice required and ask the employee to submit the resignation in writing specifying the last day of work and the reason for leaving.

Appropriate notice for an hourly employee is 2 weeks before separation.

Appropriate notice for an exempt or community-based employee is 4 weeks before separation.

The department coordinator/manager will submit the letter of resignation and completed employee termination paperwork to the respective human resources department to process records and benefits in a timely basis. If the employee is community-based, the department coordinator/manager will notify the community site leadership and will address the replacement process.

If the resignation is retirement, the employee should be referred as early as possible to the human resources department for pension and other related counseling.

DISCHARGE:

A department coordinator/manager may discharge an employee anytime without notice during the introductory period. If the employee is community-based, the department coordinator/manager will notify the community site leadership and address the replacement process.

A department coordinator/manager may discharge an employee without notice for misconduct as outlined in the performance action policy. If the employee is community-based, the department coordinator/manager will notify the community site leadership and address the replacement process.

The department coordinator/manager will submit the employee's completed paperwork and any related documentation to Human Resources in order to process records and benefits on a timely basis.

Title: Termination of the Parish Nurse (Department Policy)

Here is an example of termination of the parish nurse department policy, using the same organizational policy as a reference.

POLICY/PURPOSE STATEMENT:

The purpose is to provide guidelines to facilitate termination of the parish nurse.

PROCEDURE:

The Parish Nurse Department will refer to the organizational policy and termination of employment, and will adhere to the following procedure.

Appropriate notice for a parish nurse is 4 weeks.
The parish nurse will inform the parish nurse coordinator in writing with the following information: name of congregation, last day that the parish nurse will work, reason for resignation, and when or if the congregational leadership was informed of the resignation.
The parish nurse coordinator will notify the congregational leadership and address the replacement process.
The parish nurse coordinator will arrange for an exit interview with the department coordinator/manager and congregational leadership, as appropriate.

Title: Termination of the Parish Nurse (Site Policy)

This policy example is adapted even further to address parish nurse termination in a congregational-supported parish nurse program through the development of a site (congregational) policy.

POLICY/PURPOSE STATEMENT:

The purpose is to provide guidelines to facilitate resignation or discharge of the parish nurse.

PROCEDURE:

The congregation personnel committee will refer to the policy, termination of employment, and will adhere to the following procedure.

RESIGNATION:

Appropriate notice for a parish nurse is 4 weeks.

The parish nurse will inform the congregation personnel committee in writing with the following information: last day that the parish nurse will work and reason for resignation.
The congregational personnel committee will notify the congregational leadership and address replacement.
The congregation personnel committee will arrange for an exit interview, as appropriate.

DISCHARGE:

The congregational personnel committee may discharge a parish nurse anytime without notice during the 3-month introductory period and for misconduct that would potentially cause harm to an individual within the congregation.

APPENDIX 22C

Examples of Table of Contents

Client's Rights and Responsibilities
Communicable Disease Reporting
Continuing Education Requirements
Death in the Home
Documentation
Emergency, Medical
Environment, Unsafe
Fire Safety—Office, Church, and Home
Fiscal responsibility
Health Committee
Incident Reporting
Insurance
Mentoring
Orientation
Parish Nurse Roles
Policy/ Procedure Development
Referrals by PN to Other Providers
Safety—Home
Transportation of Clients
Universal precautions

Example: *A Hospital with Unpaid Parish Nurses (Paid Coordinator)* model
Nursing (NR) = Development and Education Of Parish Nurse Coordinator
Duties of the Parish Nurse
Health Ministry Staffing Protocol
Patient's Rights (RI) = Parish Nurse Coordinator Consultation
Maintenance of Client Record
Family Presence During Resuscitation
Performance Improvement (PI) = Management of the Parish Nurse Program
Meetings of Professional Development for the Parish Nurse
Assessment of Patient (PE) = Assessment of Client, Blood Pressure Screening Protocol, Documentation, Health Education, Health Counseling, Integration of Health and Faith Protocol
Education (PF) = Health Educator
Continuum of Care (CC) = Bereavement Follow-up, Coordinator of Volunteers, Resolve Through Sharing
Infection Control (IC) = Infection Control Protocol for Parish Nurses
Procedures (PRO) = Development of a Parish Nurse Program within the Congregation

Example: *A Church Paid Parish Nurse* model (One Parish Nurse)
Administration:
Fiscal
Parishioner Rights and Responsibilities
Reporting of Abuse, Neglect, Exploitation
Confidentiality of Parishioner Information and Records
Unusual Occurrence/Incident Reporting
Committees:
Health Ministry Committee
Personnel Committee
Parish Nurse Ministry Services:
Definition of a Parishioner
Criteria for Providing Services
Parish Nurse Ministry Services
Referrals
Medical Emergency
Death in the Home
Documentation
Clinical Records
Scope of Practice:
Parish Nursing Practice
Safety and Infectious Disease:
Safety Plan
Infection and/or Communicable Disease
Personnel:
Appointment to Position
Liability
Health Standards
Orientation to Position
In-Service Requirements
Work Schedule/Equipment
Personnel Records
Compensation/Employee Benefits

Example: *A Church with Unpaid Parish Nurse* model
Liability
Work Schedule
Documentation
The Parish Nurse Practice
Referrals
Medical Emergencies
Health Committee

Building a Parish Nurse Network: A Case Study

23

Annette D. Stixrud

In her 2000 Westberg Symposium keynote address, "Parish Nursing at a Kairos Moment," Judith Ryan worked with the participants to craft a statement defining where we were at that moment in time. Under "purpose" were three challenges:

- To challenge the nursing profession to reclaim the spiritual dimension of nursing care
- To challenge the healthcare system to provide whole person care
- To challenge the faith community to restore its healing mission

Parish nurse networks weave elements from the nursing profession, the healthcare system, and the faith community to provide an infrastructure that supports the mission of parish nursing and makes the strategic vision, access to a parish nurse ministry in every faith community, possible (Ryan, 2000).

A Compelling Case for Networking

We generally use the term *network* to mean an interconnected group or system. In parish nursing it is about connecting the three institutional cultures—the nursing profession, faith communities, and healthcare—to achieve the best whole-person health possible for every individual. Realizing the strategic vision is difficult when these cultures do not interact in a way that fosters a network of understanding, resources, and support. The task of a networker is to build bridges so that a larger vision emerges; leaders in faith communities, nursing, and healthcare find they need each other.

Effective coordination of agencies and resources produce better results than individual efforts. Jimmy Carter (1996) gives a wonderful illustration of the effects of successful coordination when writing about the Task Force for Child Survival:

> A few years ago, leaders of the World Health Organization, UNICEF, the World Bank, the UN Development Program, and the Rockefeller Foundation were all striving in their own ways to immunize children throughout the world. However, they were never able to reach more than 20 percent of the total, primarily because they were not cooperating with one another. The Task Force for Child Survival was created and located at the Carter Center so that all five organizations could work as a team. Within only 5 years, with no appreciable increase in funding or personnel, 80 percent of the world's children were immunized against polio, measles, and other contagious diseases. (p. 173)

Of course, measurement of a single outcome like childhood immunization rates is a much easier task than quantifying illness prevention and health promotion outcomes through interventions such as prayer, visitation, education, advocacy, referrals, and screenings; however, the theory still applies. We can get more done with fewer resources by sharing, organizing, and pooling our best practices. Our efforts multiply quickly when we teach and encourage our faith communities to have both a spiritual and communal approach to societal problems.

An Experience of Building a Regional Parish Nurse Network: Initial Steps

In 1989, a group of people in Portland, Oregon, met to discuss how to begin parish nursing in the Northwest. They invited Granger Westberg, founder of parish nursing; Ann Solari-Twadell, director of the International Parish Nurse Resource Center at Lutheran General Hospital, Park Ridge, Illinois; and the Reverend James Wylie, senior vice president of Lutheran General Health System, to come to Portland as keynote speakers for a conference on this topic. This initial conference attracted about 80 people, and a task force to continue efforts in creating a parish nurse ministry was formed.

The groundwork for a feasibility study was laid by Chaplain William Adix, who at the time was director of the Pastoral Care Department at Emanuel Hospital and Health Clinic; Marianne Gallagher, oncology nurse at Emanuel and Diaconal Minister in the United Methodist Church; Judith Andersen, nursing instructor at Clackamas Community College; Jane Hagan, at the time a graduate student at Oregon Health Sciences University (OHSU) who worked with the Oregon Geriatric Education Center; Reverend Martin Dasler, pastor of Resurrection Lutheran Church; and Reverend Darrel Lundby, assistant to the bishop of the Evangelical Lutheran Church in America (ELCA), Oregon Synod. This group of people became the original board of directors for Northwest Parish Nurse Ministries (NPNM).

In January of 1991, Barbara Connors was hired by the board to do a feasibility study among churches in the area to identify interest in parish nursing. Connors had graduated from the nursing program at Emanuel Hospital in Portland and returned to our community after serving as a parish nurse in Boston. After 10 months of speaking to pastors, congregations, and women's groups, she had a list of over 100 churches interested in beginning a parish nurse ministry.

As a result of the feasibility study, the NPNM Board saw as its greatest need an effort to educate nurses about the concept of parish nursing. To accomplish this, Connors—along with Judith Andersen and in consultation with the International Parish Nurse Resource Center—worked with Ann Widmer (a NPNM Board member), director of Health Care Administration at Concordia College, Portland, Oregon to plan the first parish nurse class in the Northwest. The curriculum was developed with the help of directors of other parish nurse education programs offered throughout the United States.

The second annual NPNM conference was held in October, 1991. Its purpose was to further educate pastors and nurses about parish nursing and the upcoming class planned for January, 1992. Judith Ryan, Ann Solari-Twadell, and Dorothy Klinegartner, a parish nurse from California, were the keynote speakers. In November, 1991, before the first class, Barbara Connors had decided to pursue other avenues of ministry, and the board invited this author to coordinate NPNM on a part-time basis.

The first parish nurse class in the Northwest was offered through Concordia College one weekend a month for 3 months beginning in January, 1992. Thirty nurses from a 350-mile radius attended this class.

The response to the first class was overwhelmingly positive. However, the need for continued support and ongoing education of these new parish nurses became evident early on. The class only scratched the surface of parish nursing. In addition, their pastors and congregations had many preconceived ideas about what these nurses would/could/should do. Monthly networking and ongoing education groups for pastors and parish nurses were started in the Portland area. A newsletter was created to keep the parish nurses, congregations, schools of nursing, and hospitals informed about NPNM activities. Education for faith communities and healthcare systems about the roles and functions of the parish nurse was—and continues to be—a priority. The NPNM board saw its focus as the education and support of parish nurses by providing the basic parish nurse class and ongoing services of support for the participants.

The Institutional Cultures that Constitute the NPNM Networking Infrastructure

The Nursing Profession and Nursing Education

The American Nurses Association has recognized parish nursing as a specialty in nursing practice since 1997. The *Scope and Standards of Parish Nursing Practice* (1998) is available through the Health Ministries Association or the American Nurses Association. The real genius of parish nursing is that it takes professionally qualified nurses who believe that we care for others as well as ourselves as an expression of God's love and prepares them to work in faith communities that, for the most part, already know and trust them.

Education of parish nurses and parish nurse coordinators (PNCs) through schools of nursing can impact nursing education at its core. To offer the basic parish nurse curriculum, nursing faculty are often involved either as prepared facilitators trained through the IPNRC to teach the curriculum or as experts who work with faculty members to bring their expertise to teach one of the modules in the curriculum.

Reclaiming the spiritual dimension of nursing care is taught through the curriculum but manifests itself in the working world through individual parish nurses and their effect on the nurses with whom they work. Since the first parish nurse class in the Northwest was offered through Concordia University in 1992, NPNM has worked with over 20 schools of nursing in the Northwest to offer the parish nurse class. Most of these schools of nursing continue to work with NPNM and their local healthcare systems to offer the class on an annual basis.

In 1993, after offering the class only in the Portland area, the NPNM Board heard that Chaplains Art Schmidt (a NPNM Board member) and Kathryn Olson at St. Joseph Medical Center, as well as several churches in Tacoma, Washington, were interested in starting parish nursing. Judith Andersen and I approached Cynthia Mahoney, associate professor and director of Continuing Nursing Education, and Carolyn Schultz, professor at Pacific Lutheran University (PLU) School of Nursing. They quickly embraced the idea of working with us to bring a class to their area. Shortly after the PLU meeting, I was invited to speak about parish nursing at a gathering of pastors at St. Leo's Catholic Church in Tacoma to encourage them to help recruit some nurses for the class set for January, 1994.

For me, going to Tacoma and working with PLU, St. Joseph Medical Center, and St. Leo's has remained one of the most enlightening and significant moments in my work in the development of a regional network. Two specific insights regarding network building came together for me in a powerful way. The first was that offering a class in a community meant bringing people together from that community—healthcare, faith communities, and the school(s) of nursing—to work together to teach the class. When I went back to Portland, that core community—made up primarily of those who helped to teach the class—would continue to tend and nurture the parish nurses in that community. These were the people the nurses could count on who knew at least some things about this new ministry and had learned even more about parish nursing in the process of preparing to give a class.

My second insight was that parish nurse coordinators were needed in each area where I taught classes. These coordinators could then work with me to build a network. St. Joseph Medical Center became the first healthcare system in the Northwest to hire a parish nurse coordinator. The coordinator, Sister Margaret Whelan, was, in fact, the one who continued to make sure that Tacoma-area parish nurses were provided with the support necessary to begin their programs. Building community in local areas through offering the class and ongoing support of the nurses by healthcare systems through the coordinators became two of the basic structures of the network.

It quickly became clear that to grow a network, classes needed to be moved geographically closer to the nurses interested in being trained. As an individual with a long-term commitment to missionary work, I was more than familiar with the concept. Any faith's missionary society will promulgate the fact that to make a message or program known means that you go to the people and not expect them to come to you. Although there are those nurses who, once having heard about parish nursing, will go to almost any lengths to learn more, there are many more who will respond to the call when the information is closer at hand. Bringing the basic parish nurse class to a community is a philosophical belief that makes sense and accounts for the fact that NPNM has started parish nursing in Utah, Alaska, California, Idaho, Washington, and Oregon.

In the beginning months of training parish nurses, one of my own struggles was that not all of the nurses who completed the coursework started programs in their churches. There were and continue to be a variety of reasons for this, ranging from the lack of acceptance by the individual pastor and/or congregation to the nurse's own personal reasons. However, an informal survey I conducted of nurses who took the class offered through NPNM but did not become parish nurses showed that the class changed how these nurses were practicing nursing in their healthcare settings. Participants reported that the awareness of the spiritual needs of their patients and their ability to see their patients as a whole people was increased.

In my experience as a nurse for over 40 years, the nursing profession seems to have drawn generally ethical and compassionate people to its ranks. Nursing practice is, at its core, both a strong, scientific, problem-solving discipline and an art that specializes in mending broken bodies, minds, and spirits. With high medical costs, diagnostic related groups (DRGs are a system of reimbursement used for Medicare payments for hospital services), and the early release of patients from hospitals, schools of nursing recognize the need to prepare nurses for an ever-changing climate and site of healthcare. As a result, nursing education is in a good position to subsume ideas like parish nursing into their curriculum and planning. The basic preparation classes for parish nurses and parish nurse coordinators offered through schools of nursing are—and will remain—fundamental to building a parish nurse network.

The Healthcare System

We have entered an era of healthcare that can be described as fragmented and expensive, resulting in 40 to 50 million uninsured and underinsured. The system is enmeshed in a climate of mistrust of Western medicine that has led to a rise in alternative care. Language and cultural barriers between medical personnel and patients have created misunderstandings and negative consequences. Poor patient care in institutions that face critical staff shortages have resulted in patient safety concerns.

In tandem with other basic societal changes, healthcare has become highly technical, expensive, and impersonal. Most of us would not want to be without a system that can increase the life expectancy of the most vulnerable among us. However, we need to learn, both as individuals and members of society, to understand the implications of current healthcare practices and return to the original meaning of the word *health* as wholeness. With this understanding, healthcare would include faith communities, schools, political structures, and medical communities as a part of a healthcare system. We would see prevention and health promotion as central and illness care as what we do when healthcare does not work.

NPNM would not exist were it not for the generosity of one particular healthcare system, Legacy Health System. Chaplain Bill Adix at Legacy Emanuel Hospital knew and respected Granger Westberg. Adix had been a chaplain at Emanuel Hospital (now one of the Legacy hospitals) for almost 30 years when NPNM was established. Emanuel had been a Lutheran hospital and remains connected to the Oregon Synod of the Evangelical Lutheran Church in America (ELCA). Legacy continues to provide office space and other amenities for NPNM, housing the executive director, administrative assistant, and the Portland metro parish nurse coordinator. In addition, it has made grant monies available on an annual basis to continue a ministry that extends far beyond its own boundaries. Legacy continues to be represented on the NPNM Board by chaplain Patrick Tomter, director of Spiritual Care at Legacy Good Samaritan Hospital, and Judith Andersen, president of the NPNM Board, who is also a member of the Legacy Health Care Board. When I asked Sonja Steves, vice president of Human Resources why Legacy would continue its generous support, Steves replied, "Because it is the right thing to do."

Other start-up funds for NPNM came through a grant from Wheat Ridge Ministries (see Wheat Ridge Ministries Grants Program, Seeding Health and Hope, http://www.wheatridge.org, in Itasca, Illinois), the United Methodist Church of Oregon and Idaho, and the Oregon Synod of the ELCA. Adequate and continued funding to keep a regional program afloat is an ongoing challenge. Currently, in addition to Legacy Health System, we receive funding from Providence Health Care Systems both in Portland, Oregon, and Spokane, Washington. We also receive funding from Tuality

Health Care in Hillsboro, Oregon. Additional support comes from over 500 hospital, congregational, and individual memberships and other gifts.

Over 20 parish nurse coordinators in the Northwest are funded either part time or full time by a healthcare system in their communities. The funding of parish nursing is an investment in the community that buys a great deal of good will and ultimately saves the community money. Thus far, only scattered studies show what parish nursing can do to bring health and wellness to communities. There need to be many more to prove its effectiveness (Northwest Parish Nurse Ministries 1995; Tri-Cities Chaplaincy, 2003).

I cannot overstate the need for healthcare systems to see faith communities as partners. During the past 13 years I have had an opportunity to work with dozens of hospitals in towns and cities with hundreds of faith communities. Out of four outstanding examples of what can happen when hospitals and faith communities work together, two of the hospitals are faith-based, and two are secular. I have a friend who works with a variety of healthcare systems and who visited in one of these hospitals. He commented about the wonderful atmosphere he experienced. Needless to say, I was excited to tell him about the terrific parish nurse program there! The parish nurse is included in several departments within the hospital to bring about positive changes, as well as working with their community outreach. Healthcare, as it relates to the building of a parish nurse network, needs to be viewed in the broadest possible context.

Faith Communities

Reverend Granger Westberg pondered why we would let people end up in a hospital in crisis rather than doing something when they were a little bit sick. As a result, he saw faith communities as logical venues—places where we talk about and act on values and beliefs around stewardship of ourselves and our earth—for addressing health issues and whole person health.

Kinast and Seidl (1995) have pointed out, "There are 52.3 churches for every hospital in America. They represent an enormous resource for healthy living, but that resource will not be utilized if the health delivery system functions in isolation from the churches [faith groups]" (p. 1).

Faith communities vary in their acceptance of parish nursing. In my experience, if the concept of parish nursing is understood at the highest level of the church leadership, pastors are quick to embrace this ministry. The Oregon Synod of the Evangelical Lutheran Church in America (ELCA), under the leadership of Bishop Paul Swanson and former assistant Darrel Lundby (current and past board member), has parish nurses in 40 of the 120 congregations in a period of 12 years, many of them paid.

Faith communities are where the parish nurse and healthcare meet. Healthy congregations understand that God's intention for creation is to bring about wholeness through the health and healing of body, mind, heart, and spirit. In modern English, the term *religion* is understood to mean the reconnection of the human and the divine. *Salvation* and *shalom* are words that in the broadest sense mean wholeness of the person, community, and the world. The word *religion*, in fact, is derived from the Latin *ligare* which means "to join, link, or bind," coming from the same root as ligament. The prefix re- + *ligare* means "back" or "again." Parish nursing is done in this context of restoration.

Building a parish nurse network is about making connections within an everyday secular context in a practical sense to accomplish "reconnection" within a context of a faith community. The advent of parish nursing takes place in the midst of serious dialogue about the compatibility between science and religion and an environment of earnest research on the effects of faith and health. Search engines on the Internet can find many listings for you on this topic. This is set against an ever-frustrating illness-care system and burgeoning number of homebound people unable to attend worship services even if they so wished. The tacit acceptance that faith is good for your health is ironic, coming just at a time when faith communities are wringing their hands over what to do with their incapacitated members.

The recognition that most of us can never pay for all the services needed to lubricate our social structure either individually or collectively is an important awareness. When extended families living in proximity of one another were the rule and not the exception, family members (especially women who were not employed outside the home) were, for the most part, able to fulfill needed services, free of charge, for aging family members or those with disabilities. The one social structure that still has enormous social capital capable of caring for people from birth to death is the faith community.

The ministry of parish nursing practice is becoming an essential part of the faith community landscape. Will these faith communities recognize parish nurses as an integral part of the spiritual dimension of a health and healing ministry in the church or will they simply relegate these nurses to act as medical case managers for their parishioners? This will depend, in large part, on the education and dialogue in which parish nurses and faith communities are willing to engage.

Weaving Parish Nursing into an Enduring Networking Structure

Structures Related to the Parish Nurse

Since our first NPNM class we have observed that the best-case scenario for educating and supporting the individual parish nurse is to (1) provide the basic parish nurse class, encourage ongoing education, and make networking/support groups available; (2) recognize the importance and encourage the development of a strong spiritual life; (3) encourage the support of a pastor, congregation, and family; and (4) establish a connection with a parish nurse coordinator.

The importance of our observations was substantiated by the response to a research survey conducted by Solari-Twadell (2002) and completed by 1161 parish nurses. The three most important factors that helped them in fulfilling their role were attendance at the basic preparation program in parish nursing, their personal religious beliefs, and the support of their pastor. We find that it is the PNCs that help to support the parish nurses in these three areas.

Providing Basic Parish Nurse Course, Ongoing Education, Networking/Support Group

The basic parish nurse preparation curriculum we have used to educate parish nurses since its development in 1997 comes through the International Parish Nurse Resource Center (IPNRC). Parish nurse coursework is offered in almost every state in the United States. The curriculum is based on nursing theory, practice, and research. You can find when and where classes are taught by checking on the IPNRC web site: http://www.ipnrc.parishnursing.org.

Courses offered through NPNM (http://www.parishnurseministry.org) are available in a variety of settings and through several venues. Schools of nursing, hospital or healthcare systems, regional organizations, denominations at the national level, and public health departments are sponsoring agencies. The classes are held at retreat centers, college or university classrooms, churches, or public service buildings. Most courses require between 35 and 45 contact hours and are held as week-long seminars, as regular classes during a college quarter or semester, or over the course of several weeks.

Continuing education classes in both nursing and parish nursing are also an important aspect of professional development. Local healthcare systems have been generous in including parish nurses (sometimes charging a nominal fee) in continuing education classes. Organizations periodically offer classes in cities throughout the United States or offer continuing education units for online or mail-in classes. (For classes near you, see PESI Health Care, P.O. Box 1000 Eau Claire, Wisconsin 54702, 800-843-7763, or see the PESI Health Care web site: www.pesihealthcare.com. For online or mail-in classes, see *NurseWeek* web site: www.nurseweek.com).

Parish nursing continuing education classes and conferences provide an excellent opportunity to network with parish nurses from other locations and learn about their programs and resources. Upcoming classes and conferences can be located by checking the IPNRC, regional, denominational, or local parish nurse web sites. Newsletters are often available through these same sources and can be accessed online, or you can ask to be put on their mailing list. Sometimes a membership fee or donation is requested.

Monthly or quarterly parish nurse networking/support groups are available in many places throughout the United States. A PNC generally arranges these groups. For more information about where you would find coordinators, check with the IPNRC.

Networking/support groups provide local parish nurses with an opportunity to connect and learn from each other, to participate in continuing education classes (often provided through the local healthcare system), and become acquainted with local referral sources. Recently I asked coordinators with whom I work to list a few of their favorite networking meetings. Examples of popular programs they listed are theological reflection, hearthstones (small clay hearts with words like faith, trust etc. that are drawn out of a basket and become "your" word for the day on which to ponder and find meaning), information about end-of-life issues, prayer retreats, community services (e.g.,"gatekeeper" training, hospice, public health, domestic violence prevention), an annual parish nurse recognition, CPR and blood pressure updates, current issues in healthcare (HIPAA), stroke prevention, and an opportunity for parish nurses to report on what they are doing in their congregations.

Fostering Spiritual Growth

In the Northwest it is not uncommon to have nurses without a faith community attend a parish nurse course. Hearing from parish nurses after the class who tell about reconnection to their original faith community or even pursuing studies to become pastors has been a rewarding part of my ministry. One poetic and passionate response I treasure is from a participant who wrote the following:

> I cannot begin to tell you of the impact that the parish nurse training has had in my life! It put many things into a clear perspective and affirmed many of my innermost spiritual feelings. Indeed, it was like a caterpillar which had formed its chrysalis and was waiting for … something. I do not feel that the butterfly has emerged yet, but I now know that is what the process is about. I was baptized, for the first time in my life, on the 15th of this month. I have been able to pray with a neighbor of my mother's whose husband died the day after Thanksgiving. There is much need and hurting in the world, and in our own neighborhoods and families. This is where I am needed for now, in my own community. I am learning that I can be of service to others and learn to let God work through me, even as I am

also wounded. It makes me more aware of others' pain, and it helps me to know that I cannot remove their pain. But I can offer to be their companion as they journey through it. (Klotz, 2002)

Solari-Twadell and McDermott (1999) state that "parish nursing holds the spiritual dimension to be central to the practice" (p. 3). In any job description or discussion about the selection of a parish nurse for any particular faith community, the nurse's spiritual maturity will be an important consideration. Regular worship is an important aspect of our faith journey that brings us in a meaningful and intimate way into the life of a supportive community of fellow seekers and believers. Recognition of the need for worship is a part of spiritual maturity.

Parish nurses say that their prayer and devotional life seem to become more important the more deeply they become involved in the ministry of parish nursing practice. A parish nurse will often spend the first year of practice focused on the nursing aspects of parish nursing. The second and subsequent years, as the parish nurse feels comfortable with the physical, mental, and emotional aspects of the ministry, the need for deepening spiritually and an understanding of the necessity of spiritual practices becomes more obvious. It is helpful to have a spiritual companion or director as mentioned in Chapter 4 on spiritual formation.

Spiritual retreats and days of renewal are offered through parish nurse networking groups, individual denominations, and retreat centers throughout the United States. Contacting denominational headquarters or looking in the yellow pages of the telephone book for retreat centers will provide the names of places that provide rooms and meals for individual private/silent prayer retreats.

Scripture study groups through faith communities, parish nurse support groups, college/university classes, community, or Internet groups are plentiful. Studying what other faith traditions teach from their scriptures about faith and healing is a rich, rewarding, and enlightening experience.

Gaining the Support of the Pastor, Congregation, and Family

Clergy support for the position and person of the parish nurse is crucial to the ministry.

The support starts with the faith leader and continues with the assistance of both the health team and faith members. Clergy who have parish nurses are often the best educators of clergy who do not. One of our newest strategies has been to supply badges at pastoral conferences with a picture of the pastor and parish nurse(s). Underneath the picture are the words "Ask Me About Parish Nursing in My Church!" Another strategy has been to request time at pastoral conferences and ask four or five pastors whose congregations have parish nurses to share with other interested pastors how parish nursing works in their churches.

An issue we continue to stress in our parish nurse classes is that parish nursing is about using the nursing process to help everyone become a minister of health. Parish nurses can be a catalyst for making this happen, but in every step of the process they should recognize when and how others must be involved. The most important network, when you get down to it, is the grassroots network of health ministry in the congregation.

Many of our parish nurses comment that they would not be able to practice parish nursing without the support of their spouse or children. It cannot be emphasized enough how family support makes a crucial difference in the outreach that is accomplished. In addition, they appreciate the support of a PNC.

Facilitating a Connection with a Parish Nurse Coordinator

Many parish nurses throughout the country independently manage successful parish nurse practices in their congregations without the help of a parish nurse coordinator. In building a parish nurse network, however, we felt having a trained PNC was valuable. In our experience, the PNC adds definition and legitimacy to the parish nurse role by providing another level (and voice) to the education of clergy and faith communities about parish nursing. Coordinators are able to share knowledge of the bigger picture of what is happening both locally and nationally.

The coordinators with whom we work most often list our annual parish nurse recognition event as their favorite networking program. These usually come in the form of a dinner, reception, or tea and provide an opportunity for

clergy to pay tribute to the work and dedication of "their" parish nurse(s).

Structures Related to the Parish Nurse Coordinator

Our PNC network in the Northwest has been described as a "virtual organization." We do not have legal ties with one another, but we do offer spiritual support, network, and consult with one another and learn about resources relevant to our ministries. The majority of our coordinators are paid, either as full-time or part-time employees, by a healthcare system. An encouraging sign occurred recently when a public health department hired a coordinator and subsidized the cost of a parish nurse class. Of our PNCs not employed by a healthcare system, three volunteer for their regional denominations, and one coordinates all the parish nurses in her county. All the PNCs we work with organize a parish nurse network within a certain geographic area. Other expectations vary according to the coordinator's sponsoring agency and the desired outcomes.

Parish Nurse Coordinator Accountabilities

The coordinators build and maintain networks connecting the individual parish nurses to the healthcare systems, faith communities, and the nursing profession.

Accountabilities of the PNC fall under the following categories:

1. Administration of a parish nurse program requires:
   a. Working with the organization or advisory council in the development of an infrastructure (includes reporting requirements, policies and procedures, and written agreements) to support a parish nurse program. The philosophy, purposes, mission, and vision of parish nursing articulated at the 2000 Westberg Symposium provide the underpinnings of this infrastructure
   b. Planning for the integration of the parish nurse program into the sponsoring organization's mission and continuum of care
   c. Developing a documentation system relevant for both unpaid and paid parish nurses that meets the state's scope and

standards as well as the parish nurse scope and standards of practice

d. Developing and initiating an annual evaluation of the parish nurse

e. Providing an annual written report for each faith community

f. Producing quarterly and annual reports with outcome information for the sponsoring organization

2. Parish Nurse Coordinator Educational Responsibilities

a. Recruitment of nurses for the basic parish nurse class and coordinating it with NPNM. In addition, they ensure ongoing continuing education for parish nurses.

b. Provision of materials, consultation, and education to pastors/health committees/faith communities interested in developing a parish nurse/health ministry program

c. Development of networking/support groups/theological reflection opportunities on a monthly or quarterly basis

d. Initiation and/or participation in parish nurse research

3. The PNC initiates relationships, education, and recruiting of faith communities not already involved in parish nursing.

4. Coordinators develop community relationships by:

a. Cultivating relationships with local school(s) of nursing, enlisting nursing students to work with parish nurses in helping with health surveys, blood pressure screenings, and so on

b. Working with healthcare systems in providing continuing education opportunities for parish nurses as well as resources for health fairs

c. Enlisting the expertise of the public health department to provide local benchmarks and Healthy People 2010 goals so that faith communities and public health departments can work together in their mutual efforts to create healthier communities

The coordinators each bring rich backgrounds, experiences, and gifts to this ministry, and for that reason, there are as many varieties of programs as there are coordinators. Perhaps the most important personal characteristics of these coordinators are deep faith, incredible tenacity, and a passion for nursing, especially parish nursing. Each year we update the parish nursing history that each coordinator has written about the area he or she serves and publish it in our annual conference book.

In my experience, support for parish nurse coordinators is crucial for the longevity of parish nursing. The ministry of a PNC can be the most important aspect of the network of support for the individual parish nurse outside of the support of his/her clergy. An informal survey I conducted of parish nurses who finished a parish nurse class but did not have support from a parish nurse coordinator in their community showed that the parish nurse ministries in their local churches ceased after about a year. This suggests the importance of ongoing support and encouragement from coordinators.

Structures of support for the coordinators consist of (1) the basic parish nurse coordinator class; (2) network/support groups specifically for them; (3) continuing education; and (4) organizational support.

Parish Nurse Coordinator Basic Class

Coordinators are expected to take the basic parish nurse class as a prerequisite to the coordinator class. The basic parish nurse coordinator class is offered in a limited number of places in the United States. Classes offered are posted on the IPNRC website. This class prepares coordinators to work with their sponsoring organizations in developing a supportive infrastructure for the parish nurses in their area. Because parish nursing in the Northwest is still in its beginning stages, we feel that our efforts to educate and support parish nurse coordinators are imperative.

Parish Nurse Coordinator Networking/Support Groups

Regional and denominational support/networking groups specifically for parish nurse coordinators are held throughout the United States. Some information about these groups can be found on the Internet. Parish nurse conferences often provide an opportunity for the coordinators to gather either before or after the conference to meet for several hours or a day. Inspiration and renewal experienced from attending parish nursing and health ministry conferences and the Westberg symposium are vital for the PNC and a conference allowance is an important budget item for hiring organizations to consider.

NPNM provides an opportunity for coordinators to meet at least three times each year. We pray together and share frustrations, accomplishments, and resources. We also use part of our time together for continuing education.

Parish Nurse Coordinator Continuing Education

Much of what was previously written about continuing education as well as the spiritual support of parish nurses is true for parish nurse coordinators. In addition, however, participating in at least one unit of clinical pastoral education (CPE), pursuing training as a spiritual director, or attending lay ministry training can be helpful for the PNC and help encourage parish nurses under their coordination. For further information on clinical pastoral education, see the Association of Clinical Pastoral Education, Inc. (www.acpe.edu). For spiritual direction, see the Spiritual Directors International web site (www.sdiworld.org).

In addition, as an important aspect of their calling, parish nurse coordinators should have a broad understanding of other religious traditions. Knowing more about the beliefs and rituals of other faiths is enriching and helpful in understanding more about our own beliefs. Local and Internet classes in world religions are available through many colleges and seminaries.

Parish Nurse Coordinator Organizational Support

Hospital systems, denominations, and other organizations that hire parish nurse coordinators usually offer various types of benefits and support to those they employ, such as an education/conference allowance. However, because of the nature of the job and the lack of knowledge an organization might have about what PNCs actually do, coordinators may need to educate sponsoring organizations about their specific needs. This will be especially true when it comes to the spiritual aspect of their jobs, particularly the need for spiritual retreats and theological reflection opportunities.

Five years ago, many healthcare systems hiring coordinators did not realize the importance of the training offered for them and/or the necessity of providing ongoing support through coordinator meetings and retreats. As PNCs are establishing themselves in their organizations and communities and providing the necessary education and statistics to show the difference parish nurses and coordinators are making in their communities, the barriers are being lowered. Each accomplishment of a parish nurse and parish nurse coordinator helps to ensure the continuing success of parish nursing as a whole.

Resources allocated to the parish nurse coordinator by the hiring organization are usually financial, management oversight, public relations recognition for the program, office space, and material resources. The hiring organization pays an hourly wage or salary and benefits, including a travel and education allowance, postage, and office supplies. Also included will be a budget item to help defray the costs of monthly or quarterly parish nurse networking/support meetings and an annual parish nurse recognition event.

Management oversight includes establishing a reporting system that reflects what parish nurses and parish nurse coordinators do and demonstrates progress toward the objectives and outcomes pertinent to the sponsoring organization's mission and continuum of care.

Gunderson (1997) writes:

Measuring outcomes is nothing more than deciding what to keep track of, what to pay attention to in a systematic way. This is a profoundly moral activity if it has any role in shaping real-world choices of one strategy over another, one partner over another, one technology or program over another. This is not merely a technical task that can be delegated to some instrument, no matter how refined. It is the stuff of leadership...

To understand what this means for community programs, it's important to ask:

- Is it conceivable in our bookkeeping system for the money saved from a prevented gun injury to be transferred from the ER to a community outreach program?
- Could prevention activities ever show a profit on our books?

- Is the problem caused by the answers to these questions with the prevention system or with simplistic bookkeeping? (p. 62)

The most difficult challenge we have at NPNM is showing our value in a dollar amount. Parish nursing is not an exact science. We cannot say specifically what we have prevented, so it is very hard to show its efficacy. It is not a business that shows a profit. However, of all the things that a coordinator does—and in order for parish nurse ministry to continue to garner support—demonstrating parish nursing's value to the sponsoring organization is most crucial. Studies that substantiate the important and money-saving contributions being made by parish nurses in the community are useful and necessary for this purpose. A good example of parish nurse program outcomes reports for both 2003 and 2004 is available through Tri-Cities Chaplaincy (2003). Another study done in 1995 showed a possible cost saving of $398,200 through 408 parish nurse visits (Rydholm, 1995).

One added challenge for coordinators is getting volunteer parish nurses to adequately document what they do. This partly relates to the fact that many of the parish nurses have always done a lot of work in their churches and they forget that now much of that work should count as parish nursing hours. The other reason is as volunteers, they don't feel they have time to do paperwork.

I recently talked with a church secretary and asked how parish nursing was going in her church. She went to great lengths to tell me how the parish nurse sits in the back row and watches people come into church each week. After church she spends time asking people how their doctor visit went, if they have been able to get a ride to pick up a prescription, or if they would like their blood pressure checked this week. The pastor also shared how the parish nurse had made several calls with him when people had health concerns. When I asked the nurse how her parish nursing practice was going, she told me she was not able to do any because of lack of time.

Coordinators often are discouraged because many nurses who are trained as parish nurses are not doing parish nursing. My philosophy is that we train them and provide consultation, networking

opportunities, continuing education, and resources to help them—ultimately God oversees the process.

Parish Nurse Recruitment Strategies: Think Globally and Locally

We use many strategies to find those nurses who might feel called to parish nursing and are willing to take the basic parish nurse class. One way we have done this is to run an ad about upcoming classes in the state board of nursing newsletter. We have also purchased their mailing list, which we have not found to be as helpful. The postage to send class information is expensive to send to everyone on the list, and there is no way to know who may or may not be interested.

We also contact regional denominational and religious headquarters and inquire if they have a newsletter. If they do, we ask if we can advertise parish nurse classes through them. Some even include our class information on their web page or provide a link to our web site.

The regional hospital systems, especially faith-based systems, have a network of hospitals that share information with one another. The mission directors or directors of spiritual care or chaplaincy are excellent conduits through which to contact nurses interested in a parish nurse class. One director of chaplaincy doubled our class attendance when he sent the class brochure to the home of every nurse in the hospital.

Many of the nurses who respond to being "called" to parish nurse ministry seem to learn about it through word of mouth. Either a pastor or nurse friend will ask them if they have ever heard of parish nursing. A typical response seems to be that even if they had not heard the term used before, they knew instinctively what it was. Continued education of the three natural partners (nurses, congregations, and healthcare institutions) will bring long-term results.

We find that being attached to a hospital system is a tremendous advantage when we are recruiting nurses for a class. Not only do we have access to the nurses presently employed, but also the hospital systems often continue to correspond with their retired nurses—a goldmine of experience, education, and competency in the practice of parish nursing!

Long-term care, hospice, and public health are also sources to be explored while looking for nurses who might want to be trained as parish nurses. The Internet and yellow pages are helpful in providing names and contact information of agencies.

Schools of nursing not only have faculty who are interested in the concept of parish nursing in the education of their students, but they also might be willing to sponsor/host a class, provide continuing education credits (this is a revenue stream for them), be part of the teaching faculty for the class, and use parish nurses/faith communities as community sites for their students. The schools of nursing have our future recruits! It is in the long-term interest of parish nursing that they be included as an important part of the network.

The faith community not only has the nurses needed for the parish nurse training, but they also have the two other entities that require an in-depth education and understanding of parish nursing, namely the ministerial team and the congregation. Ministerial associations, clusters, Catholic Charities, and Lutheran Social Services are all groups that comprise members who are or who know nurses interested in taking the training. These people are also in positions where, once they are educated, can be part of the education of faith communities.

Choosing a Governance Board for a Regional Network

However large or small the network, the principles for assembling a board will be the same. Who are the individuals in each group (nursing, healthcare, and faith communities) who would be committed to the mission, vision, and purposes stated earlier? What are the strengths needed to make it all happen?

Three of the NPNM board members are on the nursing faculty at three different schools of nursing. Four others represent different healthcare systems. Two are directors of spiritual care; one is a director of finance; and another is regional director of mission integration. We also have representation from a large church body, a senior program coordinator for a county department of aging services, chief operations officer for a regional social service agency, president and CEO of a visiting nurse association, and a parish nurse coordinator. Each of these people provides a strength that is partly responsible for our success.

During the past 2 years we have worked to make our board regional. We have been able to accomplish this through conference calls, and it is quite noticeable that those who join us by telephone have a history of making valuable contributions to our work despite the distance.

The initial task of the NPNM board was to conduct a feasibility study and then choose an executive director. When I began as director, the board spent their time supporting and helping me organize and build the program. I have often thought that living a short distance from the NPNM Board President Judith Andersen (former and current NPNM board member) and walking with her each morning in the early years of the program were the greatest help to me in taking those first steps in building a network. It was a great time to share my enthusiasm and perceptions and get important feedback.

During the past few years board policies were put into place to provide the structure needed for a strong future. Now that the program is established, the board's focus continues to be on governance and effectiveness, which includes strategic thinking and fund raising.

Many resources for board information and education are available on the Internet, and many communities have nonprofit board training available. The primary challenge to the development and the preservation of a parish nurse network is securing funding for the ongoing support of the organization. Funding efforts can occur at several levels, but the governing board is in the most powerful position to meet this challenge.

Conclusion

Northwest Parish Nurse Ministries has been gifted with a fine board of directors and the support of several healthcare systems; many schools of nursing; faith communities; and individuals who give of their time, talents, and financial assets. We have been especially blessed by the participants in the parish nurse classes (now over 1500) and the coordinators and faculty who make the classes possible. Reflecting on the network of people and institutions who have helped NPNM implement our mission and vision, I can respond only one way—to God be the glory!

Wouldn't it be wonderful ...
if faith groups—a Baptist church,
a Catholic mission, a Jewish congregation,
a Muslim center—adopted a close-by
geographical area and made sure ...
that every single child in the neighborhood
was immunized against the basic diseases?
... that there was no hungry person in that area?
... that every person had a basic medical exam?
... that every woman who became pregnant would
get prenatal care?

... that every elderly person was contacted daily? Suppose these congregations convinced parents and children to fight the presence of guns. Suppose they made a commitment to provide the kinds of alternatives needed to reduce the violence that afflicts the poorest among us.
These are very exciting and very redemptive options for the faith groups of our nation.
But are they possible?
We believe the answer is yes.

—Former President Jimmy Carter (1994)

REFERENCES

American Nurses Association and Health Ministries Association. (1998). *Standards of practice for parish nurses.* Washington, DC: Author.

Carter, J. (1994). *Faith and health.* Atlanta: The Carter Center.

Carter, J. (1996). *Living faith.* New York: Random House.

Gunderson, G. (1997). *Strong partners: realigning religious health assets for community health.* Atlanta: The Carter Center.

International Parish Nurse Resource Center. (n.d.). *Information for parish nurses: root assumptions.* Retrieved June 5, 2004, from http://www.ipnrc.parishnursing.org

Kinast, R. L. & Seidl L. G. (1995). Partners in healing: *healthcare organizations and parish communities.* St. Louis: Catholic Health.

Klotz N. (personal communication, November, 2002).

Northwest Parish Nurse Ministries. (1995). *Summary of visits: parish nurse project/project no. 309-95.* Portland, OR: Author. (Available from NPNM, Room 1072, 2801 N. Gantenbein Avenue, Portland, OR 97227.)

Ryan J. (2000). Parish nursing at a kairos moment. Keynote address. Fourteenth Annual Westberg Parish Nurse Symposium: Weaving parish nursing into the new millennium. September, 2000. Itasca, IL.

Rydholm, L. (1995). *Summary of visits parish nurse project.* Mankato, MN: St. Joseph's Hospital.

Solari-Twadell, P. A. (2002). The differentiation of the ministry of parish nursing practice within congregations. *Dissertation Abstracts International* 63(06) 569A. (UMI No. 3056442).

Solari-Twadell, P. A. & McDermott, M. A. (Eds.) (1999). Parish nursing: promoting whole-person health within faith communities. Thousand Oaks, CA: Sage.

Tri-Cities Chaplaincy. (2003). *Program outcomes year-end report: July 1, 2002, to June 30, 2003.* (Available from the Tri-Cities Chaplaincy, Attention: Parish Nurse Coordinator Dorothy Anderson, 2108 W. Entiat Avenue, Kennewick, WA 99336.)

Working with Underserved Congregations: A Case Study

24

Janet Wall DiLeo
Cassandra Scott Graham
Phyllis Ann Solari-Twadell

The following is a discussion of the McFarland Institute's success in addressing healthcare disparities among the underserved African-American population of metropolitan New Orleans by educating nurses to initiate the ministry of parish nursing practice in their churches. In this southern urban area rich in spiritual tradition, the development of parish nursing programs in over 50 congregations has been found to be an ideal means of addressing the whole person healthcare needs of underserved populations.

Context

The setting for this case study is New Orleans, Louisiana. The French founded New Orleans in 1718. Much of the city is below sea level, bordered by the Mississippi River and Lake Ponchatrain. Throughout its early history, the people of New Orleans suffered from epidemics of yellow fever, malaria, and smallpox. With improved hygiene, vector control, safe food, clean water, and immunizations the epidemics dissipated. New Orleans, a principal port, had a leading role in the slave trade. Today New Orleans is noted for its Creole culture and persistence of voodoo as well as music, food, architecture, and fun (Wikipedia, 2000).

The 2000 census of New Orleans noted 484,674 people; 67% were African-American and 28% were white. The medium income was $27,133; the per capita income, $17,258. Twenty eight percent of the population were below the poverty line, with 40.3% of those living in poverty under the age of 18 and 19.3% older than 65 (Centers for Disease Control, 2004). These demographics have a strong relationship to the mortality data for New Orleans with the leading causes of death listed as heart disease, cancer, diabetes, and preventable injuries. The underlying factors related to the causes of death were identified as obesity, tobacco use, limited intake of fruits and vegetables, and alcohol consumption. These factors are related to lifestyle choices, are preventable and relate to socioeconomic status, ethnicity, and access to health resources. Shaw, Dorling, Gordon, and Smith (2000) noted, "The causal relationship between poverty and ill health is now proven beyond any reasonable doubt and has been acknowledged and accepted by the world's leading authorities on health and social development" (p. 170).

Taylor and Braithwaite (2001) elaborate and focus on the African-American community noting "Much of the data presented in 1992 regarding health disparity remains unchanged. Although a few improvements have occurred in the overall health status of African-Americans the scientific body of health data shows that blacks continue to lack parity, and are not even close to parity, with their white counterparts" (p. 3). Issacs and Knickman (2002) continue, "The uneven availability of continuing medical care of acceptable quality is one of the most serious problems we face today. We need to better provide health services of the right kind, at the right time, to those who need it" (p. xiii).

However, in addition to the uneven distribution of healthcare resources, we live in the United States with disparities in paying for healthcare, especially for the poor. Issacs and Knickman (2002) report:

> Despite spending more than a trillion dollars on healthcare every year in the United States, more than 43 million Americans are still without health insurance, up from 31 million in 1987. Ten million children are uninsured. But the lack of health insurance is only part of this dismal picture. People, who are poor, lower class, minority or who live in inner cities or rural areas, continue to have trouble getting medical services from a system that has become less, rather than more, responsive to their needs. Managed care may cut costs, but often at the expense of services and avoiding people with chronic diseases and other costly conditions. (p. xiii)

Social position and ethnicity also often contribute to the health status of individuals and communities. "Our health is affected not simply by the ease with which we see a doctor … but also by our social position and the underlying inequality of our society…. Health is produced … by the cumulative experience of social conditions over the course of one's life" (Daniels, Kennedy, & Kawachi, 2000, p. 4).

The Ministry of Parish Nursing Practice and the Underserved

The parish nursing literature addressing care of the underserved and marginalized is limited. Gragnani and Corbett (1990) describe the ministry of parish nursing practice in six Chicago neighborhoods. This outreach by Missionary Sisters of the Sacred Heart of Jesus, who sponsored Columbus-Cabrini Medical Center, the sponsor of this parish nurse effort, was designed "to move closer to the marginal and disenfranchised underclass in order to offer preventative services. Parishes selected served those who do not speak English, those who may be refugees of war, poverty or political dissent, or those who are second and third generation victims of discontinued educational and social programs" (Gragnani & Corbett, 1990, p. 78). Gragnani (1999), who

dedicated the majority of her parish nurse ministry to the underserved and marginalized, again wrote a decade later of ten parish nurses who worked in urban ministry. Gragnani noted, "Inner city work takes tenacious determination because of the comprehensive life problems of the people" (p. 58).

An article written about the ministry of parish nursing practice in the African-American community is particularly pertinent to this case study. Armmer and Humbles (1995) noted,

> The role of the African-American church in the lives of the community has been a pivotal one. Issues of civil and human rights were first championed through the church. The church has been the setting for collaboration and complementary interactions of religious, civil and political leaders that have resulted in the present levels of integration and opportunity, particularly for persons of color. Given the powerful influence of the church in the lives of many African-Americans, it is logical that healthcare—and particularly health promotion—would be appropriately addressed by and through the church (p. 66).

The ministry of parish nurse practice described in this case study is in an ideal position to address a multiplicity of whole person healthcare needs for underserved African-Americans on an individual, group, and community level. The challenges are many, including working with poorly educated people or those who have a limited knowledge of mainstream healthcare practices; collaborating with congregations that have no healthcare professionals; working in a community that has limited access to healthcare delivery services; and working with church leadership who are stretched thin with numerous management responsibilities and, more often than not, a secular position in the community.

This discussion is intended to be a resource for those working to initiate changes and enhance resources in challenged communities through collaborative development of the ministry of parish nursing practice within congregations. The institution under discussion is the McFarland Institute of New Orleans, Louisiana. Through its Congregational Wellness Division, the McFarland Institute is working to unlock the potential of communities through investing in the spiritual, physical, and emotional rebuilding of congregational members in largely African-American communities. The term *church nurse* is used to describe the nurses working in the ministry of parish nursing practice as a parish in Louisiana is better known as a geographical county.

The McFarland Institute Church (Parish) Nurse Program

The sale of Mercy-Baptist Hospital in New Orleans, Louisiana, in 1966 resulted in generating the funds that were used to establish the not-for-profit organization Christian Health Ministers, also know as the McFarland Institute. The Congregational Wellness Division of McFarland Institute is dedicated to assisting congregations to reclaim their role as a place of healing—for spiritual, emotional and physical ills (www.tmcfi.org). The division's main initiative is the church (parish) nurse program. This initiative is designed to promote community wellness by educating registered nurses to provide whole person health education, health screening, and healthcare referral in their local congregations. In 1997, the McFarland Institute implemented a pilot project with three congregations of different denominations within the five civil county service areas of the McFarland Institute. The goal of the 3-year pilot program was to test the feasibility of establishing church (parish) nursing programs in congregations that had registered nurses among the membership. McFarland covered program start-up costs (office equipment and supplies, stethoscopes, etc.) and the salary of the registered nurse in decreasing amounts over the 3 years. The McFarland Institute intended that the congregations would contribute funds in the second and third years of the pilot project to supplement their funding. Two of the congregations paid salaries to the registered nurses until the funding from the McFarland Institute for this project was depleted. The third congregation elected not to continue compensating the church (parish) nurse. The lack of financial support from the third congregation was due to the congregation's limited resources. It is important to note, however, their discontinuing payment to the church (parish) nurse was not related to

lack of interest in the ministry of parish nursing practice.

The nurses in the pilot program were extremely successful, as evidenced by over 23,000 documented contacts made by the end of the third year. One of the pilot congregations under the direction of the church nurse established a "3:16 group" for men who were struggling with alcohol and drug abuse. The "3:16 group" met daily for fellowship, spiritual guidance, nourishment, assistance with seeking jobs, and assistance in accessing resources in the healthcare system. Another church nurse contacted a group of senior citizens that gathered in the congregation for bingo twice a week. The church nurse offered to establish an exercise session for them that would meet immediately before the bingo. Several years later that group of seniors is still meeting for exercise and bingo every Wednesday and Friday morning.

Based on the pilot project's success, the Congregational Wellness Division sought to provide parish nursing education and limited funding for program costs. Technical assistance and consultation regarding program development were also offered. However, the ministry of parish nursing practice became a volunteer model as the Congregational Wellness Division was unable to finance the compensation for the church (parish) nurses. Moreover, qualitative data from pastors and nurses indicated that the volunteer model was closely aligned with the mission and vision of the African-American churches.

In 2000, the program sought and received funding from the Robert Wood Johnson Foundation with matching funds from a community partner. With these monies, the Congregational Wellness Division of the McFarland Institute was able, over a 3-year period, to add an additional fifteen churches to the congregational nurse network. Start-up funds of $4000 were awarded to each church in the form of a mini-grant. Each congregation was asked to make a dedicated commitment to the initiation of the ministry of parish nursing practice. This commitment on the part of the congregation included: (1) the pastor's support for establishing a health ministry; (2) appointing a registered nurse from the congregation as the parish nurse; (3) collecting health assessments from a minimum of 20% of the active church membership; and (4) agreeing to maintain the health ministry for a period of 5 years after the initial funding. Nearly 125 registered nurses from local congregations have been educated through the McFarland Institute's basic parish nurse preparation. Many of the nurses who have completed the basic parish nurse preparation now minister in their churches as volunteer church nurses. All the churches that have sought funding and support from the Congregational Wellness Division of the McFarland Institute are predominantly African-American. Many of the churches are located in economically depressed areas of the city. Many of the congregation members can be described as working poor who are either uninsured or underinsured. Although some of the churches had the rudiments of a health ministry, often these ministries lacked structure and funding (Bihm, 2004).

Resources that are offered to churches that partner with the Congregational Wellness Division church (parish) nurse program are the following:

- An administrative structure that has a library of resources and expertise in the staff of the center who understand health promotion
- Consultation directed to the development of the church nurse and specific health promotion programs
- Assistance in assessing and analyzing the needs of the congregation
- Assistance in assessing the available talent and resources offered in the congregation
- Assistance in development of a month-to-month plan of action aimed at health promotion for the congregation
- Ongoing educational programs and spiritual retreats for the church nurse
- Providing a quarterly networking meeting for the church nurses to share resources, support each other, and pray together
- Providing policies, procedures, and guidelines for church nurses working in the congregations.

The McFarland Institute Church (Parish) Nurse Program has positively impacted the community in the following ways:

- Linking the healthcare and religious community to successfully promote health and wellness

- Providing recognized tangible benefits to the community
- Educating the community regarding access to an increasingly fragmented healthcare system.

Lessons Learned

Valuable fundamental lessons have been learned in working with the parish nurses, clergy and laypeople in the congregations and in the communities in which they reside. The following material is shared with the reader in hopes that some of these "lessons learned" will be helpful to others in their future work with underserved congregations, particularly those ministering to African-Americans.

Lesson 1: Go Where You are Invited

The president of the McFarland Institute, Reverend Dr. Gene Huffstutler, in the fashion of Reverend Granger Westberg, knocked on the doors of numerous churches in the metropolitan New Orleans area seeking churches that would be interested in offering a ministry of parish nursing practice. He was able to garner support for a church (parish) nurse program at only three churches. Over the next several years, the success of the program spread among the churches in the community. The pastors and particularly the nurses in other churches, many of whom worked full time but were highly committed to working in their churches, became interested in the church nurse program because of the experience of other congregations that had initiated the program. Eventually, the church leadership including the nurses started to seek out the services and funding offered by the McFarland Institute to get a ministry of parish nursing practice instituted in their congregations.

Lesson 2: Honor the Priorities of the Congregation

The parish nurse coordinator must listen carefully. Consideration must be given to the fact that the priorities of the parish nurse coordinator may not be the priorities of those of whom they are working with representing the congregation. It is important to first address the congregation's perceived priorities. For example, the parish nurse coordinator and/or the church nurse may determine obesity to be a key health issue when assessing the congregation's health concerns. However, the church leadership may be concerned with personal safety in the neighborhood or a leaky church roof. It is important to address their perceived concerns first. Once mutual respect and trust have been established between the parish nurse and the church leadership, the parish nurse coordinator and parish nurse will be in a better position to introduce initiatives addressing the documented health issues facing the congregation.

Lesson 3: Find a Common Language

Clear communication is a priority when an institution—whether that be a healthcare institution or foundation—is collaborating with a congregation in developing a ministry of parish nursing practice. Finding a common language from which to communicate is crucial to the development of a trusting relationship between the parish nurse coordinator from the institution, pastor, church leaders, and congregants. The development of a common language needs to take into consideration the culture, denomination, geographical location, and social dynamics such as the socioeconomic level of the congregation, as well as the sincerity of intent. This can be an ongoing process that must be tended to diligently.

Lesson 4: "Buy-in" is Critical to the Success of Any Church-Based Initiative

It is important for the parish nurse to meet with the pastor and ascertain his or her level of interest, support, and commitment to the development and sustaining of a ministry of parish nursing practice. During these conversations it is important to give the pastor and other significant leaders in the congregation an overview of the gravity of the health issues facing the community surrounding the congregation. It is key to seeking their support in addressing health promotion issues with the congregation. The pastor of one of the most active churches himself became a vegetarian after having had a myocardial infection. On numerous occasions since, he has preached to

his congregation about the importance of diet and exercise. The church (parish) nurse, following this lead, incorporated healthy nutrition practices and weight management classes into the life of the congregation. These measures have started to diminish radically the incidence of obesity and hypertension over time among church members of this congregation.

Lesson 5: Recruit Interested Spokespersons

Interested spokespersons recruited as supporters of the ministry of parish nursing practice are instrumental to the integration of the ministry into the life of the congregation. Their support is crucial to the process. It is important to determine the unofficial, as well as the official, leaders or gatekeepers of the congregation. The unofficial leaders of the congregation are those who are highly regarded among the congregation and who elicit a significant level of respect and support from other congregation members. They can be anyone from a community matriarch, to the head usher, to the director of the nurses' guild. This person is held in high regard, exudes confidence, and can conceivably be the parish nurse's entrée into the greater community, engaging respected community leaders. Given their interest and energy for health promotion activities for their congregation, many unofficial leaders of congregations have been instrumental in creating walking and weight management groups.

Lesson 6: Encourage Involvement of Spokespersons from Subgroups in the Congregation

When developing programming for the congregation, one must work with specific subgroups in the congregation. A representative of that subgroup should be a part of the planning, and his or her voice should be heard. For example, a member of the Youthful Elders group could be assigned to represent senior citizens' concerns. The same will apply to participation at events. "Do what I do," rather than "Do what I say," is an old adage that remains true in the church arena. Pastors are held in high esteem. Getting the church pastor and church leaders to attend an event will assure participation, just having them talk about the need for attendance at a given event may not necessarily result in the level of attendance you desired.

Lesson 7: Include the Concerns of the Community at Large in the Planning

Determine the health needs of the larger community and level of interest in the congregation for reaching out and working with other groups in the community in addressing health issues of a common concern. Examples include neighborhood safety, the desire for a walking track, or the need for hypertension screening. Strength in numbers applies here. Once the congregation becomes linked with other resources in the community, the congregation's commitment to sustain the designated initiative is fuller. A regular meeting with representatives from other community agencies often bolsters the intent of the congregation. Resources that were not as easily accessible previously become available, and little indicators of hopefulness begin to be apparent.

Lesson 8: Start with an Assessment of the Health Status of Congregation Members

A starting point in integrating the ministry of parish nursing practice into the life of the congregation is to develop and distribute a health assessment to members of the congregation. It is a simple tool that includes general health questions and also space for standard biometric data, including height, weight, blood pressure, pulse, respirations, and body fat percentage. Confidentiality of data must be maintained and strongly promoted upon distribution of the health assessment. This will encourage participation; obviously the larger the sample, the more data will be retrieved, providing a more conclusive report. A captive audience is crucial to assessment completion and retrieval. Distributing and retrieving the assessment at the same event is recommended. Once the results of the assessment instruments are reviewed by the parish nurse and the data have been tabulated, a "health report card" can be generated for the congregation. The results of this health assessment can be

the basis on which health promotion programming can begin providing a more conclusive report and greater service to the congregation.

Sensitivity to the congregation's concerns that may be triggered in health data collection is important. The information is personal, and congregation leadership and members typically want to know the reason for generating the data and how it will be maintained. Confidentiality is crucial to upholding congregation participation and the church (parish) nurse program's reputation. A history of abuse and betrayal of African-Americans' data, fueled by the Tuskegee studies, may create a reluctance on the part of the congregation leadership to allow such a practice. Also, congregation members fear that embarrassing personal information may reach their pastor or fellow congregation members.

Lesson 9: Use Resources External to the Congregation to Support the Development of Programming for the Congregation

Community assessment reports that have been done by the government, hospitals, or local health departments may provide information that will be useful to the congregation in program planning. This may not be as helpful in situations in which the members of the church community do not live in the vicinity of the church. Church members in some communities often have been raised in a specific church, have grown-up and moved away from the old neighborhood, but still return to the church for Sunday worship.

Lesson 10: Evaluation is the Key to Understanding, Improvement, and Development of Future Programming

Evaluation is a key component to incorporate into the planning of a parish nurse program. Evaluation assists in creating and maintaining the integrity of the ministry of parish nursing practice and ensuring a quality level of service. An instrument should be distributed to participants for retrieval at the completion of any health education program offered. An annual evaluation of the parish nurse program and church nurse should be given to the congregation. Both instruments provide valuable feedback on the programs' delivery and relevance and are helpful in future program planning and maintaining sensitivity to the foremost health issues needing to be addressed.

Lesson 11: Identify Partners in the Community

Usually numerous agencies have resources to dedicate to providing services for the underserved in a designated community. Identifying who they are, what resources they have to support programming in the community, what they are currently doing in the community, and what they would like to do in the community is important. Once these resources are identified, it is often efficient and effective to try and gather representatives from these resources at a meeting. In this way relationships are developed; splintering of resources often is discontinued; and the people of the community are served more effectively.

Lesson 12: Understand and Support the Congregation as Owner of the Church Nurse Program

Staff from the Congregational Wellness Division of the McFarland Institute always identify themselves as consultants to the development of the health ministry being supported by the congregation. It is clear from the beginning that the congregation owns the church nurse program. The McFarland Institute is a committed partner to the congregation in supporting them in their desire to sustain the church nurse in their congregation. The McFarland Institute is also a conduit for organized resources from the community to be offered to the members of the congregation in an effort to support the health of the community.

Lesson 13: Choose Culturally Sensitive Staff to Work with the Congregation

Staff from the Congregational Wellness Division of The McFarland Institute include a director, nurse coordinator, training coordinator, and a data entry specialist. Those working with the church (parish) nurses and congregation leadership are African-American. This has enhanced the cultural sensitivity of the program towards congregation concerns as well as enhanced support for and rapport with congregation leadership.

Conclusion

Working with underserved congregations presents an interesting challenge for the sponsoring institution, the congregation, the parish nurse coordinator, and the parish nurse. Developing sufficient response to the needs of the underserved is best done through coordination of available resources funneled through an established and trusted institution in the community. The McFarland Institute is a good steward of resources that were made available from the sale of a hospital and other funding agencies. The McFarland Institute provides a strong infrastructure that has a clear mission statement, dedicated professionals, and knowledgeable staff. Resources benefit the congregation and its members and drive a relationship development between other appropriate resources and agencies in the community. The McFarland Institute represents credibility and has an excellent reputation in the community and the state for its work with underserved churches. All this benefits the congregation and ultimately the community at large in addressing health disparities

May God's blessing come to you in your work in assisting underserved congregations in retrieving their mission of health and healing. In doing so, you are exercising justice and supporting resolution to the problems of equal access for all to health resources.

REFERENCES

Armmer, F.A. & Humbles, P. (1995). Parish nursing: extending health care to urban African-Americans. *Nursing and Health Care: Perspectives on Community*, 16(2): 64-68.

Bihm, B. (2004). Church nurse: building on a proud tradition. *Journal of Christian Nursing*, Spring, pp. 16-17.

Centers for Disease Control. *National Center for Health Statistics: New Orleans parish profile*. Retrieved July 28, 2004 from http://www.oph.dhh.state.la.us/php/reg1/orleans/chronic.pdf

Daniels, N., Kennedy, B., & Kawachi, I. (2000). *Is equality bad for our health?* Boston: Beacon Press.

Gragnani Boss, J.A. (1999). Parish nursing practice with underorganized, underserved, and marginalized clients. In P.A. Solari-Twadell & M.A. McDermott (Eds.). *Parish nursing: providing whole-person health within faith communities*. Thousand Oaks, CA: Sage.

Gragnani Boss, J.A. & Corbett, J. (1990). The developing practice of the parish nurse: an inner city experience. In P.A. Solari-Twadell, A.M Djupe, & M.A. McDermott (Eds.). *Parish nursing: the developing practice*. Park Ridge, IL: Lutheran General Health Care System.

Issacs, S. & Knickman, J. (2002). *To improve health and health care: The Robert Wood Johnson Foundation anthology* (vol. v). San Francisco: Jossey-Bass.

The McFarland Institute. Accessed March 25, 2005 from www.tmcfi.org

Shaw, M., Dorling, D., Gordon, D., & Smith, G.D. (2000). *The widening gap: health inequities and policy in Britain*. Bristol, England: The Policy Press.

Taylor, S.E. & Braithwaite, R.L. (2001). African-American health. In R.L. Braithwaite, & S.E. Taylor, (Eds.). *Health issues in the black community*. San Francisco: Jossey Bass.

Wikipedia (2000). Greater New Orleans. Accessed July 28, 2004 from http://en.wikipedia.org/wiki/greater_new_orleans

Grant Writing for Parish Nurses and Parish Nurse Coordinators

JoVeta Wescott
Faith Bresnan Roberts

"Give and it will be given to you; good measure, pressed down, shaken together, running over, they will pour into your lap. For whatever measure you deal out to others, it will be dealt to you in return." Luke 6:38 (Holy Bible, RSV)

For many parish nurse coordinators, submitting and obtaining a constant stream of grants will be part and parcel of their positions. We hope that this chapter will assist both the new and/or established parish nurse coordinator do just that. Should the parish nurse coordinator not be asked to obtain grant funding, it is a given that the individual congregations in their program will be asking about this process. This chapter has been written with both coordinator and parish nurse in mind, and we strive to demystify this topic for anyone actively pursuing a grant.

You're a new parish nurse or parish nurse coordinator. You need money for your program. Everyone you talk to advises you that the best thing to do is "just write a grant." Sounds easy enough, right? You can do anything you want, and someone will pay you to do it, right? Sounds good, doesn't it? Ask any parish nurse leader what keeps them up at night and the answer will always be funding. It is the bane of our existence. Whether the program is based in an institution, church, or supported through a community organization, ongoing financial support is imperative. For the majority of parish nurse programs, dollars from grants are the initial and often continuing source of their viability.

Simply stated, a grant is a contribution of money. The good news is that money is available for selected projects. The bad news is that getting a grant isn't as easy as it sounds. It takes time, knowledge, skill, talent, and energy. Often after receiving a grant, one realizes restrictions and reporting requirements are part of the package and wonders if it is all worth the effort.

So, what is this grant writing all about? You say you've never written one before? Nor had we before entering this wonderful world of the ministry of parish nursing practice. As we've traveled this path, we've learned a few tips that might make your trip a little more pleasant and enjoyable while saving you some frustration. We have shared some of our experience previously by presenting to parish nurses locally (Wescott, 2003) and welcome this opportunity to share with a broader audience. We hope that this chapter will allay some of your fears and show you how to do your homework, how to apply for and sustain grant monies as funding sources. Too often grants are viewed as impossible to obtain or difficult to write. That is simply not the case.

Considerations in Preparing to Write

Start at the Beginning

This may sound strange when you are so excited about parish nursing and "just want to get out there and initiate or expand a program. Doesn't everyone understand the potential good you can do?"

Not unless you tell them. In order for that to happen, you must be able to articulate your program and specific needs to them. For those in the business and philanthropic world, this probably would be called your marketing plan.

We refer to this beginning as the "grant thinking" stage; it is probably the most important stage, the one that takes the longest to prepare. During this phase you will begin looking at numerous things. One can learn grant writing; grant thinking is what can exhaust your creativity. Grant seeking and writing require a lot of good planning and hard work. The most important thing you can do to ensure the funding you seek is to plan well.

Begin by thinking and talking with others, perhaps members of the health and wellness cabinet or others in the congregation. Seek out those who have written and received grants. Listen to their advice. Carefully examine your motives and what you want to accomplish. Has anyone done what you want to do? Should the grant be awarded, who will benefit? Can the program you're imagining be replicated in other churches? Will you have matching and/or in-kind support from your congregation? Do you need to collaborate with others in the community?

Seldom will you receive grant funds just to "do parish nursing." Noble as it may seem, the funder does not always see the ministry of parish nursing practice through the same lens as you do. Not every program will receive a million-dollar grant, but grant monies do continually support a significant number of small parish nurse programs. A common surprise that many a novice grant writer finds is that grant dollars are finite and require that the program put in place ways to continue funding after the grant ends. In other words, the work is never done! This is usually called *sustainability*.

Begin by looking at philanthropy in your community. Ask yourself and others questions such as: Who gives? To whom or what do they give? Why do they give? What are the common links among organizations receiving philanthropic support? Does parish nursing have a place within the philanthropic arena of your local/regional community?

According to Martha McCabe, grant writer specialist at Via Christi Foundation, Wichita, Kansas, 60,000 plus grant-making foundations exist in the United States. Eighty percent of grants are available for organizations. So, how do you get the money for your program? The process is very competitive, and you must follow all directions very carefully and correctly. Usually you will not have a face-to-face or telephone conversation to sell your program. Your written application will be the only voice the grant reviewer reads. A well written, articulate request will more likely receive funding. Be prepared to answer this question well in writing: Why does the program need funding? This is usually called *program need*.

Experts in grant writing say the success rate for receiving grant monies runs around 20% (Gitlin & Lyons, 2004). Parish nurses are not the only ones out there seeking dollars. Also keep in mind that since 9/11 many corporate and family foundations have seen their funds decrease because of the economy. This means that success is even more elusive. Foundations are looking very carefully at who will receive their limited funds. What is true in the world of healthcare is also true in the grant world: mission matters. Grantors want to give money to groups that will help both the applicant and the grantor accomplish their goals (Guyer, 2002).

Your role then during this "grant thinking" preparation stage is to investigate as many different potential funding sources as you can. The Internet offers information on various grant opportunities. An example is the federal government's website described in Appendix 25A. *Google* is also a good search engine. Talk with others who have received grants. These people can offer you a lot of valuable information about seeking and keeping grant funds. You can also check with your local library. National state-by-state directories (www.fdncenter.org) outline every grant and list past grant recipients. Take special note of how specific their parameters are. You will be wasting your time and energy to apply for money to a group whose mission and goals are not congruent with your needs. For example, say you are a Presbyterian parish nurse seeking funds for nutrition counseling in your church. During your investigative process you see that grant funds are available from several different organizations. However, their guidelines also state that no dollars are given to faith-based organizations or that their money is only given to Methodist churches.

Do *not* waste your time, energy, and money to apply for this funding.

Read the directions carefully and follow them to the letter. From personal experience we know this to be true. Recently, one of the authors was refused a grant based on the way it was titled, even though the rules had changed after the RFP (request for proposal—the application) had been distributed. Titles of grants can be extremely important. The title should not be something trendy and cutesy because your request can be misunderstood as something not serious. Short titles that describe your grant in a few words are best. You know what they say about the golden rule: those who have the gold, make the rules. The hopeful recipient is not to question but to do better the next time. Part of the whole grant thinking process is learning how to play by the rules.

Another important consideration as part of the process that needs to happen long before you begin the actual grant writing is to establish a track record with area funders. Because you will not ordinarily have a track record of funding, you will need to build relationships with those that have the available dollars. Look to their staff as a resource. These people are your friends! One of the greatest gifts one of the funders gave us was to emphasize that it is okay to ask for money— even from churches and clergy. Many foundations have project directors that are more than pleased to assist you by answering questions about grant review and how decisions are made, helping you with budget concerns, etc. Others do not offer any technical assistance. Seek out multiple potential funding sources for your project.

Learn what funders care about. Is it children, the vulnerable elderly, the poor, minority groups, or wellness? Has the foundation demonstrated a real commitment to funding in the area that you seek funding? Does it seem likely that the foundation will make a grant in your geographic area? Does the amount of money you are requesting fit within the foundation's average grant award? Does the foundation have any policy prohibiting grants for the type of support you are requesting (i.e., only Catholics, only churches whose membership is 5000 to 8000, or small rural churches with membership below 100)? Are you looking at a Christian Scientist funder for medical supplies? Read carefully and be alert to the restrictions.

Does the foundation prefer to make grants to cover the full cost of a project, or does it favor projects where other foundations or funding sources share the cost? One of the authors recently received a grant that was contingent on receiving funding from another source, as the foundation wanted to work collaboratively with the other organization. We have also received supplemental funding for lodging and food while traveling that complemented another grant to offer training on developing and facilitating support groups. Look at the big picture when seeking funding. What types of organizations does the targeted foundation tend to support? One of the authors recently received a federal grant from the Administration on Aging. Before this grant was awarded, the agency had never given this particular funding to a faith-based organization. In reviewing the RFP no mention was made that it would not fund a faith-based organization, so the risk was taken to our organization's benefit.

Other examples of untapped sources utilized by the authors' programs include the following:
1. Community dollars designated "for the good of the community," which were used to fund a "Vial of Life" program
2. Federal dollars for diabetes, which were used to send ten nurses to attend a parish nurse basic preparation course. The premise of the grant was that people would be more compliant with their treatment if asked how they were doing every week at church
3. Community dollars were used to hold a tea. All nurses in the community were invited to come and learn about parish nursing. These dollars have also been used to purchase a video from the International Parish Nurse Resource Center (IPNRC) and to provide scholarships for eight nurses to attend a basic parish nurse preparation course.

Ask yourself whether the organization has specific application deadlines and procedures or if it reviews proposals continuously. Most foundations have more grant applications than they will ever be able to fund, so if yours does not meet their requirements, it is immediately eliminated. Don't give them an excuse to discard what you have worked on so diligently.

Partnerships are a plus: Think collaboratively. Could you partner with another church in your neighborhood? Might you want to check with a local hospital and see if they would be interested in partnering with you? Today many grantors specifically require collaboration of several entities (i.e., Robert W. Johnson Foundation [RWJF] Faith in Action grants).

All the while you're building relationships, you need to become an expert in your program area. Do your homework in every area that you can. Know your program's and your own personal strengths and weaknesses. Be able to articulate those to others. You need to be persistent. Isn't that a quality that all nurses must possess? Consider that you and/or your church can offer the funder a strong commitment. Look at other projects you or your church may have participated in that would show this as a strength. A high leverage may be the matching money your church has to offer or the number of volunteers available to help with the project. Your innovative plan can be part of your strength. Play to your strengths. Tie your plan to the funder's mission and current work. If this is the year the foundation is focusing on high school youth, it would be a waste of your time to apply for the after-school kindergarten project you need funded.

Part of your preparation phase is learning to accept rejection and not taking it personally. If you cannot do this, then do not proceed past this point. Proceeding will only make you miserable and could make you lose the vision of what your ministry is all about. Because of the large number of people seeking funding and the relatively small numbers of available monies, rejection is part of the picture for which you need to prepare before you even submit the paperwork. You might seek the assistance of someone you trust to open this correspondence; then they can gently or excitedly share the joy or the sorrow with you.

Develop a Solid Plan of Action

You may want to do a large project in stages. For instance, you may apply for a grant with one foundation that will build a walkway around the lake that borders the church. You then may do another grant to provide adequate lighting for safety of walkers. Another grant could include benches and chairs. You might even want to apply for equipment to mark off the distance around

the parameter. Or maybe you want to put birdhouses and bird feeders somewhere in the area. Think creatively! Shut your eyes and do some brainstorming of what the area could look like if you had all the money you needed for this project. Then think about how it would affect the members of your congregation. Does it provide a healthier lifestyle by giving them a safe place to walk (day and night), a quiet place to meditate, a place to de-stress and feed the birds? Partner with others; involve others in your congregation in the planning. Don't forget, it's the results that count. Emphasize the outcomes of your project, not the activities that will get you to that point. This is sometimes referred to as "impact" of the program. The more ideas you have, the better chance you have of obtaining funding. It's also important to remember that seeking funding can't be about you. Your project needs to be something that addresses a need in the community. Parish nurses must always be seeking to serve the needs of the faith community as a whole and not solely their own personal needs.

Sustainability

What happens after the grant is awarded? Design a sustainable project. One of the biggest things that organizations look for is sustainability. Use leveraging to bring in more money than the grantor has to offer. Sadly, several parish nurse projects have disappeared because they were unable to provide the sustainability required by the grant. Typically funding sources give you a certain amount of time to show them how you will provide the remaining monies to keep your program going. If you tell them you will be able to raise matching funds then make sure you have people committed to raising those funds. Maximize in-kind donations when you're documenting sustainability. Examples of this would be use of the phone and computer at church, donated office space, time spent by volunteers to copy handouts, make phone calls, lay brick, plant flowers, etc.—anything with which someone could help during the grant period. Build your program size around what you can reasonably sustain. For instance, if you can only serve 100 congregants instead of 500 with an agreed-upon amount of money, make your plan fit what you can actually do. Maybe you'll need to plan a showcase fundraiser to serve the remaining 400 congregants or seek matching funds from another source.

Sometimes step-down funding structures are available. For example, the first year you receive 100%, and the church paid nothing; the second year the foundation would pay 75%, and the church would pick up 25%, with each year the funder decreasing and the church increasing their amount. Many of the paid parish nurse positions in the United States today have been initiated using this model.

Prioritize your Program

There could be many needs in a congregation: you want to start a blood pressure clinic, conduct an educational program with a speaker honorarium, have money for the church ladies to knit blankets for all the babies born in your church, build a new gym so the youth and elderly can all work and play together, and send your nurses to a parish nurse basic preparation course. You need to prioritize these needs and determine what is needed to be done first. Oftentimes parish nurses start out with so much fire that they want to do everything yesterday. Have your Health/Wellness Cabinet help you to select and prioritize. Then begin the process of seeking funding.

If you are applying for the grant through your church, they will have to have a 501(c) 3 not-for-profit status. If you are applying for grant funds through another entity, you will need to check their nonprofit status. Most grantors require this documented nonprofit status before applying for funding.

Anyone that is interested in applying for grant funding needs to become computer-savvy and familiar with the Internet because most of the RFPs are announced online. In 2005 all federal grants, along with many others, will be required to be done online. FYI: at least 50% of foundations will not reply to you as to whether they received your material. Until online submission is the rule, always send your application by FedEx or registered mail to validate its on-time arrival. It is not acceptable to call and ask about the status of a proposal. Our caveat to you: trust and pray.

Writing the Grant Proposal

After spending time digesting all of the above requirements, you may be ready to begin the actual process of grant writing. As stated earlier, this skill is learnable. One of the authors once asked an officemate who seemed to get a grant a day to help her learn to write grants. She responded that all you do is cut and paste. The statement is partially true. Once the basics of your program are outlined, the material can be pasted into several grant applications. However, generally it is wise not to assume that what one grantor wants submitted is also what another will want. All grantors will have specific requirements, formats, and for most some type of form and budget to complete. If you are not comfortable writing a grant or do not think that you have acquired the necessary skills, seek out a grant writer to either write the grant for you or assist you in the process.

When looking at the actual proposal, keep in mind it is usually divided into the following segments:

- Cover Letter or Application Form (provided by grantor)
- Project Summary or Abstract (usually less than one page)
- Table of Contents
- Need Statement
- Goals and Objectives
- Methodology or Project Design
- Evaluation
- Future Funding (Sustainability Plan)
- Budget

Don't be too proud to ask for help. Concentrate on your strengths and ask other people to share their strengths with you and your congregation. We believe the average parish nurse may not have the time to invest in learning good grant-writing skills. However, many churches have people sitting in the pew next to you that have written grants and would be happy to do it as their contribution to their church. Unfortunately, no grantor will pay the cost to hire a professional grant writer, so ask whether anyone in your congregation or community is willing to donate his or her skills to your program.

Some grants will pay for personnel salary; others will not. If you are asking for salary, confirm who will receive this money (e.g., the parish nurse, the church secretary, the pastor). Personnel compensation is very important budget information in a grant application. If several people (e.g., the project director, administrative help, or perhaps a driver to transport congregants to special events) will receive compensation, be sure to state this fact in the application and budget. Seldom will the grant pay 100% of the salary for a person to work on the grant project; therefore, one needs to decide how many hours will be spent on the grant. After these hours have been determined, you can translate this information into a percentage of your time or the person you are naming to work on the project. Keeping a worksheet in your area is wise so you can accurately track the hours spent on the grant once received. This makes grant reporting much easier and also gives you documentation if the grant should ever be audited.

Project Timetable/Timeline

Prepare a detailed timetable for implementing the grant. When will you implement the steps in your program? You may say that by May 1 you will have the first meeting of the steering committee; by July 15 you will have had your first training class; and your evaluation will be completed by September 30. Be specific. Most grantees will allow some flexibility with the timetable after the grant is funded.

Some basic essentials of the actual grant writing exist. First, as stated earlier, you need to carefully and narrowly define your project. Having selected your potential funders by reviewing their guidelines, submission dates, eligibility, evaluation process, budgets, and award levels, you now should develop your specific goals. Be able to succinctly answer the questions who, what, where, why, and when. Abide vigilantly by the guidelines and the submission deadlines.

Follow the Directions

Read the specifics of the grant application and organize your materials accordingly. If the grantor states that the funder will not accept more than a two-page proposal, then do not submit one line more than the guidelines tell you. One of the authors recently was involved in reviewing

materials for a foundation. The first way of deleting proposals was to discard all those who had submitted more material than requested. Because a funder will receive hundreds of requests, this is an easy way to begin the elimination process.

As you write your narrative, review your goals and your responses to the who, what, where, and when questions. Who will benefit from your project (elderly, children under age 14, etc.)? How exactly will their benefit be demonstrated (increased consumption of fruits, decrease in falls at home, etc.)? Is some other group in the community already providing this service and/or could some other group provide this service as well as you can? Make sure you note how your partners will add to the project. Be specific about your concerns. For instance, are you specifically targeting Vietnamese women between the ages of 40 and 64 to encourage them to have mammograms? Cite the research that proves why this project would be valuable. Are you Vietnamese, or will someone who is Vietnamese be contacting the women? Successful grant applications tend to have unique programs. The writer's ability to follow the requested format while making a strong case for their programs gives a proposal a leg up on the other applicants.

Project Outcomes and Dissemination of Outcomes: How Many People Will be Affected?

How will you know your project has been successful? Are the results measurable? All funders are looking for outcome measures, and it doesn't matter that you don't think you have time to collect these numbers. Do you want the money? Collect outcome data. To find out how the program is working, some of the possible outcomes to be monitored include the following: productivity (how many individuals participated and/or were served?) and cost-effectiveness (how much did the event cost?). In business you would be looking at the return on investment (ROI), quality (pre/post tests), and client outcomes (changes in behavior). Identify the types of records you will use to collect the necessary data to report the measurable outcomes. Surveys are the most frequent tool used for data collection.

You've worked hard; now get ready to really brag about your program. We live in an outcome-based world, and people want to hear/see results, not good intentions. Grantors are not impressed with hearing how the data will be collected. They can be impressed with what changed as a result of the program. What changed in your parish nurse practice because of the data collected? Do not hesitate to spell out for others why your program is different. This is usually called dissemination of your outcomes. Do a press release to your local newspaper or perhaps a note in your church bulletin or institutional newsletter initially to let others know you've received the money for a particular service. Later, issue another release with a brief article or human-interest story about the implementation of the program. Because we have professional responsibilities to help further our profession, consider publishing your findings in a professional journal and/or making a presentation at a national conference. When using your grantor's name in written material, be sure to follow their specific instruction for how they want it written. Make sure your partners are included in getting the information out as well. Then call your friends and supporters! Have a party! Above all, celebrate your hard work.

Project Budget

The budget for the project is how you identify the estimated costs. It should be as accurate as possible. One of the authors had a funder challenge the budget projection she had made. The funder could not believe that the parish nurse could accomplish what she said she planned to do with the amount of money requested. The author had researched it so thoroughly that she knew she could and was just stubborn enough to prove it to them. Grantors are accustomed to knowing what the line-item budget should look like, so you can't get by with just putting numbers in the slots. They will ask if the cost is too high or too low for the local market. You absolutely must know what your market is, not the market of a parish nurse friend who lives 500 miles from your city. Make sure you give sufficient budget information including details and explanations. More detail in your budget is better than less detail. If you are going to be printing booklets at the end of the grant period that detail everything, then make sure you include all personnel costs,

paper, copying/printing, binding, etc. Don't forget to list in-kind and matching revenue dollars. Know where you can be flexible if needed. Some vendors will negotiate costs. What happens if the funder chooses to fund only a portion of what you have requested? What adjustments could you make and still continue with your project?

Comprehensiveness and Accuracy

You may be asked to provide supporting letters from community leaders that you have worked with in the past. You may not. Some funders will request resumés from everyone whose name is listed as a participant in the grant. Others do not. One may want you to submit additional information on a floppy disc; others want nothing more than the two pages of answered questions. Again, do as they request. Following directions is of the utmost importance. Don't submit what is not asked for by the grantor. Box 25-1 presents 10 common errors to avoid in grant writing developed by a grant writing consultant (ward, 2002).

Before submitting the grant, make sure that it is complete and accurate. Edit, edit, edit! Make sure every word is used correctly. Make sure nothing can be misunderstood. The grant reviewers know nothing about your program except what is on the paper. Your story must be true, accurate, succinct, and to the point. Check your spelling and grammar. Don't use jargon. The finished product needs to be as close to perfect as you can make it. Submit it on time or before the due date. Make sure you have included all requested documentation (Burgener, 2003). Remember, if the guidelines request six copies, then you must send six copies. Again, read the directions carefully before submitting. Make sure you have the proper authorized signature on your grant. If you are in an organization, it may be someone at the vice presidential level; in the congregation, it will probably be your pastor.

As a last suggestion, we would advise you to have someone outside your program review your grant before submission. After you have worked so hard, you will not be the best proofreader. Most communities have several nonprofit agencies that are also writing grant proposals. Offer to read and review their submission in exchange for their reading yours. Often after receiving monies

---

BOX 25-1   10 Common Errors to Avoid in Grant Writing

Deborah Ward, a grant-writing consultant based in Lancaster, Pennsylvania, developed a list of 10 common errors to avoid in grant writing. The following are her recommendations.

1. The writing isn't succinct or intelligible. As a result, the proposal just doesn't make sense. To avoid this situation, give the finished proposal to someone outside your field of expertise to read before you submit it. This will help you to identify parts that needed to be clarified.

2. The estimated costs for the proposal are inaccurate, incorrect, or inflated. In a grant proposal, never guess at the cost of any item. Chances are that a reviewer or a staff person will identify the inaccuracy, which will affect the credibility of your entire proposal.

3. The proposal contains typographical and grammatical errors. Although a proposal with such errors will be read, what kind of message do you suppose it sends to a reviewer? Take time to have at least two people proofread your proposal before you submit it.

4. The proposed budget doesn't match the narrative, or there are costs in the budget that are not mentioned or explained in the narrative. Always be sure that the budget accurately reflects the costs of the project's activities. Otherwise, the reviewers are likely to suggest that unexplained costs not be included in the grant award.

5. The objectives are too vague and open to individual interpretation. Repeat the following mantra every time you write a grant proposal: objectives must be measurable! Objectives that are not specific or measurable will lead to vague evaluations and, in all likelihood, rejection of your proposal.

6. The proposal was hastily assembled. In most cases, reviewers can easily spot proposals that were written at the last minute. Items are missing; budgets are incomplete; and the proposal sounds choppy and unfinished. Never underestimate the time needed to develop a project idea and complete the paperwork.

7. The proposal is filled with jargon and acronyms. Don't assume that grant reviewers are experts in the subject area and that they understand your jargon and acronyms. In fact, the reviewer may not be working in health care at all. Command of the language is important; make sure that your proposal has substance and clarity, and that you explain what you mean.

8. The proposal is full of buzzwords and clichés. See number 7! What may seem perfectly clear to you may be mystifying to the reviewers.

9. The writer ignores instructions. Every grant has rules and directions that must be followed. If you want your proposal to be read and considered, read and reread the directions. Otherwise, you risk having your proposal disqualified without being read.

10. The proposal doesn't match the funders' objectives. Sometimes individuals are more interested in the funding than what the funding is supposed to accomplish. Just because a funder has a lot of grant money doesn't mean your project will get any. Don't expect funders to depart from their objectives just because you have a good project idea. In fact, if your project doesn't match a funder's interest, your proposal will likely go unread. So be sure you do your research and find a funder that closely matches your project idea.

---

from a foundation, you can expect to be invited to serve on a grant review panel. Accept the invitation. Your grant writing skills will improve each time you submit and/or review a grant.

Conclusion

Every day, in congregations across the globe, parish nurses serve as a vital link between congregations and healthcare entities. They assist fractured families to see past their pain and lift up to God thanks and praise and endless requests in prayer. The ability of a parish nurse program to maintain its visibility and viability can often be tied directly to a constant source of funding. Our prayer is that you will find a grant source to keep your ministry vibrant and alive.

REFERENCES

Burgener, S. (2003). *Grant writing*. Presentation for Community Parish Nurse Program's Basic Preparation Course, Champaign, IL (November 7, 2003).

Gitlin, L.N. & Lyons, K.J. (2004). *Successful grant writing: strategies for health and human service professionals.* New York: Springer.

Guyer, M. (2002). *A concise guide to getting grants for nonprofit organizations.* Hauppauge, NY: Nova Science.

Holy Bible: Revised Standard Version, Catholic Edition (1966). Camden, NJ: Thomas Nelson for Ignatius Press.

Ward, D. (2002). The top 10 grant-writing mistakes. *Principal,* 8(5): 47.

Wescott, J. (2003). *Grant Writing* (presentation and handouts). Presentation for Parish Nurse Basic Preparation Course, Wichita, KS (August 9, 2003).

APPENDIX 25A

Simplify the Federal Government's Grants Management Process

Since October 2003, a new website promises to "simplify the grants management process and create a centralized, online process to find and apply for over 600 grant programs from the 26 federal grant-making agencies." It is www.grants. gov. You can go to this site to view information loaded (up to the present) and to read general information. U.S. Dept. of Health and Human Services is one of the managing partners for the www.grants.gov program, along with 10 additional partners listed on the website. Some facts that the HHS representative highlighted to the authors of this chapter include the following:

- All grant-making agencies will participate in grants.gov over time.
- This program is one of the 24 federal cross-agency e-government initiatives focused on improving access to services via the Internet.
- The first stage of grants.gov, a pilot program, is successfully completed.
- You will be able to search for a word or phrase to identify grant opportunities, and the list will show a range of grant opportunities for that topic.
- Once a match is found, download an electronic application to apply for the grant.
- After completing the application, submit it through the grants.gov site.
- Application is time-stamped, and the appropriate federal agency has immediate access to it.
- Agency will receive application, sending confirmation back to the applicant through grants.gov.
- Process will accelerate without handling paper applications.

The Waterwheel Model of Spiritual Leadership

Phyllis Ann Solari-Twadell

26

Parish nurse coordinators (PNCs) are in leadership positions. Parish nurses by the very nature of their ministry are also in leadership roles. The position, however, only presents the opportunity; it does not provide the knowledge, capacity, or ability to be a leader. To be a leader and actualize the functions of a leader often requires additional learning. One who is interested in enhancing her or his potential as a leader may begin by reflecting on what natural gifts, abilities, and capacities she or he currently brings to a leadership position. Once personal leadership strengths are assessed, areas for further development will become clear. This is a starting point of continuous learning in improving leadership capabilities. Spiritual leadership is only one conceptualization of leadership. However, the very dynamics of this leadership model make it fitting for those in ministry to consider.

Spiritual leadership is a dynamic concept that is discussed primarily in recent business literature. Fairholm (1997, 1998) was one of the first leadership scholars who combined spirituality and leadership. This author states that "spiritual leadership is a holistic approach that considers the full capacities, needs, and interests of both leader and led: spiritual leaders see leadership as a contextual relationship in which all participants want to grow and help others in their self-development activities" (p. 11). Spiritual leaders create an environment where those that are led are encouraged to reflect upon their work experiences in order to find a deeper meaning in those experiences. Fairholm (1998) suggests further that the "spiritual leadership process includes building community within the group and a sense of spiritual wholeness in both leader and led. Spiritual leaders have and live by a higher moral standard and ask others to share that standard" (p. 40). "Spirituality transcends the ordinary; and yet, paradoxically it can be found only in the ordinary. Spirituality is beyond us, and yet it is in everything we do. It is extraordinary, and yet it is extraordinarily simple" (Kurtz & Ketcham, 1992, p. 35). A number of dissertations are directed to understanding and fostering spiritual leadership (Marinoble, 1990; Jacobson, 1994; Walling, 1994; Larkin, 1995; Santerre, 1996; Yoder, 1998).

The intention of this chapter is to describe spiritual leadership through the construct of a waterwheel. A waterwheel was used in earlier times to generate power, often at a mill to grind grain or at a foundry. The waterwheel is constructed with buckets at the perimeter of the wheel to catch the flowing water. Spokes reach out from a central core or hub supporting the perimeter of the wheel. As the water flows, the buckets fill with water. As the buckets fill with water they become heavy, forcing the wheel to move circularly. The wheel is in continuous motion because of the water's ceaseless movement. The water that flows out from the buckets forms ripples in the water. These ripples keep moving out from the waterwheel. The Waterwheel Model of Spiritual Leadership and the assumptions that correspond with the model are displayed in Figure 26-1 and Appendix 26A. The model will be described in this chapter through the use of eight assumptions.

The Framework of the Waterwheel

Assumption 1: Spiritual Leaders Have Foundational Life Experiences that Impact the Development of their Core Beliefs and Values

In Bolman and Deal (1995) the main character works with a spiritual director to "reclaim and rekindle his spiritual center" (p. 41). In one discussion with the spiritual director, he says, "I got lost at a carnival once. I was panicked. Terrified. I still dream about it. Remember Hansel and Gretel? In new places I still leave crumbs" (p. 46). Foundational life experiences leave footsteps. Some things that happened to us as children may be very vivid in our minds and can shape our responses today. However, foundational experiences may also—though never thought consciously—leave trailers: beliefs about how something should or shouldn't be, how someone should or shouldn't behave, or the expected outcome from a given experience. These beliefs are the fodder for personal values that are lived out in the current day. All human beings have foundational life experiences. Unless they are explored, these experiences can unknowingly provide the makings of core beliefs and values that may help or hinder what we are trying to do or be today. These core beliefs and values are the hub of the waterwheel construct.

Nouwen (1994, pp. 27-28) presents another reflection on the "hub." He writes

> Wheels help me to understand the importance of life lived from the center. When I move along the rim, I can reach one spoke after the other, but when I stay at the hub, I am in touch with all the spokes at once. To pray is to move to the center of all life and all love. The closer I come to the hub of life, the closer I come to all that receives its strength and energy from there. My tendency is to get so distracted by the diversity of the many spokes of life, that I am busy but not truly life-giving, all over the place but not focused. By connecting to the heart of life, I am connecting with its rich variety while remaining centered. What does the hub represent? I think of it as my own heart, the heart of God, and the heart of the world. When I pray, I enter the depth of my own heart and find the heart of God, who speaks to me of love. And I recognize, right there, the place where all of my sisters and brothers are in communion with one another.

The great paradox of the spiritual life is, indeed, that the most personal is most universal, that the most intimate is most communal and that the most contemplative is the most active.

Assumption 2: Spiritual Leaders Have the Capacity for Self-Awareness that May Support or Alter their Core Beliefs and Values

Self-awareness is discussed in most literature that addresses spiritual leadership. As individuals our internal selves are constantly interfacing with the external reality. Interaction is continuous; each influences the other. We are not necessarily being formed by what is occurring external to us as often as "we are helping to create the circumstances of our lives" (Conger, 1994, p. 72). "Self-awareness is key to self-knowledge. Leaders thrive by understanding who they are as well as what they believe and value, by becoming aware of unhealthy blind spots or weaknesses that can derail them and by cultivating the habit of continuous self-reflection and learning" (Lowney, 2003, p. 27). Life's events, as discussed earlier, can impact a person's core beliefs. Over time it is important to have an awareness of how a person, place or event has changed a person or their beliefs. Without self-awareness, decisions and judgments could be made without understanding how they were formed or what they mean to the individual. Fairholm (2003) notes, "Tools and behaviors used in spiritual leadership uniquely focus on self-awareness, other awareness and the need to develop both" (p. 4).

Assumption 3: Spiritual Leaders Have Core Beliefs and Values Made Visible through their Actions and Decisions

People generally live life or at least are more at peace living life according to their core beliefs and values. Observing a leader over time or in times of crisis will give a clear message as to whether the leader can make decisions aligned with his or her core beliefs and values or whether compromise occurs and actions conflict with who they believe themselves to be. "Core beliefs and values are nonnegotiable; they are the centering anchor that allows for purposeful change" (Lowney, 2003, p. 29). "A leader's most compelling tool is who he or she is. Leadership behavior develops naturally once this internal foundation is laid" (Lowney, 2003, p. 19). However, if this internal foundation of core beliefs and values either has not been formed or contains beliefs that are not consistent with respect, honesty, trust, and integrity, techniques of leadership can never compensate. Followers do not have a high regard for leaders whose core beliefs and values are flawed, and they will in most instances not continue to follow them. Maxwell (1999) states, "we have no control over a lot of things in life. We don't get to pick our parents. We don't select the location or circumstances of our birth and upbringing. We don't get to pick our talents or IQ. But we do choose our character" (p. 4). Character is based on our core beliefs and values as well as the ability to live them out in life.

Assumption 4: Spiritual Leaders Build Relationships and Tell Stories that Transmit New Ways of Thinking, Being, and Doing

Spiritual leaders create environments by developing relationships that take the time for telling stories. Telling stories requires listening to the underlying culture of the surroundings. "People trudging into the hospital also bring with them varying capacities for spiritual awareness, a wide range of abilities to be open to the spiritual and to see things from a spiritual point of view. During the course of the day, these capacities will be tapped. They will come into play in the midst of the rules, roles, responsibilities, and systems. The deeply personal will emerge to influence the socially structured relationships" (Shea, 2000, p. 115). Spiritual leaders are highly relational people who understand that connection to others allows the most profound understandings to be shared and that relationships foster not only personal transformation but also community transformation.

The people most in touch with the spiritual dimension and thereby most able to communicate it may not be at the top of the social and organizational ladder (Shea, 2000, p. 116). The phenomena of relationship development and storytelling can occur throughout an organization and emphasize the understanding that spiritual leaders can exist at every level within an organization. To tell their stories, spiritual leaders must be able to

self-remember. Self-remembering is remaining in touch with the soul as you become more in touch with the world (Shea, 2000, p. 138). So the spiritual leader moves within and out repeatedly in forming relationships and telling the story.

Assumption 5: Spiritual Leaders Have a Connectedness with a Power Greater than Themselves

History repeatedly has shown that people hunger for something larger than themselves. Leaders who offer that will have no shortage of followers. In fact, "*higher purpose* is such a vital ingredient to the human psyche that scripture says, 'Where there is not vision, the people perish'" (Jones, 1995, p. 177).

People want to feel connected to each other at work in the pursuit of a transcendent purpose (Ashmos & Duchon, 2000). Knowing that work is not just to earn money or to be given credit for accomplishing a specific task but is designed to contribute to a worthwhile pursuit can be a significant motivator. Rosner (2001) noted that "the purpose of spirituality is not to serve work; rather the purpose of work is to serve spirituality. It is about experiencing a sense of purpose and meaning in work beyond performance of tasks and a sense of contributing to the greater community" (p. 83). Nadesan (1999) presented evidence that a spiritually sensitive work environment enhances productivity by encouraging commitments to the goals of the organization.

The Driving Force that Makes the Waterwheel Function: Continuous Learning

Assumption 6: Spiritual Leaders are Continuous Reflective Learners

Just as the waterwheel is moved by the continuous flow of water, continuous learning stimulates and challenges the spiritual leader to be open to new ideas. Learning means to study, to accumulate knowledge and experience. The second understanding is to practice constantly. These two definitions combined can be understood as "mastery of the way of self-improvement." The roots of the English word *learning* suggest a similar meaning: "to learn came to mean gaining experience following a track-presumably for a lifetime" (Senge, Kleiner, Roberts, Ross, & Smith 1994, p. 49). Senge, et al (1994) defines learning within organizations as "the continuous testing of experience and the transformation of that experience into knowledge-accessible to the whole organization and relevant to its purpose" (p. 49). They suggest that four questions regarding learning processes for an organization be asked: Do you constantly test your processes? Are you producing knowledge? Is the knowledge shared? Is the learning relevant?

Continuous reflective learning molds spiritual leaders. "The spiritual leader takes the time to reflect, pausing and practicing inner listening. Inner listening is centering and dwelling in such a way that the deeper levels can emerge into consciousness with both their wisdom and folly" (Shea, 2000, P. 139). Once spiritual leaders become conscious of how they learn, think, and interact and begin developing capacities to think and act differently, they have begun to change organizations for the better. Those changes will ripple out and reinforce a growing sense of capability and confidence (Senge et al, 1994, p. 48).

Maxwell (1999) refers to continuous reflective learners as "teachable": "As a teachable leader, you will make mistakes. Forget them, but always remember what mistakes taught you. If you don't, you will pay for them more than once" (p. 146).

Spiritual Leaders Actualize Sustaining Capacities: The Buckets

The buckets in the waterwheel model of spiritual leadership must be present if the wheel is to function continuously. If one of the buckets is missing, the continuous movement of the wheel is threatened. Just as the buckets are a necessity for the uninterrupted function of the waterwheel, the sustaining capacities are key to the function of the spiritual leader. It is important that a leader recognizes if she or he does not have strength in an identified capacity. Can a deficiency in a leadership capacity be nurtured or developed? Can a capacity not able to be actualized by a leader be represented through another person in the leadership team? Many scenarios probably could be related to deficiency in a sustaining capacity. The important factor is an awareness or knowledge of the lack of

a sustaining capacity. The order in which the sustaining capacities are arranged on the waterwheel holds no significance. Each of the buckets must be present in order for the wheel to function as the water is flowing.

Assumption 7: Spiritual Leaders Actualize Sustaining Capacities

This author has chosen the term "capacities" to reflect the significance of the buckets in the waterwheel model of spiritual leadership. Both the terminology and the specific naming of the buckets was the result of an extensive literature review.

Service Oriented

Greenleaf (2002) states there is a difference in leaders who perceive that they are a "leader first" and those leaders who "want to serve first" (p. 27). Leaders who want to serve first are "making sure that other people's highest priority needs are being met" (Greenleaf, 2002, p. 27). Greenleaf goes on to say that the "best and most difficult test is: Do those served grow as persons? Do they, *while being served* become healthier, wiser, freer, more autonomous, more likely themselves to become servant? *And,* what is the effect on the least privileged in society? Will they benefit or at least not be further deprived?" (p. 27).

Wheatley (2002) states "service brings joy" as one of eight spiritual principles she identified. She speaks to "the joy and meaning of service found in every spiritual tradition" (p. 6). The real leader serves the people and their best interests. This may not always be the most popular position, the easiest, the most impressive, but it is the most loving. This posture of service reflects a loving concern for others rather than a desire for personal glory.

Self-Disciplined

Self-discipline is not a popular subject. It is much easier to see where someone else would benefit from being more disciplined than to recognize one's own need for discipline. Self-discipline is an exercise of the spirit in relationship with the mind and body. It is truly a whole person experience. If the body is not willing, the mind provides the rationalization, and the spirit dissipates. If the spirit is waning, the mind lags in quickness, and the body becomes more lethargic. If the mind is wanderlust, the spirit often is wishy-washy and the body fatigued. It is difficult to get the whole person "in sync" and willing to be "in tune" to a discipline. Maxwell (1999) makes the following suggestions for improving self-discipline: "(1) develop your priorities and follow them; (2) list the reasons or benefits of being more disciplined, making a disciplined lifestyle your goal; (3) get rid of excuses by challenging them; and (4) remove rewards until the job is done" (p. 128-129).

Ethical

Wolf (2004) discusses a model of spiritual leadership in healthcare administration. She emphasizes ethical values and behavior. An ethical posture is of great value because it exercises discernment and judgment needed to unravel the paradoxes in a work environment. One does not have to go far in contemporary news to hear of business leaders' breeches of ethical behavior. Catastrophic results for employees of these businesses often result. Pensions are lost as individuals are faced with not only finding new employment due to closure of a company, but also more profoundly dealing with a chronic sense of hopelessness. What was trusted and committed disappears because of a lack in the ethical behavior of leadership and ultimately of the company involved. Kanungo & Mendonca (1994) note that the "ability to distinguish between morally good and evil acts is critical to the formation of character. Knowing ethical principles alone (as criteria for distinguishing between good and evil acts) is of little value unless we make an effort to habitually incorporate these principles in our behavior" (p. 170).

Intuitive

Spiritual leaders are able to listen on many levels. They have the capacity to use their feelings and conceptualizations as a way of listening while interpreting the external activities in a context different from the one that may be presented. Through experience spiritual leaders have come to know and appreciate the message communicated by the feelings that are surfaced within. This may provoke a more critical examination of the matter at hand. Minimally, intuitive thinking will often encourage the raising of questions that might otherwise not be asked. The line of questioning may lead to a manner of thinking that promotes new perspectives on a presenting problem or issue.

Creative

New learning brings different insights and perspectives to a problem or situation. Being able to creatively solve a problem or gain a new perspective on a situation is energy-producing. Research netted the observation that one of the byproducts of practicing spirituality at work is creativity (Neck & Millman, 1994). Continuous learning—opening the mind to new perspectives and knowledge—feeds a person's capacity for creativity. Working in a team environment where others are approaching work from an open-minded perspective can also feed one's capacity for creativity.

Open-minded

Maintaining an open mind is difficult; it is often scary and forces a person to abandon her or his prejudices. Being open-minded is based on accepting that life is uncertain and change is constant. Understanding this intimates that movement from the old to the new passes through a cycle of chaos. It is hard to let go of the old not knowing exactly what "new" will mean (Wheatley, 2002). However, often there is no better choice; to stay with the same process, procedures, or perspectives would be a sure demise of what already is available and assists people. Assuming a posture of open-mindedness is an invitation to becoming, renewing, and stretching yourself.

Grateful

An attitude of gratitude is the healthiest attitude that an individual can have in life. It is the opposite of resentment. Gratitude encompasses the realization of giftedness, contribution, participation, and accomplishment. People in a work setting that are grateful reach out in a positive spirit to others. Continuous reflective learning can inspire gratitude. The opportunity to learn, seen as a gift with the new learning supporting participation and accomplishment, can contribute to the gratitude of the community. I have the opportunity to learn. I learn. I contribute the new learning to my work, which is part of the work of the community. The new learning leads to accomplishment. I am grateful, and so is the community and/or team of people with whom I work.

Faith-filled

People who are faith-filled often relate to their work as "vocation" or "call." This notion of vocation or call denotes that work is given to us, that we are meant to do it. Vocation is not decided upon; it is something that is received. It originates from outside us and reminds us that we are part of something beyond our narrow sense of self. We are part of a larger purpose (Wheatley, 2002). Many will say that their vocation is a gift from God. Faith believes in the not yet seen. Certainly working toward a vision, which is not yet visible, is an act of faith.

Wisdom Seeker

In *One Minute Wisdom* De Mello (1985) writes:

Is there such a thing as One Minute Wisdom?
'There certainly is' said the Master.
'But surely one minute is too brief?'
'It is fifty seconds too long.'

To his puzzled disciples the Master later said,
'How much time does it take to catch sight of the moon?'

"Then why all these years of spiritual endeavor?"
'Opening one's eyes may take a lifetime.
Seeing is done in a flash' (p. 1).

Wisdom is not a commodity. It cannot be digested through an educational program. Wisdom is a spiritual gift and pursuit—one said to be more valuable than gold (Brown, 1995). Insight and learning about self can often appear through the "willingness to plumb the depths of inner wisdom" (Klenke, 2003, p. 57). Living life with an attitude of openness and then reflecting on one's life experience often can produce wisdom. Continuous reflective learning can be a stimulus to wisdom. New learning can cause reflection on meaning and purpose. Insight can be obtained from the reflection on the new learning. This new insight may be a source of wisdom in the future. Vision comes from wisdom. The lessons of life and experience are fertile soil for wisdom and the creation of vision.

Open to Surrender

Surrender is a spiritual phenomenon. Surrender is not acceptance. I can accept that something will change and still not fully give in to the meaning and significance of this change. The following reading is a good representation of what it is to surrender.

Changes
Any real change implies the breakup of the world as one has already known it. The loss of all that gave one identity, the end of safety. And at such a moment, unable to see and not daring to imagine what the future will now bring forth, one clings to what one knew, or thought one knew; to what one possessed or dreamed that one possessed. Yet it is only when persons are able, without bitterness or self-pity, to surrender a dream they have long cherished or a privilege they have long possessed that they are set free—they have set themselves free—for higher dreams, for greater privileges. All people have gone through this; go through it, each according to their degrees, throughout their lives. It is one of the irreducible facts of life.

-Author Unknown

This reading emphasizes that in order to survive real change one needs to surrender to what is occurring and accept the reality that is presenting. Only in surrender and acceptance is there the opportunity to be free, creatively responding to the presenting change.

Discerning

Discernment is a reflective process. Discernment is the ability to find the root of the matter through contemplation. In *The Spiritual Exercises of Saint Ignatius: A Literal Translation & A Contemporary Reading* Fleming (1991) notes that discernment is "an ability to recognize ever earlier the direction of certain movements or feelings in our lives, and so to be able to follow or reject them almost in their very sources" (p. 203). Discernment relies on intuition as well as rational thought (Maxwell, 1999). Often discernment is not done alone or in isolation but with a trusted colleague, spiritual director, or spouse. Discernment can provide a structured process invoking both the rational and the spiritual dimension of the decision maker to improve decision quality.

Inquisitive

Spiritual leaders inquire. They seek. They inquire of themselves, their God, and others around them. They ask the hard questions. They ask the important questions, ones that may have no answer but require that one live out the mystery before them. Being inquisitive is a push to continuous reflective learning. Without the desire for inquiry the manner of things tends to stay the same. Often the questions that arise for the spiritual leader have to do with the meaning of the work being done. Without being inquisitive what goes on is left unchallenged and may occur without the true meaning being understood. Wheatley (2002) notes that leaders must help others remember why they are doing the work they are doing. What are we hoping to accomplish? Who are we serving by doing this work?

Christians believe that God gives God's self away to humans in a twofold way that is ultimately one: through the inner world of our human wondering and desiring, thinking and planning, and our outer world of nature and human history (McDermott, 1994). An inquisitive mind serves well in coming to know God. "Jesus asked question after question. Perhaps he asked so many questions because one of his mottos was 'You shall know the truth, and the truth shall make you free'" (Jones, 1995, p. 94).

Spiritual Leaders Foster Capacity Building in Others: The Ripples

Assumption 8: Spiritual Leaders Foster Capacity Building in Others

As the continuous flow of water fills the buckets, forcing the movement of the waterwheel, the water in the buckets empties out creating ripples in the pool of water. These ripples are concentric circles that move reaching out to far ends of the pool of water. These ripples create a particular environment for the pool. The spiritual leader who lives out her or his capacities on a daily basis models for others new and different ways of being. The more consistent the actualization of the capacities the clearer the lessons are to those who interact or observe the spiritual leader. The result is an environment that projects a particular way of thinking, behaving, and responding. Those working in this environment experience and absorb a manner of relating that in turn reinforces the nature of the environment.

This author believes the following are characteristics identified as a result of the leader's spiritual posture.

Inspiration

Followers can be inspired by the leadership provided to them. If individuals are inspired, they can renew interest, pride and productivity in their work. Klenke (2003) noted "some evidence that spiritually anchored organizations add shareholder value" (p. 57). Thompson (2000) reported that "organizational performance and financial success can depend on the spiritual enrichment of the workplace and that 'spirited workplaces' have done better with respect to profitability and therefore have added shareholder value" (p. 19).

Values

As discussed above values clearly communicated from leadership and seen as consistent with an individual's values can provide a framework for relating and performing. These values may mirror ethical behavior when the spiritual leader demonstrates ethical mindedness to those around them. Those within the workplace may adopt these values over time. The adoption of different values over time may alter the work climate, the way people relate to each other, and the productivity of the work community.

Vitality

Work understood as "calling" orients an individual. Work resonates with her or his faith life and adds a sense of vitality and purpose to work (Delbecq, 1999). This idea relates to the previous discussion regarding productivity. For a person filled with vitality is likely to be more filled with energy and productive in her or his work.

Respect

"Each person is unique, valuable, and deserving of respect. Each has a set of strengths, weaknesses, needs, fears, experiences, values, beliefs—in unique combination. Some aspects of these resources work toward wholeness, others toward disintegration" (Tubesing, 1977, p. 6). Leadership that can understand this and live it out in their interactions with others will set the tone that all persons can be affirmed for the uniqueness and life within. If the leader is respectful, she or he will be respected and set that tone within the whole of the organization.

Integrity

Integrity relates to the manner in which the individual or the organization adheres to the stated values. An organization may have clearly professed values on their materials but not live them out in day-to-day operations. Such an organization is quite different from one that not only professes values but also lives them out vigorously in their work. Therein lies the integrity. Is there a truth in what is professed? Or is it a perfunctory "lingo"?

Trust

Trusting the authority person is linked with trusting the group (McDermott, 1994). If the leadership is trustworthy but the work group is not, there is dissonance within the organization. If the work group is not trusted but the leadership is, there is still dissonance in the organization. The goal is trust throughout the organization. For example, if the leadership is trustworthy, trustworthiness will also usually be demonstrated in the work group or team. Trust contributes to a peace-filled work environment that functions with respect for all.

Courage

Courage comes from the old French word for *heart* (*coeur*). We have to engage the heart to portray courage (Wheatly, 2003). Courage is the ability to go on anyway despite obstacles and fears (Bolman & Deal, 1995). Often the greatest courage is needed in just being true to one's personal values and beliefs in the midst of decision making. Tough decisions require courage on the part of leaders. The payoff of courage is often values made visible, inspiration, vitality, trust, respect, and integrity.

Wholeness

Perspective on the whole is a requirement for development of a vision. The idea that nobody wins until we all do is powerful in giving followers the message that everyone is considered and is part of the whole (Jones, 1995). Each person is given a mandate to be responsible for self, for other persons, and for the world all inhabit (Droege, 1979). One cannot honestly profess to understanding caring for the whole without considering the importance of stewardship. The idea of stewardship is an important spiritual concept. It is hard at times to acknowledge the whole. However, not considering the whole eliminates the possibility of community respect, integrity, and vitality.

Vision

Leaders must continually strive to lead through a vision that is bold and courageous yet remain flexible to accommodate continual change (Delbecq, 1999). A leader's courage to fulfill the vision comes from passion, not position (Maxwell, 1999). Vision is intended to inspire others to take initiative and move toward realization of the vision.

Understanding Vision

Vision leads the leader.
Vision starts from within.
Vision draws on your history.
Vision helps gather resources.

(Maxwell, 1999, pp. 150-51)

Honesty

Honesty is to foster truth seeking in all interactions and work. Honesty can call upon courage to make itself visible. However, if the leader cannot be honest with self, she or he will have trouble in being honest with others inside or external to the organization. Pride often leads to failure because it can lead to impatience, an unwillingness to build consensus, the inability to receive criticism, and the unwillingness to endure periods of trial and uncertainty (Delbecq, 1999). If leadership fails to display honesty with themselves or others, there is likely to be little basis for honesty to be displayed among followers.

Communication

Relational people are usually good communicators. Credibility precedes great communication as a person is more likely to listen to someone they believe to be credible than not (Maxwell, 1999). The following relates to reflection on considerations related to all people.

All Things People Have in Common

They like to feel special, so sincerely compliment them.
They want a better tomorrow, so show them hope.
They desire direction, so navigate for them.
They are selfish, so speak to their needs first.
They want to trust, so show them responsibility.
They want to experience security, so show them how it looks.
They desire to be loved, so show them you care.

They get low emotionally, so encourage them. They want success, so help them win.

(Maxwell, [as adapted by Solari-Twadell] 2000, p. 107)

Community

Palmer (1998) offered the following definition of community: "An outward and visible sign of an inward and invisible grace, the flowing of personal identity and integrity into the world of relationships" (p. 90). If a leader has a picture of the whole and is relational, respected and respectful, and honest with self and others, leaders and followers will share a sense of community.

Hope

Hope encourages each to believe that tomorrow will be a better day, that whatever burden is present in this time will pass, and that peace and joy will return or come to fill the future. Leadership can build up people's hopes: maybe this person who is leader will make a difference, change the course, lift the burden, and bring new insights to the work at hand.

Prayer

The more that individuals and groups come to see themselves and their work as part of something greater than themselves and the work of the collective as contributing to the benefit of the whole, the greater the understanding that the "spirit" is larger than any one person. Naturally people may begin to pray. Pray for the well-being of the other, the work, the leader, the output, and the community. Prayer encourages humility, which is needed for all to work together in peace.

Conclusion

Spiritual leadership is a dynamic process that has the capability to unlock the potential of the individual as well as the whole of the organization to achieve a stated vision, providing meaning and purpose to the work, while giving those involved in the experience a connection with something greater than self. Spiritual leadership is anchored through identified core values and foundational life experiences, actualized through self-awareness, service, intuitive thinking, ethical behavior, creativity, gratitude, open-mindedness, gratitude, faith, surrender, discernment, inquisitiveness, and wisdom. Clear communication of values and discernment enhanced by a connection to a power greater than oneself allows the spiritual leader to foster values, vitality, inspiration, community courage, respect, wholeness, integrity, trust, vision, honesty, hope, and prayer and a high value on relationship building among followers.

The Waterwheel Model of Spiritual Leadership construct provides a visual of the important dynamics of this complex phenomenon. The intention is that this model will provoke discussion, continued study and further understanding of spiritual leadership. The long-range work is to have leaders such as parish nurse coordinators, parish nurse educators, parish nurses, and others in ministry understand how they can strive to develop within themselves the capacities to model spiritual leadership to others.

REFERENCES

Ashmos, D. & Duchon, D. (2000). Spirituality at work. *Journal of Management Inquiry,* 9(2), 134-45.

Bolman, L.G. & Deal, T.E. (1995). *Leading with soul: An uncommon journey of the soul.* San Francisco: Jossey-Bass.

Brown, T. (1995). Jesus CEO?: Laurie Beth Jones sees "omega principles" as the answer to contemporary management problems. *Industry Week,* March 6.

Conger, J.A. (1994). *Spirit at work: discovering the spirituality in leadership.* San Francisco: Jossey-Bass.

Delbecq, A.L. (1999). Christian spirituality and contemporary business leadership. *Journal of Organizational Change Management,* 12(4): 345-49.

De Mello, A. (1985). *One-minute wisdom.* New York: Image Books, Doubleday.

Droege, T. (1979). The religious roots of wholistic health care. In G.E. Westberg (Ed.). *Theological roots of wholistic health care.* Hinsdale, IL: Wholistic Health Centers, Inc.

Fairholm, G. (1997). *Capturing the heart of leadership.* Westport, CT: Praeger.

Fairholm, G. (1998). *Perspectives on leadership: from the science of management to its spiritual heart.* Westport, CT: Quorum.

Fairholm, M.R. (2003). Leading with spirit in public organization. *PA Times,* 26(11) November: American Society for Public Administration.

Fleming, D.L. (1991). *The spiritual exercises of Saint Ignatius: a literal translation and a contemporary reading.* St. Louis: The Institute of Jesuit Sources.

Greenleaf, R.K. (2002). *Servant leadership: a journey into the nature of legitimate power and greatness.* New York: Paulist Press.

Jacobson, S.E. (1994). *Spirituality and transformational leadership in secular settings: delphi study.* Unpublished doctoral dissertation. Seattle University: Seattle, WA.

Jones, L.B. (1995). *Jesus, CEO: using ancient wisdom for visionary leaders.* New York: Hyperion.

Kanungo, R.N. & Mendonca, M. (1994). What leaders cannot do without: the spiritual dimensions of leadership. In J. Conger (Ed.). Spirit at work: discovering spirituality in leadership. San Francisco: Jossey-Bass.

Klenke, K. (2003). The "S" factor in leadership, education, practice, and research. *Journal of Education for Business,* September/October.

Kurtz, E. & Ketcham, K. (1992). The spirituality of imperfection: modern wisdom from classic stories. New York: Bantam.

Larkin, D.K. (1995). Beyond self to compassionate healer: transcendent leadership (Doctoral dissertation, Seattle University: Seattle, WA, 1995). UMI 9527055.

Lowney, C. (2003). *Heroic leadership: best practices from a 450-year-old company that changed the world.* Chicago: Loyola Press.

Marinoble, R.I. (1990). Faith and leadership: the spiritual journeys of transformational leaders. Unpublished doctoral dissertation, University of San Diego: San Diego, CA.

Maxwell, J.C. (1999). The 21 indispensable qualities of a leader: becoming the person others want to follow. Nashville: Thomas Nelson, Inc.

McDermott, B.O. (1994). Partnering with God. In J. Conger. Spirit at work: discovering the spirituality in leadership. San Francisco: Jossey-Bass.

Nadesan, M. (1999). The discourses of corporate spiritualism and evangelical capitalism. *Management Communication Quarterly,* 13(1): 3-43.

Neck, C. & Millman, J. (1994). Thought self-leadership: finding spiritual fulfillment in organizational life. *Journal of Managerial Psychology,* 9(6): 9-16.

Nouwen, H.J. (1994). *Here and now: living in the spirit.* New York: Crossroad.

Palmer, P. (1998). *The courage to teach: exploring the inner landscape of a teachers life.* San Francisco: Jossey Bass.

Rosner, J. (2001). Is there room for the soul at work? *Workforce* 80(2): 82-83.

Ross, R., Smith, B., Roberts, C., & Kleiner, A. (1994). *Core concepts about learning in organizations.* In P.M. Senge, A. Kleiner, C. Roberts, R.B. Ross, & B.J. Smith. The fifth discipline fieldbook. New York: Currency Doubleday.

Santerre, B.G. (1996). *Numinous leadership: stories of educational leaders integrating spirituality and practice.* Unpublished doctoral dissertation, University of St. Thomas: St. Paul, MN.

Senge, P.M., Kleiner, A., Roberts, C., Ross, R.B., & Smith, B.J. (1994). *The fifth discipline field book: Strategies and tools for building a learning organization.* New York: Doubleday Publishing Group.

Shea, J. (2000). *Spirituality and health care: reaching toward a holistic future.* Park Ridge, IL: The Park Ridge Center for the Study of Health, Faith, and Ethics.

Thompson, D. (2000). Can you train people to be spiritual? *Training and Development,* 54(12): 18-19.

Tubesing, N.L. (1977). Philosophical assumptions: assumptions underlying wholistic health care with implications for implementation and research. Hinsdale, IL: Wholistic Health Centers, Inc.

Walling, D.M. (1994). Spirituality and leadership. Unpublished doctoral dissertation. University of San Diego: San Diego, CA.

Wheatly, M.J. (2002). Spiritual leadership. *Executive Excellence,* 19(9): 5-6.

Wolf, E. (2004). Spiritual leadership: a new model. *Healthcare Executive,* 19(2): 22.

Yoder, N.A. (1998). *Inspired leadership: exploring the spiritual dimension of educational administration.* Unpublished doctoral dissertation. University of Wisconsin—Madison: Madison, WI.

The Waterwheel Model of Spiritual Leadership

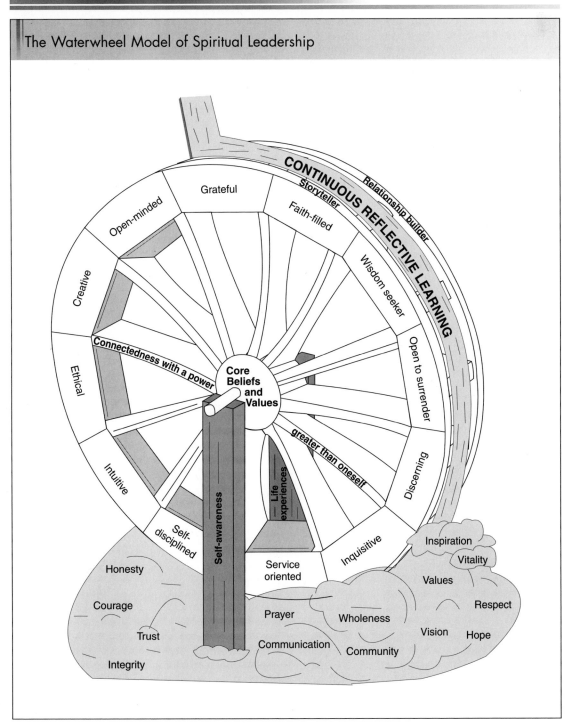

Figure 26-1 The Waterwheel Model of Spiritual Leadership. (Copyright © Phyllis Ann Solari-Twadell, PhD, RN, MPA, FAAN, Loyala University Chicago, Chicago, IL.)

Continued

The Waterwheel Model of Spiritual Leadership—cont'd

Assumptions:

1. Spiritual leaders have foundational life experiences that impact the development of their core beliefs and values.
2. Spiritual leaders have the capacity for self-awareness that may support or alter their core beliefs and values.
3. Spiritual leaders have core beliefs and values made visible through their actions and decisions.
4. Spiritual leaders build relationships and tell stories that transmit new ways of thinking, being, and doing.
5. Spiritual leaders have a connectedness with a power greater than themselves.
6. Spiritual leaders are continuous reflective learners.
7. Spiritual leaders actualize sustaining capacities.
8. Spiritual leaders foster capacity building in others.

Challenges to the Administration of the Ministry of Parish Nursing Practice

27

Phyllis Ann Solari-Twadell

Mary Ann McDermott

Good stewardship necessitates thoughtful reflection on proper administration of resources for the ministry of parish nursing practice. Start-ups and pilot projects deal with a myriad of unknowns, thus attention to an infrastructure to ensure program sustainability is often lacking. Tolerance for ambiguity and ability to adapt and change are key skills in such an endeavor. Once the Chief Executive Officer of Lutheran General Hospital made the decision to fund the parish nurse pilot project, the determination was made to house the program under the Director of the Department of Pastoral Care, Reverend Larry Holst. An internal multidisciplinary advisory group wisely was selected to work with the program. The group consisted of Dr. Greg Kirschner, MD; Reverend Lee Joeston, a Lutheran Chaplain; Anne Marie Djupe, RNC, MA, a member of the Staff Development Department; Chaplain Florence Smith, a Catholic chaplain who was also a nurse; and Reverend Granger Westberg. Reverend Holst chaired the advisory group.

To their credit, some years later senior management adapted and changed the administrative infrastructure. Initially an add-on responsibility for Holst, it was eventually acknowledged as a fulltime position and a person was designated to develop and manage an infrastructure for the program. In the late 1980s, Anne Marie Djupe was designated Director of Parish Nursing Services, and a separate cost center was established for the program. That office's fostering relationships with parish nurses, clergy, and congregations to enhance services was paramount to the future success of parish nursing services, which still exist today within Advocate Health Care.

Administration of this ministry is often viewed and implemented as an add-on responsibility to an existing administrative role in the hospital, network, or system. Although this view is understandable during the set-up of a new program, this mentality, while cost-effective, in itself challenges the long-term administration of the ministry of parish nursing practice and also creates a myriad of additional challenges.

Because of the impact of several of the challenges that emerged in the other two units of this book, we have included them in our discussion of challenges to the administration of the ministry of parish nursing practice.

Challenge: Role Clarity, Mindset, Communication

Communicating What You Do Is Difficult Without Role Clarity

The role confusion presented by different management configurations, titles, and responsibilities given to those responsible for the coordination or management of a ministry of parish nursing practice is well presented by Zerull in Chapter 19. The grassroots development of parish nursing encourages the creation of roles and position titles that fit the unique perspectives of the diverse settings of the ministry of parish nursing practice. This diversity in administrative positions in parish nursing has been addressed

327

directly in a number of articles in the parish nurse literature. As the movement matures, however, reviewing current titles and responsibilities and communicating the benefits of consistent language for positions will be imperative. Role clarity regarding the administration of parish nursing by institutions, coalitions, and congregations nationally will provide 1) the potential to learn more effectively from one another; 2) clear justification for consistency in salaries for the parish nurse management position; 3) more consistency in responsibilities for designated position titles; 4) justification for the responsibilities of the parish nurse administrator; responsibilities not to be added onto another already established position; and 5) clear communication of the parameters of different administrative roles needed for different organizational frameworks or infrastructures related to the ministry of parish nursing practice.

In public forums, those in managerial parish nurse positions have been reluctant to address the titling, responsibilities, and salary issues related to their positions, thus communicating a mindset of intimidation and/or vulnerability. This vulnerability is fed by the fear that if attention is paid to the discrepancies between responsibilities and accountabilities of the position and/or the time and salary allotted, the entire program may come under question and be threatened and/or discontinued. Even if the responsibilities are unclear or the position title not commensurate with the work or time allotted, a position evidently must seem better than no position at all. Coming from a more altruistic perspective, to struggle along with lack of clarity and/or being underpaid for management services provided or having added-on management responsibilities to another position is better than not having the opportunity to serve in this capacity at all. All these are very logical human responses to the identified problem. However, do they really serve the congregations or people in the congregations well? Do they serve the next administrator for the program or the long-term viability of the program well? More likely this mindset enables the problem to continue, creating obstacles to the maturation of the movement. Possibly, it may be a necessary step until the ministry of parish nursing practice substantiates the value rendered. Every circumstance has its special issues, but in most instances role

ambiguity usually does not serve well the person, the people that work with the role, or the people who depend on the role. Learning even from other administrators within the same system—but certainly with other parish nurse administrators across the country—becomes difficult, if not impossible. However, this challenge will be with us until significant merit and funding are given to the ministry of parish nursing practice. Merit and funding follow value. Value is determined by documented differences evident in the presence of the service. Many parish nurses and parish nurse manager/coordinators still do not appreciate or value documentation of services. Without documentation, a challenge elaborated on in Chapter 8, there is little story to communicate the value of the ministry of parish nursing practice and the differences that are being made in the lives of people served.

Challenge: Inspiration, Vision, and Mission for Parish Nurse Coordinators/Managers

Creation of a Vision and Mission, Collective or Otherwise, for Parish Nurse Coordinators/Managers

"Where there is no vision, the program will perish" is a theme of several chapters in this section as well as other sections of this book that must be echoed here. Vision provides inspiration; minimally it provides some direction. A shared vision "builds a sense of commitment in a group by developing shared images of the future that could be created as well as the identification of principles and guiding practices by which to get there" (Senge, Kleiner, Roberts, Ross, & Smith, 1994, p. 6). Minimally, development of a personal vision and mission statement encourages the identification of what *you* want to "create of yourself and the world around you" (Senge et al, 1994, p. 201).

Solari-Twadell, in Chapter 26, proposes a model to assist our understanding of spiritual leadership. After reviewing the model, we are each challenged to reflect on our individual capacities of spiritual leadership. Personal reflection and clarification can be a powerful exercise as a source for personal inspiration in one's work. As for a collective vision, this is an ongoing challenge for development and continuous review. A shared vision statement developed by the collective of parish nurse managers/coordinators would start with the identification of shared values. Creation of shared values is the foundation to the creation of a shared vision. When completed, this developmental work provides a source of energy, clarity, and basis for quality. For most, individual or collective, mission and vision statements do not stay exactly the same over time. Perhaps engaging in such an exercise by the collective of parish nurse managers/coordinators may assist in the clarification of roles and future implications for these roles. This would have a profound impact on the maturation of the administration of the ministry of parish nursing practice. It certainly would provide an energy and direction for the future both personally and collectively.

Challenge: Is It No Margin, No Mission? Or No Mission, No Margin?

Creative Allocation of Resources

Lutheran General would have never considered piloting the idea proposed by Lutheran clergyman Granger Westberg to sponsor and support the placement of a nurse on the staff of a local congregation without a very strong sense of mission. Mission is that sense of working on what is the faith-filled thing or the right thing to do. Today's healthcare environment offers little room for such an altruistic idea. It gets harder and harder to justify the dollars spent on a health promotion, whole person–oriented program.

In Chapter 24, DiLeo and Graham provide us with a strategy employed in one part of our country where churches, nurses, institutions, and communities have found a way to provide parish nursing services to underserved congregations. For those institutions where the ministry of parish nursing practice is tightly woven into the strategic plan, a partnership with a congregation to support the ministry of parish nursing practice is 1) a concrete and direct way for the healthcare institution to extend its mission and resources to the community; 2) an opportunity to be in relationship with people in the community in their episodes of wellness as well as their episodes of illness; 3) a way the people in the community can get to know the healthcare institution through the

parish nurse without any entry to the healthcare system itself; 4) one way the institution can demonstrate commitment to extending their benefit to the community; 5) a method of communicating to the people in the congregation and community at large the whole-person orientation of the healthcare system in partnering with a faith community; 6) a tangible experience of a continuum of care that members of a congregation can experience; 7) a cost-effective way of intervening early in episodes of illness; and 8) a strategy for ministering to people with chronic illness, possibly reducing the number of hospitalizations.

However, if the ministry of parish nursing practice is seen as a token effort to gain market share, the program is very likely to be compromised or eliminated if referrals made by the nurse to the hospital cannot be documented. The intention of the healthcare institution can be determined by investigating the integration of the ministry of parish nursing practice into their strategic plan and the consequential funding and infrastructure provided to the program as well as the leadership given to the program. One way of determining the depth of the infrastructure is to review policies and procedures that are in place to guide the program. In Chapter 22, Ziebarth provides an excellent foundation with many examples for anyone interested in establishing policies and procedures for the ministry of parish nursing practice.

For healthcare institutions to be good stewards of their resources, external funding for parish nursing is often sought. A number of grants have been written to foundations to assist in program startup and/or for special projects within a program. Two successful grantees, Wescott and Roberts, challenged us in Chapter 25 to develop strategies for creatively building a philanthropic base to supplement hospital, health system, or congregational resources for the ministry of parish nursing practice.

Challenge: Keeping It All Together

Creating and Sustaining a Parish Nurse Network

Connectiveness is a fundamental concept for any movement that has spirituality at its core. However, maintaining connection with others given geographical obstacles and limited resources is a challenge. Stixrud in Chapter 23 shares the experience of developing a parish nurse network over an extended period of time. Dedication, faith-filled intention, and an unfailing trust in God accompanies this work. Often the success or failure of such work falls on the capacities of the leader or leaders that are doing this work. Spiritual leadership becomes a very important subject for all involved in the ministry of parish nursing practice. Their association with the people who walk with them and the spirit that guides them transforms individuals committed to parish nursing. The transformation doesn't occur overnight but one day at a time.

Keeping it all together is not really the work of one individual. It takes a committed cadre of people who believe parish nursing is the answer to some of the most serious problems in the healthcare system and in churches. Fortunate are we who have the opportunity to be a part of connecting with others who believe that the ministry of parish nursing practice holds the key for a healthier tomorrow for many.

Challenge: Learning How to Develop and Sustain Relationships with Congregations in an Environment of Constant Change

Appreciating the Significance of Relationships

Solari-Twadell and Burke discuss the intricacies of working with congregations in Chapter 21. For the parish nurse coordinator this can be the most challenging perspective of administering the ministry of parish nursing practice. Congregations are ever-changing. Certainly the leadership, both religious and lay, is in constant transition. Parish nurse coordinators can maintain relationships with a limited number of congregations if a true relationship is formed. The exact number of congregational relationships that one parish nurse coordinator can effectively maintain has many variables associated with that determination. The important item is that there is a limit, and that fact should be recognized by the parish nurse coordinator and sponsoring institution. This is a factor that must be considered in strategic planning for the management of a parish nurse network

or program. Good relationships take time and commitment. When a pastor or parish nurse leaves, it takes a commitment of time on the part of the parish nurse coordinator, pastor, and parish nurse to build the relationships that will best sustain the ministry of parish nursing practice. However, building and sustaining these relationships is by far not the only work that any of these parties has to do. This is one reason that being a highly relational person is part of the essential makeup of a parish nurse coordinator. Caring about the pastors and parish nurses as significant people, not just in the context of work but in life from an overall perspective, brings the power of these relationships into position. Relationships, over time, can create life-changing opportunities for the parish nurse coordinator. This is when the phenomena of work as a "call" is often experienced.

The work with congregation requires irregular schedules for the parish nurse coordinator. With the congregation being a voluntary organization, most meetings occur in the evenings or on the weekends. The intrusion of these meetings on family time can present a challenge. Managing all with dedication and commitment can often challenge anyone's energy, thus the importance of a good sense of self, self-care and balance. The demands of the parish nurse coordinator role are dynamic and demanding. Those who survive and eventually thrive over an extended period of time in this role learn about themselves, their capacity for relationship building, and the movement of the spirit in very dynamic ways.

Challenge: Identifying What Constitutes Quality in the Ministry of Parish Nursing Practice

At Which End Are You Standing When You Are Blindfolded and Describing the Elephant?

Burkhart and Solari-Twadell present an in-depth discussion regarding quality in an outcomes environment for the ministry of parish nursing practice in Chapter 20. Many readers may want to skip this chapter, feeling that it is too much or questioning "is it really necessary to get into this?" However, it is most important that we all enter into this discussion of what constitutes quality for the ministry of parish nursing practice. We may be "walking around the elephant blindfolded." The more of us involved, however, in describing what it is we are feeling or doing, the better picture we will all have about the whole. Ignoring the subject is risky; it will not go away. Some may discount the need for this in-depth treatment of quality for a "ministry." It is almost implied that anything done in the name of ministry is guaranteed to be a quality experience! We know this is not true. However, quality is a desired goal! No congregation would not desire it so.

Investigating quality for parish nursing practice may stimulate systems to identify quality for other congregational ministries. Parish nursing always acknowledges that the benefits gained through this ministry are intended to affect others: the nursing profession, congregational and denominational organizational life, delivery of healthcare, communities, and the overall health status of people in the communities served by the parish nurse. We must never forget that the ministry of parish nursing practice is intended to be a catalyst for change. When we commit ourselves to this ministry, we are committing ourselves to a life of coming to know change, experiencing change, and being changed.

REFERENCE

Senge, P.M., Kleiner, A., Roberts, C., Ross, R.B. & Smith, B.J. (1994). *The fifth discipline fieldbook: strategies and tools for building a learning organization.* New York: Currency Doubleday.

Postscript: A Future Vision for the Ministry of Parish Nursing Practice

Phyllis Ann Solari-Twadell
Mary Ann McDermott

Happy twentieth birthday, parish nursing! According to the growth and development literature, a twentieth birthday marks a level of maturity achieved both physically and psychosocially. The physical structure is just about complete, as are the ability to view and act on problems from a comprehensive and long-range perspective. Identity is established; roles are identified and articulated. Has parish nursing matured to this level of functioning? Some commentary from our point of view, related to several inherent issues for the ministry of parish nursing practice, may assist the reader in thinking about and perhaps answering that question.

The important work of integrating the ministry of parish nursing practice into the continuum of care must be tended to with careful diligence. This integration has several significant tentacles that reach into significant other related issues. Integration into the continuum of care cannot occur without addressing the financing of the ministry of parish nursing practice. This endeavor must be carried out with the utmost attention to the essence of this whole person service so that the integrity and intent of the practice is not compromised. The nature of this kind of work on behalf of the ministry of parish nursing practice will push the congregations, as well as the sponsoring healthcare institutions and funders, to the table. This will force otherwise reluctant congregations to be better informed and move with serious intention and grounding into advocacy initiatives for equal access for all to basic healthcare services. Institutions will need to examine the benefit and cost of mission over margin. Are we there yet?

Educational preparation for parish nurses, parish nurse coordinators, and parish nurse educators will remain an ongoing and significant issue for the maturation of the ministry of parish nursing practice. Access to this preparation remains geographically challenged. Some geographic areas have an overabundance of programs, whereas other areas have none. Where parish nurse educational programs are overly abundant, continued collaboration is required to prevent competition among providers. That behavior is not congruent with the nature of the ministry of parish nursing practice. Basic parish nurse education is often economically unreasonable, especially for volunteers who are exploring or about to begin their ministry. Distance education can be one solution, but that method has yet to be fully implemented nor is access economically feasible for all. Scholarship funding needs to be made more available in these instances.

Who will be the next generation of parish nurse educators? Do the parish nurse educators of today have the parish nurse education of tomorrow in their long-range view? A very real threat of a decrease in available parish nurse education programs exists as the current education coordinators retire. Are current parish nurse educators mentoring nurses that they consider able to assume these responsibilities? Have the parish nurse education programs been well enough

333

integrated into the infrastructure of their educational institutions so that they are not person-dependent? These questions need to be faced proactively, not in a passive posture, if the ministry of parish nursing practice is to continue to mature. Are we there yet?

History has a way of continuing to surface decisions from the past that impact the present and the future. The impetus for an organization for parish nurses spawned what is now the Health Ministries Association. Files in the Westberg Archives housed at the Cudahy Library of Loyola University Chicago document the formation of that Association. The organization grew out of the work of the Advisory Board of the Parish Nurse Resource Center in the late 1980s. That board was concerned that Lutheran General Hospital possibly would not, over time, be able to finance the work of the Center. Reverend Westberg suggested that an organization of parish nurses be formed to carry out the work that was being done by the center at that time. Once the organization of parish nurses was strong enough and the Parish Nurse Resource Center was not financially able to carry on its work, the organization of parish nurses could assume the function of the center. On September 29, 1988 the advisory committee voted unanimously to recommend to those assembled that an organization of parish nurses be developed. The decision was a bit premature for the movement. Few parish nurses existed in the late 1980s. Then, as now, many were not being paid in their roles. Resources simply were not sufficient to form a parish nurse association. The idea to have what was to have been a parish nurse organization become an organization for all those interested in health ministries was driven largely by finances. An organization dedicated to health ministry would embrace larger numbers of people and organizations and provide a stronger financial base for such an organization. It was also believed that such an organization would provide a larger context for parish nursing in its development. So what began as a parish nurse association was to become the Health Ministries Association. The editors of this book remained advisors for many of the formative years of the organization.

As the ministry of parish nursing matured, some within its ranks did not perceive the Health Ministries Association as a professional nursing organization, and there was some movement toward starting a professional parish nurse organization. This movement, however, did not surface until after the American Nurses Association had designated the Health Ministries Association as the representative organization for the specialty of parish nursing practice, as the ANA worked through the first set of standards for the ministry of parish nursing practice.

Other nurses, such as those interested in or providing parish nursing services in Wisconsin, have developed a different professional organizational model by forming a special interest group within the Wisconsin Nurses Association. This special interest group encompasses parish nurse coordinators and educators as well. This professional organizational model is serving both local and national representation for parish nursing through the American Nurses Association. Still other parish nurses looking for an affiliation have done so through their religious denominations. These movements now have history, dedicated resources, and committed membership, yet none really represents a whole. It appears that the ministry of parish nursing practice is plagued with a cultural perspective of nursing—the formation of multiple professional groups rather than the ability to come together as one voice.

Through the collaborative work of the International Parish Nurse Resource Center following the 2004 Westberg Symposium, the World Forum on Parish Nursing has been formed. This is an effort to have some mechanism to provide a meeting place for those in all countries that are developing the ministry of parish nursing practice to meet, share information, collaborate on research, gain support, and further develop the body of knowledge related to this practice from an international perspective. This is a natural outgrowth of the maturation of this faith-filled movement. It will be interesting to see in 20 more years how the work of this group will have impacted world health. If the ministry of parish nursing is going to continue to grow and mature, a place where the collective can be represented and speak as one voice—representing diverse communities of faith, geography, ethnicity, and socioeconomic status as one—must exist. If this possibility can become a reality, it will come about with voices that have no stake in anything but the integrity of the ministry of parish nursing practice and are able to follow the fine whisper of the Holy Spirit that guides all that is of God. Are we there yet?

Once again, happy twentieth birthday to the ministry of parish nursing practice! May you grow and flourish into full maturity. Peace be with all who read this book and continue to take risks and break new ground. The editors respectfully invite comments, discussion, and response to the ideas and visions put forth in this text.

Index

Page numbers followed by f indicate figures; t, tables; b, boxes.

Wisconsin
    parish nursing in, 261, 262t
    public-private partnership in, 88
Wisconsin Nurses Association, 334
Wisdom, in waterwheel spiritual leadership model, 320
Women, Infants, and Children, public-private partnership with, 89

Work-study covenant, in financial support, 140-141
World Forum on Parish Nursing, 334-335
World movements, collaboration with, 79-80
Writing. *See also* Grant writing.
    agreements in, in public-private partnerships, 85-86
    journal, in spiritual formation, 48